MULTIPLE MYELOMA:
A TEXTBOOK FOR NURSES

EDITED BY

JOSEPH D. TARIMAN, PHC, MN, APRN-BC, OCN®

Oncology Nursing Society
Pittsburgh, Pennsylvania

ONS Publishing Division
Publisher: Leonard Mafrica, MBA, CAE
Director, Publications: Barbara Sigler, RN, MNEd
Managing Editor: Lisa M. George, BA
Technical Content Editor: Angela D. Klimaszewski, RN, MSN
Staff Editor: Amy Nicoletti, BA
Copy Editor: Laura Pinchot, BA
Graphic Designer: Dany Sjoen

Cover illustrations: Top left image by Lydia Kibiuk and courtesy of the National Cancer Institute (public domain). Top right image from Wikimedia Commons, January 2007 (open access artwork used under the terms of the GNU Free Documentation License [http://commons.wikimedia.org/wiki/Commons:GNU_Free_Documentation_License] and the Creative Commons Attribution ShareAlike 3.0 [http://creativecommons.org/licenses/by-sa/3.0]).

Library of Congress Cataloging-in-Publication Data

Multiple myeloma : a textbook for nurses / edited by Joseph D. Tariman.
　　p. ; cm.
Includes bibliographical references and index.
ISBN 978-1-890504-93-9 (alk. paper)
1. Multiple myeloma–Nursing. I. Tariman, Joseph D. II. Oncology Nursing Society.
　[DNLM: 1. Multiple Myeloma–nursing. WH 540 M9605 2010]
　RC280.B6M85 2010
　616.99'418–dc22

2010016023

Publisher's Note
This book is published by the Oncology Nursing Society (ONS). ONS neither represents nor guarantees that the practices described herein will, if followed, ensure safe and effective patient care. The recommendations contained in this book reflect ONS's judgment regarding the state of general knowledge and practice in the field as of the date of publication. The recommendations may not be appropriate for use in all circumstances. Those who use this book should make their own determinations regarding specific safe and appropriate patient-care practices, taking into account the personnel, equipment, and practices available at the hospital or other facility at which they are located. The editor and publisher cannot be held responsible for any liability incurred as a consequence from the use or application of any of the contents of this book. Figures and tables are used as examples only. They are not meant to be all-inclusive, nor do they represent endorsement of any particular institution by ONS. Mention of specific products and opinions related to those products do not indicate or imply endorsement by ONS. Web sites mentioned are provided for information only; the hosts are responsible for their own content and availability. Unless otherwise indicated, dollar amounts reflect U.S. dollars.
ONS publications are originally published in English. Publishers wishing to translate ONS publications must contact the ONS Publishing Division about licensing arrangements. ONS publications cannot be translated without obtaining written permission from ONS. (Individual tables and figures that are reprinted or adapted require additional permission from the original source.) Because translations from English may not always be accurate or precise, ONS disclaims any responsibility for inaccuracies in words or meaning that may occur as a result of the translation. Readers relying on precise information should check the original English version.

Printed in the United States of America

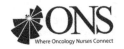

Integrity • Innovation • Stewardship • Advocacy • Excellence • Inclusiveness

To my mother, Narda, for her unconditional love,
To my siblings, especially Dina, for her unwavering support,
and Leonila, for her loving discipline,
To my partner, Todd, for his enviable sensitivity and modesty,
To my nieces and nephews, for providing the inspiration,
To all my relatives, friends, and colleagues,
for providing the encouragement,
This book is whole-heartedly dedicated.

Joseph D. Tariman

Contributors

EDITOR

Joseph D. Tariman, PhC, MN, APRN-BC, OCN®
Predoctoral Fellow
University of Washington
Seattle, Washington
Chapter 1. Introduction; Chapter 14. On the Horizon: Future Considerations

AUTHORS

Elizabeth Bilotti, MSN, RN, ANP-BC
Nurse Practitioner
Division of Myeloma
The John Theurer Cancer Center at Hackensack University Medical Center
Hackensack, New Jersey
Chapter 12. Survivorship Issues

Beth Faiman, RN, MSN, APRN-BC, AOCN®
Nurse Practitioner
Cleveland Clinic, Taussig Cancer Institute
Predoctoral Fellow, Case Western Reserve University
Cleveland, Ohio
Chapter 6. Treatment of Newly Diagnosed, Transplant-Ineligible Patients; Chapter 8. Treatment of Relapsed or Refractory Multiple Myeloma

Charise Gleason, MSN, NP-BC, AOCNP®
Nurse Practitioner
The Winship Cancer Institute of Emory University
Atlanta, Georgia
Chapter 4. Epidemiology

Patricia A. Mangan, MSN, APRN-BC
Nurse Lead, Hematologic Malignancies and Stem Cell Transplant Program
Abramson Cancer Center at the University of Pennsylvania
Philadelphia, Pennsylvania
Chapter 5. Patient Assessment

Kena Miller, RN, MSN, FNP
Nurse Practitioner
Department of Medicine, Lymphoma/Myeloma Division
Roswell Park Cancer Institute
Buffalo, New York
Chapter 10. Management and Evaluation of Patients Receiving Novel Agents

Kimberly Noonan, RN, ANP, AOCN®
Nurse Practitioner
Department of Medical Oncology
Jerome Lipper Multiple Myeloma Center
Dana-Farber Cancer Institute
Boston, Massachusetts
Chapter 2. Anatomy and Physiology; Chapter 3.
Pathophysiology

Tiffany Richards, MS, ANP-BC, AOCNP®
Nurse Practitioner
Department of Lymphoma/Myeloma
University of Texas M.D. Anderson Cancer
Center
Houston, Texas
Chapter 13. Nursing Research

Anna Liza Rodriguez, RN, MSN, MHA, OCN®
Director
Oncology Nursing and Oncology Service Line
Mount Sinai Hospital
Chicago, Illinois
Chapter 7. Treatment Modalities of Newly
Diagnosed, Transplant-Eligible Patients;
Chapter 9. Management and Evaluation of
Patients Receiving High-Dose Chemotherapy
With Stem Cell Transplantation

Sandra Rome, RN, MN, AOCN®, CNS
Hematology/Oncology Clinical Nurse
Specialist
Cedars-Sinai Medical Center
Assistant Clinical Professor
School of Nursing
University of California, Los Angeles
Los Angeles, California
Chapter 11. Patient Teaching

DISCLOSURE

Editors and authors of books and guidelines provided by the Oncology Nursing Society are expected to disclose to the participants any significant financial interest or other relationships with the manufacturer(s) of any commercial products.

A vested interest may be considered to exist if a contributor is affiliated with or has a financial interest in commercial organizations that may have a direct or indirect interest in the subject matter. A "financial interest" may include, but is not limited to, being a shareholder in the organization; being an employee of the commercial organization; serving on an organization's speakers bureau; or receiving research from the organization. An "affiliation" may be holding a position on an advisory board or some other role of benefit to the commercial organization. Vested interest statements appear in the front matter for each publication.

Contributors are expected to disclose any unlabeled or investigational use of products discussed in their content. This information is acknowledged solely for the information of the readers.

The contributors provided the following disclosure and vested interest information:

Joseph D. Tariman, PhC, MN, APRN-BC, OCN®: Millennium Pharmaceuticals, Inc., speakers bureau

Elizabeth Bilotti, MSN, RN, OCN®, APN-C: Celgene Corp. and Millennium Pharmaceuticals, Inc., consultant, speakers bureau; Merck & Co., Inc., consultant

Beth Faiman, RN, MSN, APRN-BC, AOCN®: Celgene Corp. and Millennium Pharmaceuticals, Inc., speakers bureaus

Charise Gleason, MSN, NP-BC, AOCNP®: Merck & Co., Inc. and Millennium Pharmaceuticals, Inc., consultant

Patricia A. Mangan, MSN, APRN-BC: Celgene Corp. and Millennium Pharmaceuticals, Inc., speakers bureaus

Kena Miller, RN, MSN, FNP: Celgene Corp. and Cephalon, speakers bureaus; Millennium Pharmaceuticals, Inc., advisory board

Anna Liza Rodriguez, RN, MSN, MHA, OCN®: Celgene Corp., speakers bureau

Contents

Foreword

For our patients, multiple myeloma (MM) presents challenges on every front. They must adapt to the new and unfamiliar diagnosis of what used to be thought of as "bone cancer." They must adapt to the unfamiliarity of big words for which they have no context but know the impact of these words on shaping the medical context of their futures. They must adapt to dramatic changes to their world view of health and illness, life and death. They will experience shifts in their psychosocial, emotional, physical, social, and possibly spiritual domains. They will endure extensive medical evaluations (some painful), uncertainty of next steps and the future, many treatments, and the threat of treatment-related morbidity and mortality. Treatment side effects may be arduous to manage and compromise quality of life. Given the prevalence of MM late in life, it is certain that the majority of patients will have one or more comorbidities at the time of diagnosis, thereby potentially compounding the difficulties of treatment.

For nurse clinicians, the gift of caring for our patients with MM presents us with many opportunities to experience the "transpersonal caring moment" (Watson, 1998, 2008). The gift allows us to connect with our patients at a vulnerable time, to experience a more full presence with our patients and a richer therapeutic relationship, and to participate fully in the caring-healing aspects of our profession.

The disease itself, as well as the treatments, provides clinicians with excellent learning opportunities to appreciate the effects of the disease presentation and management on potentially every organ system, in every domain of the patient's well-being, and in every aspect of the patient-nurse relationship caring environment.

The authors of this book have given a sound, scientific, and sophisticated summary of the disease entity, its pathophysiology and natural history, the advancements in diagnostics, evaluation, treatment, and supportive measures, as well as the psychological and emotional support of patients with MM. The vulnerability of our patients can be tremendous. We need to help them interpret and integrate vast amounts of knowledge into their own decision making and self-care. We need to take a whole systems approach and engage their families, caregivers, and local and extended communities in their support and care. We need to keep our patients at the center of our focus as we provide care.

Joseph Tariman and his colleagues have done just this, and they have done it with a caring ethos.

In 2004, I was contacted by a nurse in Bogota, Colombia. She had read a paper I wrote in 2001 on the nursing care of patients with MM as a paradigm for the needs of special populations. She was calling to invite me to present the paper at the occasion of the 70th anniversary of her country's national cancer institute. That was the first year that there was a "nursing" day at the otherwise established, annual international conference. This story reminds me that we never know the full extent (if at all) of how our work might touch our patients, families, and colleagues. Take this moment, then, to care deeply and fully for our patients with MM, and take the extensive knowledge that we have about this disease and its management to help our patients care for themselves and continue the fullest possible lives as they manage their disease trajectory and own integration of the meaning of the disease.

David Rice, RN, PhD, AOCNP®
Director, Quality Management and Magnet Program
Department of Nursing
Memorial Sloan-Kettering Cancer Center
New York, New York

REFERENCES

Watson, J. (1988). *Nursing: Human science and human care: A theory of nursing* (pp. 58–59). New York, NY: National League for Nursing.

Watson, J. (2008). *Nursing: The philosophy and science of caring* (Revised ed., pp. 82–83). Boulder, CO: University Press of Colorado.

Preface

Novel chemotherapeutic agents have revolutionized the treatment approaches for patients with multiple myeloma (MM) in the past decade. In contrast with conventional chemotherapies used in the 1960s through the late 1990s, novel agents offer improved clinical outcomes and better quality of life for patients with MM. However, along with the advent of novel agents in 2000s came new, not-so-well-described side effects and clinical challenges from the lack of evidence-based nursing interventions that abrogate untoward effects from chemotherapies.

This book features a comprehensive review of nursing care of patients with MM in the era of novel agents. This is the first book on MM written *by nurses, for nurses.* Sections centered on nursing assessment, novel therapies, patient education, nursing management of side effects, survivorship, and nursing research in the context of MM provide comprehensive materials that are relevant to day-to-day nursing practice.

The contributors of this book are nurses who work in the top myeloma centers in the United States. These nursing experts work unremittingly to advance the art and science of myeloma care and endlessly dedicate their time and effort to disseminate important therapeutic breakthroughs to their nursing colleagues.

Despite the huge time commitment and rigorous timeline, each contributor has successfully completed and delivered excellent manuscripts while actively providing clinical care to patients with MM. Without the hard work and professionalism of all contributors, this book would not be a reality.

Lastly, patients who participated in clinical trials that led to the U.S. Food and Drug Administration approval of novel agents have left a lifelong legacy— better treatment options for patients with MM. This book is enriched by the insightful views and opinions shared by patients with MM to their oncology nurses.

Acknowledgment

The timely completion of this book would not have been possible without the editorial support of Jonathan Tucker.

CHAPTER 1

Introduction

Joseph D. Tariman, PhC, MN, APRN-BC, OCN®

WHAT IS MULTIPLE MYELOMA?

Multiple myeloma is a B-cell neoplasm of the plasma cells. Its three hallmarks include the presence of a serum or urine monoclonal immunoglobulin, monoclonal plasmacytosis, and osteolytic lesions (Lokhorst, 2002). The clinical features of myeloma include bone pain, easy fatigability, polyuria, nausea and vomiting, recurrent infections, and neurologic symptoms, such as confusion, paraplegia, or polyneuropathy (Munshi & Anderson, 2005).

Multiple myeloma accounts for approximately 10% of all hematologic cancers (Jemal et al., 2009), with an annual incidence of 4.3 per 100,000, age-adjusted to the 2000 U.S. population (Kyle et al., 2004). In the United States, myeloma is twice as common in African Americans compared to Caucasians and is slightly more common in men than women (Jemal et al., 2009; Kyle et al., 2004).

HISTORICAL ACCOUNTS

Drs. Robert Kyle and S. Vincent Rajkumar from the Mayo Clinic in Rochester, MN, described more than 160 years of multiple myeloma and its treatment advances in a paper celebrating the 50th anniversary of the American Hematology Society (Kyle & Rajkumar, 2008). This paper began with the description of the first case of myeloma in 1844, then discussed the evolution of drug therapy and stem cell transplantation, culminating with the most recent concepts of diagnosis and therapy. According to the authors, the first few documented patients with myeloma received treatment using rhubarb pills, steel, quinine, infusion of orange peel, or the application of leeches to painful bony areas as "maintenance therapy" (Kyle & Rajkumar, 2008). No one today would think that such therapies were used, but they were. It was not until 1958 that patients started receiving the chemotherapeutic agent known as D- and L-phenylalanine mustard, otherwise called sarcolysin (Blokhin, Larionov, Perevodchikova,

Chebotareva, & Merkulova, 1958). Subsequently, it was discovered that the L-isomer of phenylalanine (melphalan) was responsible for the antimyeloma activity of sarcolysin (Munshi & Anderson, 2005). By 1962, melphalan became the first chemotherapeutic agent with a documented benefit for patients with myeloma (Bergsagel, Sprague, Austin, & Griffith, 1962).

Since the early 1960s, the need for novel therapeutic agents that could prolong and improve overall survival (OS) for patients with multiple myeloma has remained high. The median OS of 37.4 months in patients receiving conventional chemotherapies is quite dismal, with only 12% of patients making it to the fifth year compared to 52% in patients receiving high-dose chemotherapy (HDC) with autologous stem cell transplantation (ASCT) (Attal et al., 1996). These survival data were later confirmed by a meta-analysis that showed conventional chemotherapy had similar OS as treatment with melphalan and prednisone, with only 27% (age 50–64), 21% (age 65–74), and 12% (age 75 and older) of patients surviving through the fifth year, regardless of the type of chemotherapy (Myeloma Trialists' Collaborative Group, 1998).

In the 1980s, HDC with ASCT was a major breakthrough for myeloma therapy. Initial reports from phase I and II trials of HDC with ASCT showed promising clinical outcomes that led to large randomized clinical trials (Barlogie et al., 1987; McElwain & Powles, 1983; Osserman et al., 1982). By the mid-1990s to early 2000s, two large randomized, controlled studies confirmed the superiority of HDC with ASCT over conventional chemotherapies (Attal et al., 1996; Child et al., 2003), cementing HDC with ASCT as an important part of the standard frontline therapies for patients with newly diagnosed disease.

Initial reports on double (two autologous transplants) or tandem (two autologous transplants performed within a six-month period) ASCT showed OS benefits (Attal et al., 2003; Galli et al., 2005; Putkonen et al., 2005). However, other studies only showed better response rates and event-free survival, not better OS (Cavo et al., 2007; Goldschmidt, 2005). Based on these equivocal findings, large prospective, randomized, controlled studies are needed in the context of novel agents.

With the advent of novel agents such as thalidomide in 1999 (Singhal et al., 1999), bortezomib in 2003, lenalidomide in 2006, and pegylated liposomal doxorubicin in 2006, the Mayo group has reported a newly documented 50% improvement in OS in patients diagnosed during the past decade (Kumar et al., 2008). These new survival figures create "reasonable hopefulness" among patients with myeloma in achieving a better OS with a good quality of life, despite myeloma's long history of poor survivability. In the arena of HDC, the introduction of novel agents during the induction and postconditioning periods also has improved response rates and OS (Barlogie et al., 2006, 2007, 2008; Zangari et al., 2008).

The improvements in OS and event-free survival can also be attributed to some of the major advances seen in the management of patients with multiple myeloma in the past decade. Recent discoveries and advances in imaging, immunology, cytogenetics, molecular biology, stem cell transplantation, tumor microenvironment, and gene microarray expression profiling have contributed to a better understanding of the disease and improvement in its management and outcomes (Braggio, Sebag, & Fonseca, 2008; Mulligan et al., 2007; Raab & Anderson, 2008; Shaughnessy, Zhan, Barlogie, & Stewart, 2005; Shaughnessy et al., 2007). Lastly, the refinement in the delivery of HDC with growth factor support with or without stem cell transplantation, the use of bisphosphonates, and the use of supportive care also have significantly improved patient outcomes (Kyle et al., 2007; Mehta & Singhal, 2007, 2008; Tariman & Faiman, 2010).

NURSING CONTRIBUTIONS TO MYELOMA CARE

Oncology nurses are key healthcare team members during early recognition of disease complications and management of treatment-related toxicities (Bertolotti et al., 2008). They provide patient and family education regarding the disease, review conventional and novel treatment options, and assess signs and symptoms of disease or treatment complications. Oncology nurses play an important role not only as direct caregivers but also as patient advocates and educators. Nursing research demonstrates that specific nursing interventions contribute to patients' quality of life and perhaps affect event-free survival and OS of patients with myeloma (Coleman, Coon, et al., 2003; Coleman et al., 2008; Coleman, Hall-Barrow, Coon, & Stewart, 2003; Coon & Coleman, 2004a, 2004b; Poulos, Gertz, Pankratz, & Post-White, 2001). However, more nursing studies are direly needed to strengthen evidence-based nursing care.

COLLABORATION AND PARTNERSHIP

The International Myeloma Foundation (IMF), a nonprofit organization dedicated to improving the lives of patients diagnosed with multiple myeloma, has recognized the need for collaboration and partnership with oncology nurses. With the leadership of Susie Novis, IMF's president and cofounder, the Nurse Leadership Board (NLB) was created to develop guidelines in managing the side effects associated with novel therapies (Durie, 2008). This is the first major collaboration and partnership between professional nurses and a patient advocacy group in the area of myeloma care. Through the support of IMF, the NLB successfully published nursing guidelines for the management of peripheral neuropathy (Tariman, Love, McCullagh, & Sandifer, 2008), myelosuppression (Miceli, Colson, Gavino, & Lilleby, 2008), deep vein thrombosis (Rome, Doss, Miller, & Westphal, 2008), steroid-related side effects (Faiman, Bilotti, Mangan, & Rogers, 2008), and gastrointestinal side effects (Smith, Bertolotti, Curran, & Jenkins, 2008). These guidelines have been disseminated through national and regional oncology nursing conferences and in several continuing nursing education programs across the United States. The NLB is developing several other projects for future implementation, including survivorship care and long-term care guidelines.

FORGING AHEAD

Moving onward, the therapeutic options for patients with myeloma have significantly increased, patient outcomes have improved, and further insight has been gained into the biology and genetics of the disease (Barlogie et al., 2004). It has been suggested that a stepwise approach in targeting not only myeloma cells but also its microenvironment, using novel biologically based therapeutic agents alone or in combination with conventional chemotherapy, can overcome drug resistance and may further improve survival (Anderson, 2003; Barlogie et al., 2004). ASCT using high-dose melphalan as the conditioning regimen is now considered standard therapy for myeloma, at least for younger patients or those age 70 and younger with no significant comorbidities (Attal et al., 1996; Barlogie et al., 2004; Child et al., 2003; Harousseau, 2008; Mehta & Singhal, 2007).

Researchers continue to heavily investigate the role of immunotherapy in multiple myeloma, and future immune strategies will eventually lead to improved OS (Qian et al., 2005; Wang et al., 2006; Yi, 2003). The systematic application of cytogenetics and molecular genetics, especially gene expression profiling, has led to biology-based classification and staging of myeloma; wide clinical utilization of this new classification and staging needs to continue to increase among community-based healthcare providers (Chng & Bergsagel, 2008). The major challenge for clinicians is to maximize the therapeutic benefits of every novel agent. Translating all these advances to better patient care that could lead to longer OS accompanied with a good quality of life remains a big challenge in clinical practice.

REFERENCES

Anderson, K.C. (2003). Moving disease biology from lab to the clinic. *Cancer, 97,* 796–801. doi:10.1002/cncr.11137

Attal, M., Harousseau, J.-L., Facon, T., Guilhot, F., Doyen, C., Fuzibet, J.G., ... Bataille, R. (2003). Single versus double autologous stem-cell transplantation for multiple myeloma. *New England Journal of Medicine, 349,* 2495–2502. doi:10.1056/NEJMoa032290

Attal, M., Harousseau, J.-L., Stoppa, A.M., Sotto, J.J., Fuzibet, J.G., Rossi, J.F., ... Bataille, R. (1996). A prospective randomized trial of autologous bone marrow transplantation and chemotherapy in multiple myeloma. Intergroupe Français du Myélome. *New England Journal of Medicine, 335,* 91–97. doi:10.1056/NEJM199607113350204

Barlogie, B., Alexanian, R., Dicke, K.A., Zagars, G., Spitzer, G., Jagannath, S., & Horwitz, L. (1987). High-dose chemoradiotherapy and autologous bone marrow transplantation for resistant multiple myeloma. *Blood, 70,* 869–872.

Barlogie, B., Anaissie, E., van Rhee, F., Haessler, J., Hollmig, K., Pineda-Roman, M., ... Shaughnessy, J.D., Jr. (2007). Incorporating bortezomib into upfront treatment for multiple myeloma: Early results of total therapy 3. *British Journal of Haematology, 138,* 176–185. doi:10.1111/j.1365-2141.2007.06639.x

Barlogie, B., Pineda-Roman, M., van Rhee, F., Haessler, J., Anaissie, E., Hollmig, K., ... Crowley, J. (2008). Thalidomide arm of Total Therapy 2 improves complete remission duration and survival in myeloma patients with metaphase cytogenetic abnormalities. *Blood, 112,* 3115–3121. doi:10.1182/blood-2008-03-145235

Barlogie, B., Shaughnessy, J., Tricot, G., Jacobson, J., Zangari, M., Anaissie, E., ... Crowley, J. (2004). Treatment of multiple myeloma. *Blood, 103,* 20–32. doi:10.1182/blood-2003-04-1045

Barlogie, B., Tricot, G., Rasmussen, E., Anaissie, E., van Rhee, F., Zangari, M., ... Crowley, J. (2006). Total therapy 2 without thalidomide in comparison with total therapy 1: Role of intensified induction and posttransplantation consolidation therapies. *Blood, 107,* 2633–2638. doi:10.1182/blood-2005-10-4084

Bergsagel, D.E., Sprague, C.C., Austin, C., & Griffith, K.M. (1962). Evaluation of new chemotherapeutic agents in the treatment of multiple myeloma. IV. L-Phenylalanine mustard (NSC-8806). *Cancer Chemotherapy Reports, 21,* 87–99.

Bertolotti, P., Bilotti, E., Colson, K., Curran, K., Doss, D., Faiman, B., ... Westphal, J. (2008). Management of side effects of novel therapies for multiple myeloma: Consensus statements developed by the International Myeloma Foundation's Nurse Leadership Board. *Clinical Journal of Oncology Nursing, 12*(Suppl. 3), 9–12. doi:10.1188/08.CJON.S1.9-12

Blokhin, N., Larionov, L., Perevodchikova, N., Chebotareva, L., & Merkulova, N. (1958). Clinical experiences with sarcolysin in neoplastic diseases. *Annals of the New York Academy of Sciences, 68,* 1128–1132. doi:10.1111/j.1749-6632.1958.tb42675.x

Braggio, E., Sebag, M., & Fonseca, R. (2008). Cytogenetic abnormalities in multiple myeloma: The importance of FISH and cytogenetics. In S. Lonial (Ed.), *Myeloma therapy: Pursuing the plasma cell* (pp. 57–76). Totowa, NJ: Humana Press.

Cavo, M., Tosi, P., Zamagni, E., Cellini, C., Tacchetti, P., Patriarca, F., ... Baccarani, M. (2007). Prospective, randomized study of single compared with double autologous stem-cell transplantation for multiple myeloma: Bologna 96 clinical study. *Journal of Clinical Oncology, 25,* 2434–2441. doi:10.1200/JCO.2006.10.2509

Child, J.A., Morgan, G.J., Davies, F.E., Owen, R.G., Bell, S.E., Hawkins, K., ... Selby, P.J. (2003). High-dose chemotherapy with hematopoietic stem-cell rescue for multiple myeloma. *New England Journal of Medicine, 348,* 1875–1883. doi:10.1056/NEJMoa022340

Chng, W.J., & Bergsagel, P.L. (2008). Biologically-based classification and staging of multiple myeloma. In S. Lonial (Ed.), *Myeloma therapy: Pursuing the plasma cell* (pp. 41–56). Totowa, NJ: Humana Press.

Coleman, E.A., Coon, S., Hall-Barrow, J., Richards, K., Gaylor, D., & Stewart, B. (2003). Feasibility of exercise during treatment for multiple myeloma. *Cancer Nursing, 26,* 410–419. doi:10.1097/00002820-200310000-00012

Coleman, E.A., Coon, S.K., Kennedy, R.L., Lockhart, K.D., Stewart, C.B., Anaissie, E.J., & Barlogie, B. (2008). Effects of exercise in combination with epoetin alfa during high-dose chemotherapy and autologous peripheral blood stem cell transplantation for multiple myeloma [Online exclusive]. *Oncology Nursing Forum, 35,* E53–E61. doi:10.1188/08.ONF.E53-E61

Coleman, E.A., Hall-Barrow, J., Coon, S., & Stewart, C.B. (2003). Facilitating exercise adherence for patients with multiple myeloma. *Clinical Journal of Oncology Nursing, 7,* 529–534, 540. doi:10.1188/03.CJON.529-534

Coon, S.K., & Coleman, E.A. (2004a). Exercise decisions within the context of multiple myeloma, transplant, and fatigue. *Cancer Nursing, 27,* 108–118.

Coon, S.K., & Coleman, E.A. (2004b). Keep moving: Patients with myeloma talk about exercise and fatigue. *Oncology Nursing Forum, 31,* 1127–1135. doi:10.1188/04.ONF.1127-1135

Durie, B.G. (2008). Oncology nurses take the lead in providing novel therapy guidelines for multiple myeloma. *Clinical Journal of Oncology Nursing, 12*(Suppl. 3), 7–8. doi:10.1188/08. CJON.S1.7-8

Faiman, B., Bilotti, E., Mangan, P.A., & Rogers, K. (2008). Steroid-associated side effects in patients with multiple myeloma: Consensus statement of the IMF Nurse Leadership Board. *Clinical Journal of Oncology Nursing, 12*(Suppl. 3), 53–63. doi:10.1188/08.CJON.S1.53-62

Galli, M., Nicolucci, A., Valentini, M., Belfiglio, M., Delaini, F., Crippa, C., ... Barbui, T. (2005). Feasibility and outcome of tandem stem cell autotransplants in multiple myeloma. *Haematologica, 90,* 1643–1649.

Goldschmidt, H. (2005). Single versus double high dose therapy in multiple myeloma: Second analysis of the trial GMMG-HD2. *Haematologica, 90*(Suppl. 1), 38.

Harousseau, J. (2008). Role of autologous stem cell transplantation in multiple myeloma. In S. Lonial (Ed.), *Myeloma therapy: Pursuing the plasma cell* (pp. 79–90). Totowa, NJ: Humana Press.

Jemal, A., Siegel, R., Ward, E., Hao, Y., Xu, J., & Thun, M.J. (2009). Cancer statistics, 2009. *CA: A Cancer Journal for Clinicians, 59,* 225–249. doi:10.3322/caac.20006

Kumar, S.K., Rajkumar, S.V., Dispenzieri, A., Lacy, M.Q., Hayman, S.R., Buadi, F.K., ... Gertz, M.A. (2008). Improved survival in multiple myeloma and the impact of novel therapies. *Blood, 111,* 2516–2520. doi:10.1182/blood-2007-10-116129

Kyle, R.A., & Rajkumar, S.V. (2008). Multiple myeloma. *Blood, 111,* 2962–2972. doi:10.1182/ blood-2007-10-078022

Kyle, R.A., Therneau, T.M., Rajkumar, S.V., Larson, D.R., Plevak, M.F., & Melton, L.J., 3rd. (2004). Incidence of multiple myeloma in Olmsted County, Minnesota: Trend over 6 decades. *Cancer, 101,* 2667–2674. doi:10.1002/cncr.20652

Kyle, R.A., Yee, G.C., Somerfield, M.R., Flynn, P.J., Halabi, S., Jagannath, S., ... Anderson, K. (2007). American Society of Clinical Oncology 2007 clinical practice guideline update on the role of bisphosphonates in multiple myeloma. *Journal of Clinical Oncology, 25,* 2464–2472. doi:10.1200/JCO.2007.12.1269

Lokhorst, H. (2002). Clinical features and diagnostic criteria. In J. Mehta & S. Singhal (Eds.), *Myeloma* (pp. 151–168). London, England: Martin Dunitz Ltd.

McElwain, T.J., & Powles, R.L. (1983). High-dose intravenous melphalan for plasma-cell leukaemia and myeloma. *Lancet, 2,* 822–824. doi:10.1016/S0140-6736(83)90739-0

Mehta, J., & Singhal, S. (2007). High-dose chemotherapy and autologous hematopoietic stem cell transplantation in myeloma patients under the age of 65 years. *Bone Marrow Transplantation, 40,* 1101–1114. doi:10.1038/sj.bmt.1705799

Mehta, J., & Singhal, S. (2008). Current status of autologous hematopoietic stem cell transplantation in myeloma. *Bone Marrow Transplantation, 42*(Suppl. 1), S28–S34. doi:10.1038/ bmt.2008.109

Miceli, T., Colson, K., Gavino, M., & Lilleby, K. (2008). Myelosuppression associated with novel therapies in patients with multiple myeloma: Consensus statement of the IMF Nurse Leadership Board. *Clinical Journal of Oncology Nursing, 12*(Suppl. 3), 13–20. doi:10.1188/08.CJON.S1.13-19

Mulligan, G., Mitsiades, C., Bryant, B., Zhan, F., Chng, W.J., Roels, S., ... Anderson, K.C. (2007). Gene expression profiling and correlation with outcome in clinical trials of the proteasome inhibitor bortezomib. *Blood, 109,* 3177–3188. doi:10.1182/ blood-2006-09-044974

Munshi, N.C., & Anderson, K.C. (2005). Plasma cell neoplasms. In V.T. DeVita Jr., S. Hellman & S.A. Rosenberg (Eds.), *Cancer: Principles and practice of oncology* (7th ed., pp. 2155–2188). Philadelphia, PA: Lippincott Williams & Wilkins.

Myeloma Trialists' Collaborative Group. (1998). Combination chemotherapy versus melphalan plus prednisone as treatment for multiple myeloma: An overview of 6633 patients from 27 randomized trials. *Journal of Clinical Oncology, 16,* 3832–3842.

Osserman, E.F., DiRe, L.B., DiRe, J., Sherman, W.H., Hersman, J.A., & Storb, R. (1982). Identical twin marrow transplantation in multiple myeloma. *Acta Haematologica, 68,* 215–223. doi:10.1159/000206984

Poulos, A.R., Gertz, M.A., Pankratz, V.S., & Post-White, J. (2001). Pain, mood disturbance, and quality of life in patients with multiple myeloma. *Oncology Nursing Forum, 28,* 1163–1172.

Putkonen, M., Rauhala, A., Itala, M., Kauppila, M., Pelliniemi, T.T., & Remes, K. (2005). Double versus single autotransplantation in multiple myeloma: A single center experience of 100 patients. *Haematologica, 90,* 562–563.

Qian, J., Wang, S., Yang, J., Xie, J., Lin, P., Freeman, M.E., 3rd, & Yi, Q. (2005). Targeting heat shock proteins for immunotherapy in multiple myeloma: Generation of myeloma-specific CTLs using dendritic cells pulsed with tumor-derived gp96. *Clinical Cancer Research, 11,* 8808–8815. doi:10.1158/1078-0432.CCR-05-1553

Raab, M.S., & Anderson, K.C. (2008). Basic biology of plasma cell dyscrasias: Focus on the role of the tumor microenvironment. In S. Lonial (Ed.), *Myeloma therapy: Pursuing the plasma cell* (pp. 23–39). Totowa, NJ: Humana Press.

Rome, S., Doss, D., Miller, K., & Westphal, J. (2008). Thromboembolic events associated with novel therapies in patients with multiple myeloma: Consensus statement of the IMF Nurse Leadership Board. *Clinical Journal of Oncology Nursing, 12*(Suppl. 3), 21–28.

Shaughnessy, J., Jr., Zhan, F., Barlogie, B., & Stewart, A.K. (2005). Gene expression profiling and multiple myeloma. *Best Practice and Research: Clinical Haematology, 18,* 537–552. doi:10.1016/j.beha.2005.02.003

Shaughnessy, J.D., Jr., Zhan, F., Burington, B.E., Huang, Y., Colla, S., Hanamura, I., … Barlogie, B. (2007). A validated gene expression model of high-risk multiple myeloma is defined by deregulated expression of genes mapping to chromosome 1. *Blood, 109,* 2276–2284. doi:10.1182/blood-2006-07-038430

Singhal, S., Mehta, J., Desikan, R., Ayers, D., Roberson, P., Eddlemon, P., … Barlogie, B. (1999). Antitumor activity of thalidomide in refractory multiple myeloma. *New England Journal of Medicine, 341,* 1565–1571. doi:10.1056/NEJM199911183412102

Smith, L.C., Bertolotti, P., Curran, K., & Jenkins, B. (2008). Gastrointestinal side effects associated with novel therapies in patients with multiple myeloma: Consensus statement of the IMF Nurse Leadership Board. *Clinical Journal of Oncology Nursing, 12*(Suppl. 3), 37–52. doi:10.1188/08.CJON.S1.37-51

Tariman, J.D., & Faiman, B. (2010). Multiple myeloma. In C.H. Yarbro, D. Wujcik, & B.H. Gobel (Eds.), *Cancer nursing: Principles and practice* (7th ed., pp. 1518–1545). Sudbury, MA: Jones and Bartlett.

Tariman, J.D., Love, G., McCullagh, E., & Sandifer, S. (2008). Peripheral neuropathy associated with novel therapies in patients with multiple myeloma: Consensus statement of the IMF Nurse Leadership Board. *Clinical Journal of Oncology Nursing, 12*(Suppl. 3), 29–36.

Wang, S., Hong, S., Yang, J., Qian, J., Zhang, X., Shpall, E., … Yi, Q. (2006). Optimizing immunotherapy in multiple myeloma: Restoring the function of patients' monocyte-derived dendritic cells by inhibiting p38 or activating MEK/ERK MAPK and neutralizing interleukin-6 in progenitor cells. *Blood, 108,* 4071–4077. doi:10.1182/blood-2006-04-016980

Yi, Q. (2003). Immunotherapy in multiple myeloma: Current strategies and future prospects. *Expert Review of Vaccines, 2,* 391–398. doi:10.1586/14760584.2.3.391

Zangari, M., van Rhee, F., Anaissie, E., Pineda-Roman, M., Haessler, J., Crowley, J., & Barlogie, B. (2008). Eight-year median survival in multiple myeloma after total therapy 2: Roles of thalidomide and consolidation chemotherapy in the context of total therapy 1. *British Journal of Haematology, 141,* 433–444. doi:10.1111/j.1365-2141.2008.06982.x

CHAPTER 2

Anatomy and Physiology

Kimberly Noonan, RN, ANP, AOCN®

THE IMMUNE SYSTEM

The immune system plays an important role in multiple myeloma (a cancer of the plasma cells) pathogenesis. A solid knowledge of the immune system's fundamentals, particularly adaptive (acquired) immunity, is required to better understand multiple myeloma. Specifically, understanding how lymphocytes, plasma cells (the mature form of B cells), and immunoglobulins, as well as cytokine interactions, relate to each other can lead to a better understanding of the pathophysiologic changes in patients with multiple myeloma.

A functional immune system is essential to maintain good health. Without a healthy immune system, life can be difficult, compromised by infections. The immune system is able to protect the body against viral and bacterial infections, as well as cancer and many inflammatory diseases, because of its capability to differentiate self from nonself. Moreover, the immune system is unique in that a response to an initial encounter of a pathogenic antigen occurs successfully with clear evidence that memory of this antigen is present with future encounters (Alam & Gorska, 2003; Carter, 2006).

INNATE AND ACQUIRED IMMUNITY

Immunity develops as two specific types: innate and acquired. Although innate and acquired immunity often are described as separate entities, they often act together and can be dependent on each other. Innate immunity represents the first line of defense, and acquired immunity responds after several days. Innate immunity is also called natural or native immunity. This type of immunity exists in healthy individuals from birth. The cells responsible for innate immunity include phagocytic cells (neutrophils, monocytes, and macrophages), cells that release inflammatory mediators (basophils, mast cells, and eosinophils), and natural killer (NK) cells. The molecular components of innate responses include complement, acute phase proteins, and cytokines such as interferons (Delves & Roitt, 2000). Epithelial barriers that line the mucous membrane and skin block the entry of the microbes; they are considered the first line of defense in innate immunity. If microbes do break through the epithelial cells, other cells such as phagocytes, NK cells, dendritic cells, and plasma proteins, including the complement system, are activated to destroy the foreign agent (Abbas & Lichtman, 2009; Sommer, 2005).

The second type of immunity is adaptive, or acquired, immunity. *Adaptive* means that this type develops at a slower and more deliberate pace than innate immunity. The cells responsible for adaptive immunity include B and T cells (lymphocytes) and antigen-presenting cells (APCs). Lymphocytes and lymphocyte products are involved in adaptive immunity by recognizing substances known as antigens, while APCs display the antigen to lymphocytes and collaborate with them in the response to antigen. Adaptive immunity involves specificity for its target antigen that has specific receptors, which are expressed on T and B lymphocyte surfaces (Chaplin, 2006). Adaptive immune responses are generated in the lymph nodes, spleen, and mucosa-associated lymphoid tissues, which include the tonsils, adenoids, and Peyer patches. T and B cells develop from pluripotent stem cells in the fetal liver and in bone marrow and then circulate throughout the extracellular fluid. B cells reach maturity within the bone marrow, but T cells must travel to the thymus to complete their development (Delves & Roitt, 2000).

ADAPTIVE IMMUNITY: HUMORAL AND CELLULAR

Humoral Immunity

Humoral immunity is the main function of the B lymphocytes. It is mediated by antibodies that are made of molecules including heavy- and light-chain immunoglobulins. Mature B cells (plasma cells) secrete antibodies into the peripheral blood and mucosal fluids. Their functions include recognizing extracellular microbial antigens and neutralizing and eliminating microbes that may be present outside host cells, in the blood, and in the mucosal lumens. Antibodies do not have access to microbes living inside infected cells.

Cellular Immunity

Cellular immunity, or cell-mediated immunity, is primarily a function of the T lymphocytes, which defend the body against microbes such as viruses. Some T cells activate phagocytes to destroy microbes that have been ingested by phagocytes into intracellular vesicles. Other T cells kill host cells that are harboring infectious microbes in the cytoplasm (Abbas & Lichtman, 2009). Figure 2-1 differentiates the roles of B and T cells in adaptive immunity.

Figure 2-1. B and T Cells' Roles in Adaptive Immunity

Humoral Immunity	Cell-Mediated Immunity
• B lymphocytes	• T lymphocytes
• Mature in the bone marrow	• Mature in the thymus
• Defend against extracellular microbes	• Defend against intracellular microbes
• Recognize many different molecules such as proteins, carbohydrates, and lipids	• Recognize only protein antigens

Note. Based on information from Abbas & Lichtman, 2009; Sommer, 2005.

ORGANS OF THE IMMUNE SYSTEM

The organs of the immune system consist of the lymph nodes, bone marrow, thymus, spleen, tonsils, and appendix. Bone marrow and the thymus create an environment for immune cell production and maturation. Lymph nodes have the typical structure of peripheral lymph nodes, with defined T- and B-cell–dependent compartments (Crivellato, Vacca, & Ribatti, 2004). They are encapsulated organs, presenting distinct cortical and medullary regions, and are composed of lymph tissue located throughout the body. Lymph nodes remove foreign material from the lymph before entering the bloodstream and provide an environment for immune responses as well as lymphocyte proliferation. In a normally functioning immune system, 99% of all lymphocytes reside in the lymph (Sommer, 2005). The spleen is a secondary lymphoid organ and is essential in fighting infections and filtering antigens from the blood. Other secondary lymphoid tissues include the tonsils, Peyer patches in the intestine, and the appendix. These tissues contain the essential B and T lymphocytes needed to mount an immune response (Sommer, 2005).

CELLS RESPONSIBLE FOR INNATE IMMUNITY

Neutrophils, Monocytes, and Macrophages

White blood cells that are essential in the immune response include neutrophils, monocytes, and macrophages, which play an important role in innate immunity. Each cell is highly phagocytic in destroying microbes. Neutrophils produce substantial amounts of cytokines such as tumor necrosis factor (TNF) and interleukin (IL)-12. All of these cells are essential for the process of inflammation and infection clearance.

Eosinophils, Basophils, and Mast Cells

Eosinophils are needed to combat parasitic and allergic responses, whereas basophils and mast cells are similar cells with high affinity receptors for immunoglobulin E. They are key initiators of immediate hypersensitivity responses, releasing histamine and producing quantities of mediators that stimulate tissue inflammation, edema, and smooth muscle contraction (Chaplin, 2003). All of these cells are important in releasing inflammatory mediators (Delves & Roitt, 2000).

CELLS RESPONSIBLE FOR ADAPTIVE IMMUNITY

The immune system has many types of specialized cells, with lymphocytes as the main type. The other important immune system cells are the APCs and effector cells. Lymphocytes are the key mediators of adaptive immunity. They are also the only cells that produce specific receptors for antigens.

Antigens are substances foreign to the host, and they stimulate a response from the immune system. They can be microbial or nonmicrobial. Microbial antigens include bacteria, fungi, viruses, protozoa, and parasites. Examples of nonmicrobial antigens are resin (such as plant pollen), insect venom, and transplanted organs. The smallest identifiable section of an antigen bound by a receptor is known as an epitope, which is also referred to as an antigenic determinant (Harvey et al., 2008). Surface proteins located on lymphocytes, called CD (or cluster of differentiation), are used to identify a specific cell type or stage of cellular differentiation. For example, B lymphocytes have surface proteins that are CD20+, and T lymphocytes have surface proteins that are identified as CD4 or CD8. More than 260 defined CD types exist (Abbas & Lichtman, 2009; Chaplin, 2003).

Lymphocytes

Lymphocytes represent 25%–35% of blood leukocytes. B lymphocytes comprise 10%–20% of circulating lymphocytes (Sommer, 2005). B lymphocytes are derived from the bone marrow and mature into plasma cells through programmed steps (hence, myeloma is often referred to as cancer of the bone marrow by lay people). They synthesize antibodies and provide defense against microorganisms, including bacteria and viruses. Hematopoietic stem cells begin in the bone marrow where they mature in progenitor (pro-) B cells, precursor (pre-) B cells, and immature B cells. Figure 2-2 describes B-cell development. Immature B cells enter into circulation as transitional B cells, migrating to secondary lymphoid organs. These cells become naïve B cells again when entering the blood (Carter, 2006).

B lymphocytes are the only cells capable of producing antibodies, and they are responsible for creating humoral immunity. Humoral immunity prevents viral infections, eliminates bacterial invaders, neutralizes bacterial toxins, and responds to certain allergic reactions. This type of immunity is mediated by proteins called antibodies, which are secreted by plasma cells into peripheral blood and mucosal fluids. It is important to note that B cells

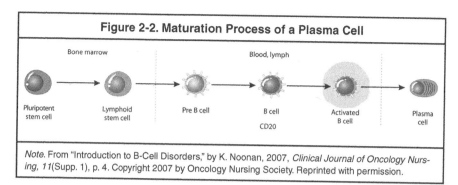

Figure 2-2. Maturation Process of a Plasma Cell

Bone marrow

Blood, lymph

Pluripotent stem cell

Lymphoid stem cell

Pre B cell

B cell
CD20

Activated B cell

Plasma cell

Note. From "Introduction to B-Cell Disorders," by K. Noonan, 2007, *Clinical Journal of Oncology Nursing, 11*(Supp. 1), p. 4. Copyright 2007 by Oncology Nursing Society. Reprinted with permission.

recognize membrane forms of antibodies that become receptors for antigens and ultimately initiate the activation process. Their function is to neutralize and eliminate microbes that may be present outside host cells, in the blood, and in the mucosal lumens, such as the respiratory or gastrointestinal system. Their main function is to recognize extracellular microbial antigens, but this does not include microbes living inside infected cells.

T lymphocytes have a unique capability of recognizing a processed antigen peptide in association with a self-recognition protein called the major histocompatibility complex (MHC) molecule. MHC is crucial for lymphocytes to differentiate self from foreign. The role that MHC plays in the human body is to recognize and accept cellular interactions between immune cells and body cells. MHC molecules are often discussed in the setting of graft rejection in an organ or tissue transplant (Chaplin, 2006). Class I MHC molecules are found on all nucleated cells in the body and are capable of alerting the immune system of any cell changes such as viruses, intracellular bacteria, or cancer. Class II MHC molecules are found on APCs such as macrophages, dendritic cells, and B lymphocytes. Class II MHC molecules communicate with the antigen receptor and CD4 molecule on the helper T lymphocytes (Chaplin, 2006).

NK cells, another type of lymphocyte, are functionally and phenotypically different from T and B lymphocytes. The function of the NK cell is to destroy tumor cells, virus-infected cells, and intracellular microbes. The NK cell is thought to be programmed to kill foreign cells automatically, in contrast to the CD8 T cells, which require activation to become cytotoxic (Chaplin, 2003).

Antigen-Presenting Cells

APCs are located in the epithelium and capture antigens so that they are presented to the lymphocytes. Dendritic cells, macrophages, and B cells are examples of APCs. APCs are often located in the skin (fibroblast), gastrointestinal tract (pancreatic beta cells), and respiratory tract (certain activated epithelial cells).

Effector Cells

Effector cells consist of lymphocytes and other leukocytes that are primarily responsible for eliminating microbes. In humoral immunity, activated B cells produce effector cells called plasma cells, which secrete protein molecules called antibodies or immunoglobulins (Sommer, 2005).

Two types of T lymphocyte effector cells exist. The first type is CD4, or helper, T cells, which produce cytokines. These specific cytokines activate B cells and macrophages. The second type is CD8 T lymphocytes, which have the ability to kill infected host cells. Both B and T effector cells generally are short-lived, with the exception of a few. Table 2-1 is a partial list of the significant cells that are essential in creating immunologic responses.

Memory Cells

Memory cells are generated from antigen-stimulated lymphocytes and survive for long periods of time. Memory cells increase with age as more infections occur. Memory cells remain inactive until they encounter the same

Table 2-1. Cells of Immunity	
Cells	**Function**
Lymphocytes: B cells, T cells, and natural killer (NK) cells	**Lymphocytes recognize antigens.**
B cells mature in bone marrow.	B cells become plasma cells, which create antibodies or immunoglobulins.
T cells mature in the thymus.	Responsible for humoral immunity T cells are the mediators for cell-mediated immunity. Two types of T lymphocytes: helper and cytotoxic T cells NK cells are involved in innate immunity.
Antigen-Presenting Cells (APCs): macrophages, B cells, and dendritic cells, specifically follicular dendritic cells	APCs capture antigens for lymphocytic display. Dendritic cells: Initiate T-cell responses.
Effector cells: T lymphocytes, macrophages, and granulocytes	**Effector cells eliminate antigens.** T lymphocytes: CD4, or helper, T cells and CD8, or cytotoxic, T lymphocytes Macrophages and monocytes: Part of the mononuclear-phagocyte system Granulocytes: Europhiles, basophils, and eosinophils

Note. Based on information from Abbas & Lichtman, 2009; Sommer, 2005.

antigen that stimulated their development. When this occurs, they rapidly respond and give rise to a secondary immune response. Naïve lymphocytes are responsible for the interaction of the primary immune response (Abbas & Lichtman, 2009; Chaplin, 2006). One of the most important functions of memory B cells is antigen presentation. Memory B cells are known to be long-lived, but they undergo homeostatic self-renewal (Ahuja, Anderson, Khalil, & Shlomchik, 2008; Carter, 2006; Dorner, 2006).

T Cells

Two types of T cells exist. The first type is helper T cells, which are CD4 cells. These cells help B cells produce antibodies and help phagocytes destroy ingested microbes. The second type is the cytotoxic T lymphocytes (CTLs), which are CD8 cells. CTLs destroy target cells by releasing cytolytic enzymes or toxic cytokines or by inducing apoptosis.

B Cells

B cells are precursors to plasma cells deriving from the bone marrow. They can mount a rapid antibody response to typical bacterial antigens. Other B cells require help from T cells that form highly selective antibodies. APCs regulate both the rapid antibody response and T-cell dependent pathways. The T-cell dependent pathway cells may differentiate into memory B cells or into antibody-producing plasma cells.

B cells play an important role in immunity independent of antibody production. B lymphocytes link innate and acquired adaptive immunity by using specific receptors expressed only on B cells. As described previously, class II MHC molecules are found on APCs and, specifically, B lymphocytes to stimulate T cells. B cells allow for optimal development of memory in the CD4 T-cell population. These cells also are capable of producing cytokines (e.g., interleukin, TNF), which regulate the effects of other APCs such as dendritic cells or mononuclear cells. Another important function of B lymphocytes is their involvement in orchestrating the inflammatory processes via proinflammatory cytokines such as TNF-alpha and IL-6. Cytokine production by B cells contributes to certain steps in immune activation and has been implicated in certain autoimmune diseases, such as rheumatoid arthritis and systemic lupus erythematosus (Carter, 2006; Dorner, 2006).

One activated B cell may generate up to 4,000 plasma cells and produces approximately 10^{12} antibody molecules per day (Abbas & Lichtman, 2009). This calculation helps to explain why humoral immunity can defend against rapidly dividing microbes. Different chemical structures, including proteins, polysaccharides, lipids, and small chemicals, activate B lymphocytes. Protein antigens are processed in APCs and require the assistance of helper T lymphocytes.

The role of B cells independent of antibody production is crucial to a normal immune response. B cells are not only responsible to B-lymphocyte activity, but also to T-cell responses in the immune system. They aid in the activation, anergy (no response to antibody or antigen), differentiation, and expansion of T cells. B-cell receptors (BCRs) are composed of monomeric immunoglobulin with disulfide-linked heterodimers called Ig alpha (Igα) and Ig beta (Igβ). When a BCR binds to an epitope, B-cell activation is initiated because of the Igα and Igβ intracellular signaling cascade.

Plasma Cells

Plasma cells are the effector cells that originate and develop from the B lymphocytes. They are antibody-producing cells and have the same specificity as the naïve B-cell membrane receptors that are responsible for antigen recognition that initiate response (Abbas & Lichtman, 2009). Plasma cells appear larger on a peripheral smear with abundant cytoplasm, which also distinguishes them from T and B lymphocytes. The nuclei of normal, mature plasma cells have no nucleoli, but the nuclei of neoplastic plasma cells such as those seen in multiple myeloma have conspicuous nucleoli (Cruse & Lewis, 2009). Figure 2-3 demonstrates how the plasma cells become aberrant in multiple myeloma.

Plasma cells synthesize immunoglobulin in response to stimulation by an antigen. An immunoglobulin is a characteristic four-polypeptide structure consisting of at least two identical antigen binding sites. Antibodies are applied to an immunoglobulin molecule with specificity for an epitope of molecules that make up antigens. Antibodies bind to antigens to immobilize them, render them harmless, or tag the antigen for destruction. The antigen is removed by another component in the immune system (Harvey et al., 2008). Immunoglobulins are divided into five classes and often function as BCRs.

Antibody responses are differentiated into T-cell dependent and T-cell independent and are determined by where the B cells are located in the lymphoid. The majority of B lymphocytes live in the follicle of the lymphoid organ and are appropriately labeled *follicular B cells*. These B cells constitute the bulk of T-cell dependent antibodies and are long-lived plasma cells (Abbas & Lichtman, 2009).

Marginal-zone B cells located in the marginal zone of the splenic white pulp respond to blood-borne polysaccharide antigens and to nonprotein antigens in the mucosal tissues and peritoneum. Marginal-zone antigens do not require T-cell help to create an antibody. These antibodies are short-lived when compared to the follicular type of B cells (Abbas & Lichtman, 2009).

B-1 B cells respond to nonprotein antigens in the mucosal tissues and peritoneum. These cells represent a transitional lymphocyte that bridges the innate and adaptive immune systems. Marginal-zone and B-1, cells express antigen receptors, have limited functionality, and are predominantly responsible for immunoglobulin-M-type responses (Abbas & Lichtman, 2009). Immunoglobulin-M will be discussed in the next section.

Figure 2-3. Plasma Cells in Multiple Myeloma

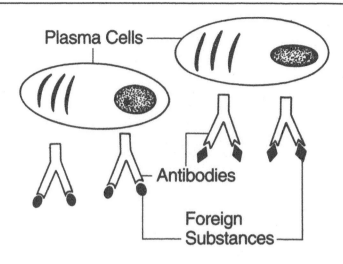

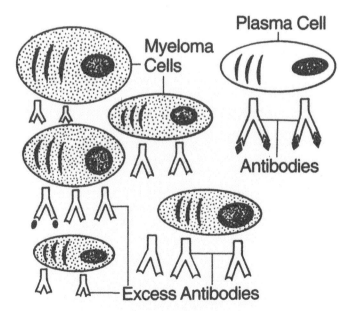

One diagram shows plasma cells producing antibodies and attaching to foreign substances to fight infection and disease. The other diagram shows the body making too many plasma (myeloma) cells. These cells produce antibodies that the body does not need.

Note. Figure courtesy of the National Cancer Institute. Retrieved from http://visualsonline.cancer.gov/details.cfm?imageid=2718.

IMMUNOGLOBULINS

Understanding the concept of immunoglobulins, what they are, and how they work is essential in relating to the pathophysiology of multiple myeloma. Antibody and immunoglobulin definitions are used interchangeably because antibody molecules are immunoglobulins of defined specificity produced by plasma cells. Immunoglobulin molecules are multifunctional tools used by cells to mediate interactions of antigen molecules with a variety of cellular and humoral effector mechanisms. Immunoglobulins are composed of four polypeptide chains. These chains include two identical heavy chains (H) and two identical light chains (L). The four chains are assembled to form a Y-shaped molecule and are linked by disulfide bonds to form a monomeric unit. Each chain consists of one variable region with each light chain attached to one heavy chain. The two heavy chains are attached to each other, and each individual heavy and light chain can be subdivided into regions known as immunoglobulin domains (Harvey et al., 2008). Five types of H chains exist: mu (IgM), delta (IgD), gamma (IgG), epsilon (IgE), and alpha (IgA). They are all encoded on chromosome 14. Light chains contain one constant and one variable domain. This differs from a heavy-chain structure, which consists of one variable and four constant domains (Abbas & Lichtman, 2009).

Immunoglobulins are divided into fragments, with each fragment determining the biologic properties that are characteristic of a particular class of immunoglobulin. Figure 2-4 will aid in the explanation of light and heavy chains, as well as fragments of immunoglobulin. The components of a full immunoglobulin structure (Abbas & Lichtman, 2009; Harvey et al., 2008; Sommer, 2005) are as follows:

- **Fab** or antigen-binding fragment; each fragment has an epitope binding site.
- **Fc**, or constant fragment, is responsible for many biologic activities that occur following engagement of an epitope.
- **Fd** is the heavy-chain section of Fab.
- **Fd′** is a heavy-chain portion of Fab with an extra amino acid.
- **F(ab′)₂** is a dimeric molecule containing two segments with epitope-binding sites.
- **Hinge region** is the area where the disulfide bonds join the heavy chain.

Heavy-Chain Immunoglobulins

The structure of an immunoglobulin contains four polypeptides: two are identical light (L) chains, and two are identical heavy (H) chains. Each subunit is categorized into immunoglobulin domains. Light chains have two domains, whereas heavy chains have four or five domains. The molecular weight of heavy chains is approximately 55 kilodaltons (kd) (Abbas & Lichtman, 2009). See Figure 2-4 to identify the heavy chain region on the immunoglobulin. Heavy-chain isotypes determine the class, or isotype. The five types of immunoglobulin are

Figure 2-4. The Immunoglobulin Structure

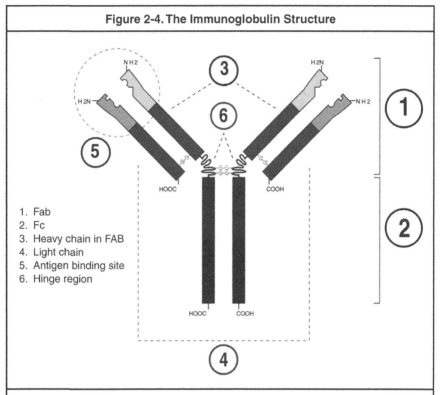

1. Fab
2. Fc
3. Heavy chain in FAB
4. Light chain
5. Antigen binding site
6. Hinge region

Note. From "Antibody," in *Wikipedia, The Free Encyclopedia*, 2010, January 4. Retrieved from http://en.wikipedia.org/w/index.php?title=Antibody&oldid=335724201.

Open access artwork used under the terms of the GNU Free Documentation License (http://commons.wikimedia.org/wiki/Commons:GNU_Free_Documentation_License) and the Creative Commons Attribution ShareAlike 3.0 (http://creativecommons.org/licenses/by-sa/3.0).

IgG, IgA, IgM, IgD, and IgE. The most abundant immunoglobulin is IgG. **IgG** is present in body fluids and can easily enter body tissue. IgG is the only immunoglobulin that crosses the placenta and transfers immunity from mother to fetus. These immunoglobulins protect against bacteria, toxins, and viruses; play a significant role in hypersensitivity; and are responsible for initiating antibody-dependent cell-mediated cytotoxicity. IgG has four subclasses, IgG1 through IgG4. **IgA** is a secretory immunoglobulin with two isoforms, alpha 1 and alpha 2. IgA can be found in saliva, tears, colostrums, and secretions found in the bronchus, gastrointestinal, prostate, and vagina. IgA prevents the attachment of viruses and bacteria to epithelial cells. **IgM** is the first immunoglobulin to be formed following antigenic stimulation. The function of IgM is to immobilize the antigen and activate the pathway of complement. IgM is the first antibody type produced by a newborn and does not cross the placenta. Most B cells display IgM on their cell surfaces. **IgD** is found on the cell membranes of B lymphocytes and serves as an antigen receptor for initiating the differentiation of B cells. Little is known about the function of IgD. **IgE** is involved in inflammation, allergic responses, and attack on parasitic infections. IgE binds to mast cells and basophils. The binding of antigen triggers cells to release histamine and other mediators that are important in the process of inflammation and allergic responses. Table 2-2 describes each immunoglobulin and the pertinent characteristics of each isotype (Abbas & Lichtman, 2009; Alam & Gorska, 2003).

Table 2-2. Types and Subtypes of Immunoglobulins and Their Functions		
Immunoglobulin	Subtype	Function
IgM	None	Naïve B-cell antigen receptor, complement activation
IgA	IgA 1, 2	Mucosal immunity and complement activation
IgD	None	Naïve B-cell antigen receptor
IgG	IgG 1–4	Complement activation, opsonization, and neutralizes microorganisms and viruses, antibody-dependent cell-mediated cytotoxicity, neonatal immunity, feedback inhibition of B cells
IgE	None	Mast cell and basophil activation triggers histamine and other inflammatory mediators needed for hypersensitivity protection, helminthic parasites.

Note. Based on information from Abbas & Lichtman, 2009; Harvey et al., 2008; Sommer, 2005.

Light-Chain Immunoglobulins

Light chains are polypeptides that are synthesized by plasma cells. Light chains unite with heavy chains to create classes of immunoglobulins. They are found on the outer portion of the immunoglobulin (see Figure 2-4). Light chains are categorized as kappa or lambda and are found on chromosomes 2 and 22, respectively. Light chains are further divided into 10 subtypes consisting of four kappa and six lambda. An individual immunoglobulin molecule possesses two light chains that are either kappa or lambda, but never a mixture of the two. This kappa or lambda restriction is helpful in determining the monoclonality of the plasma cells in multiple myeloma. Approximately 20% of patients with plasma cell disease only have an overproduction of light chains without an increase in heavy-chain production (Hillman, Ault, & Rinder, 2005). Light-chain disease is present not only in multiple myeloma but also in other diseases such as amyloidosis, POEMS syndrome (named as such for the symptoms of polyneuropathy, organomegaly, endocrinopathy, monoclonal gammopathy, and skin changes), and light-chain deposit disease (Hillman et al., 2005).

Immunoglobulins can bind to a wide variety of antigens. They can bind macromolecules as well as small molecules. The antigen-binding region on the antibody molecules form a flat surface capable of accommodating many different shapes. Epitopes or determinants located on antigens are recognized by antibodies. These determinants may be recognized by chemical sequence or shapes. The strength by which an antigen-binding surface of an antibody binds to one epitope of an antigen is known as the *affinity* of the interaction (Abbas & Lichtman, 2009).

CYTOKINES

Cytokines are low-molecular-weight regulatory proteins produced during all phases of an immune response. Cytokines play a crucial role in inflammation and immune responses, particularly during the initiation, perpetuation, and downregulation of both innate and adaptive immune responses. The immune system is dependent upon consistent and accurate intracellular communication by cytokines. As cytokines' interactions are key to myeloma cell survival, many novel therapies for multiple myeloma are now directed at interrupting cytokine pathways (Harvey et al., 2008).

Cytokines are derived from mononuclear phagocytic cells and other APCs. The antigens are taken up by APCs and are processed and presented to helper T lymphocytes. This provides one of the many pathways for this class of cytokine production. Another pathway involves monocytes, triggering the production of cytokines through the innate immune system (Borish & Steinke, 2003).

Cytokines are potent mediators of communication between immune cells. They have many important roles in immunity, including cell signaling and immune response coordination. They often are considered the hormones of the immune system. Cytokines bind to high-affinity surface receptors and are produced by nonimmune cells such as fibroblast or endothelial cells. They modulate reactions of the host to foreign antigens or injurious agents regulating the movement, proliferation, and differentiation of leukocytes as well as other cells (Sommer, 2005).

Cytokines are often described by their specific cellular interactions. Most cytokines act on cells that produce them, known as autocrines. Paracrines, on the other hand, are cytokines that act on adjacent cells. Endocrines are distant from their sites of secretion. In innate immune reactions, enough dendritic cells and macrophages may be activated to create large amounts of cytokine production that is dispersed in many body regions, thus making endocrine actions possible (Abbas & Lichtman, 2009).

Cytokines are synthesized by many cells and often are activated by T cells and macrophages. It is interesting to note that cytokines typically affect more than one cell type and have more than one physiologic cellular effect. Certain cytokines have biologic roles that overlap and develop into a cascade where one cytokine interaction is dependent upon another. Cytokines are needed to enhance or inhibit cellular interactions. In addition to positive feedback cytokine loops, many negative feedback signals regulate the immune system. Such mechanisms are essential in preventing an inflammatory response from overwhelming the host. Excessive cytokine production is associated with illnesses such septic shock, cancer, and asthma, as well as many other diseases and conditions (Sommer, 2005).

Chemokines are chemoattractant cytokines. IL-1 and TNF are examples of chemokines. Chemokines bind to glycoproteins on the surface of endothelial cells and stimulate an increase in the affinity of the leukocyte integrins for their ligands on the endothelium. Integrins are adhesion molecules that are found on leukocytes. Chemokines also stimulate the motility of leukocytes. As leukocytes accumulate at an infected area, vascular dilation and fluid accumulation occurs, along with protein buildup causing inflammation (Borish & Steinke, 2003; Harvey et al., 2008).

Cytokines have different functions in innate and adaptive immunity. Interleukins 1, 6, and 12 and TNF and interferon (IFN)-α and β are involved in innate immunity. They play an important role in inflammation, as well as in controlling viral infections and intracellular parasites. IL-12 is a key inducer of adaptive cell-mediated immunity and indirectly of inflammation and has the potential to influence the cytolytic potential of cytotoxic T cells and NK cells (Borish & Steinke, 2003).

Cytokines activate the immune cells in adaptive immunity by aiding in the proliferation and differentiation of the appropriate development of effector and memory cells. Cytokines such as IFN-gamma (IFN-γ) and IL-2, IL-4, and IL-10 are essential for these interactions. IL-2 is necessary for the proliferation and function of helper T and cytotoxic T cells, B lymphocytes, and NK cells. IL-2 also interacts with T lymphocytes by binding to specific membrane receptors present on activated T cells. Additionally, IL-2 receptors can trigger class II MHC interactions. Sustained T-cell proliferation relies on both IL-2 and IL-2 receptors. If either is missing, cell proliferation is not possible. IL-4 is a cytokine that regulates molecules that direct B cells needed to produce IgE antibodies. IL-5 is an activator of eosinophils and works with IgE antibodies to control parasitic infections. IFN-γ is the key macrophage-activating cytokine that aids both adaptive cell-mediated immunity and innate immune responses. Macrophages and NK cells are activated by IFN-γ to kill microbes more efficiently (Sommer, 2005).

Many cytokines stimulate bone marrow pluripotent stem cells and progenitor or precursor cells to produce white blood cells, red blood cells, dendritic cells, and platelets. The colony-stimulating factors, such as granulocyte progenitor cells and granulocyte-monocyte progenitor cells, were named according to the type of cell that they target. IL-11 stimulates thrombocyte production, and erythropoietin stimulates red blood cell production (Sommer, 2005). Table 2-3 lists and describes cytokines and their biologic activities.

Table 2-3. Types of Cytokines, Cell Sources, and Their Biologic Effects		
Cytokine	**Cell Sources**	**Target and Biologic Effects**
Interleukin (IL)-2	Activated T cell	Growth factor for T cells; activates cytotoxic T and natural killer (NK) cells
IL-3	Helper T cells	Growth factor for progenitor hematopoietic cells
IL-4	Helper T cells	Promotes growth and survival of T, B, and mast cells; activates B cells and eosinophils; induces IgE-type responses
IL-5	Helper T cell	Induces eosinophil growth; induces IgA production in B cells
IL-6	Mononuclear phagocytes, endothelial cells, and fibroblasts	Stimulates liver to produce acute-phase response; induces proliferation of antigen-presenting cells and especially antibody-producing B cells
IL-7	Bone marrow stromal cells	Stimulates survival and expansion of immature precursor B and T cells
IL-10	Mononuclear macrophages, dendritic cells, and some helper T cells	Decreases inflammation and inhibits activated macrophages
IL-12	Mononuclear phagocytes and dendritic cells	Mediator of the innate immune response to intracellular microbes; key inducer of cell-mediated immune responses to microbes; activates NK cells; promotes interferon-gamma production by NK and T cells
IL-15	Macrophages	NK and T-cell proliferation
IL-18	Macrophages	Interferon production in NK and T cells
Tumor necrosis factor	Macrophages and T cells	Inflammation; neutrophil activation; fever; synthesis of acute-phase proteins, fat catabolism, and apoptosis
Interferon-alpha and -beta	Dendritic cells, macrophages, and fibroblast	Antiviral; increase class I major histocompatibility complex and NK activation
Interferon-gamma	NK and T cells	Activates macrophages and stimulates antibody responses

(Continued on next page)

Table 2-3. Types of Cytokines, Cell Sources, and Their Biologic Effects *(Continued)*		
Cytokines	**Cell Sources**	**Target and Biologic Effects**
Chemokines	Macrophages, dendritic cells, endothelial cells, T cells, fibroblasts, and platelets	Increases leukocyte integrin affinity, chemotaxis, and activation
Colony-stimulating factors (CSFs) (granulocyte-CSF [G-CSF], granulocyte macrophage-CSF [GM-CSF], macrophage-CSF [M-CSF])	Activated T cells, macrophages, and endothelial cells, and bone marrow stromal fibroblast (GM-CSF and M-CSF)	G-CSF promotes growth and maturation of granulocytes. GM-CSF promotes growth and maturation of granulocytes and monocytes. Macrophage-CSF promotes growth and maturation of monocytes.

Note. Based on information from Abbas & Lichtman, 2009; Borish & Steinke, 2003; Sommer, 2005.

Cytokines are used in oncologic as well as non-oncologic practices. IFN is used for the treatment of many types of cancers, including melanoma, Kaposi sarcoma, renal cell cancer, and hematologic malignancies. IFN also is used for multiple sclerosis, hepatitis C, atopic dermatitis, and chronic granulomatous disease. Antitumor necrosis factor is used to treat rheumatoid arthritis. Cytokines continue to be studied in many clinical settings, and the use of cytokines to treat various diseases is likely to increase (Harvey et al., 2008).

CONCLUSION

The immune system is an interconnected complex system that is vital to our survival. Immunity develops in two specific pathways—innate and acquired. Innate immunity is native immunity, whereas acquired develops slowly. Acquired immunity is categorized into humoral and cell mediated. B lymphocytes are responsible for humoral immunity, and T lymphocytes are responsible for cell-mediated immunity. B and T lymphocytes are essential to the immune system. B lymphocytes are the only cell capable of producing antibody-secreting plasma cells. Antibodies produced by plasma cells secrete immunoglobulin. The role of antibodies is to bind with the antigen, immobilize the antigen, and ultimately cause antigenic destruction.

Immunoglobulins are composed of four polypeptide chains. These chains include two identical heavy chains and two identical light chains. Light chains are categorized as kappa or lambda and are found on chromosome 2 and 22, respectively. Heavy chains are more complicated, as there are five types: IgM, IgD, IgG, IgE, and IgA. Immunoglobulins are divided into fragments, and each fragment determines the biologic properties that are characteristic of a particular class of immunoglobulin. Figure 2-4 explains the immunoglobulin fragments.

Cytokines are low-molecular-weight regulatory proteins that are produced during all phases of an immune response. They play an essential role in initiation, perpetuation, and downregulation of immune responses, innate and adaptive immunity, and inflammation. Cytokines often are categorized and described by their specific cellular interactions. They are crucial to the immune system interactions.

Patients with multiple myeloma will experience a dysfunctional immune system. Understanding the immune system is critical when caring for people with multiple myeloma. Although the impact of a compromised immune system can be devastating to patients, knowledge of immunity will help nurses in identifying strategies that will aid in the care provided to these patients.

REFERENCES

Abbas, A.K., & Lichtman, A.H. (2009). Introduction to the immune system. In A.K. Abbas & A.H. Lichtman (Eds.), *Basic immunology: Functions and disorders of the immune system* (3rd ed., pp. 1–23). Philadelphia, PA: Saunders.

Ahuja, A., Anderson, S.M., Khalil, A., & Shlomchik, M.J. (2008). Maintenance of the plasma cell pool is independent of memory B cells. *Proceedings of the National Academy of Sciences of the United States of America, 105,* 4802–4807. doi:10.1073/pnas.0800555105

Alam, R., & Gorska, M. (2003). 3. Lymphocytes. *Journal of Allergy and Clinical Immunology, 111*(Suppl. 2), S476–S485. doi:10.1067/mai.2003.121

Borish, L.C., & Steinke, J.W. (2003). 2. Cytokines and chemokines. *Journal of Allergy and Clinical Immunology, 111*(Suppl. 2), S460–S475. doi:10.1067/mai.2003.108

Carter, R.H. (2006). B cells in health and disease. *Mayo Clinic Proceedings, 81,* 377–384. doi:10.4065/81.3.377

Chaplin, D.D. (2003). 1. Overview of the immune response. *Journal of Allergy and Clinical Immunology, 111*(Suppl. 2), S442–S459. doi:10.1067/mai.2003.125

Chaplin, D.D. (2006). Overview of the human immune response. *Journal of Allergy and Clinical Immunology, 117*(Suppl. 2), S430–S435. doi:10.1016/j.jaci.2005.09.034

Crivellato, E., Vacca, A., & Ribatti, D. (2004). Setting the stage: An anatomist's view of the immune system. *Trends in Immunology, 25,* 210–217. doi:10.1016/j.it.2004.02.008

Cruse, J.M., & Lewis, R.E. (2009). *Illustrated dictionary of immunology.* Boca Raton, FL: CRC Press.

Delves, P.J., & Roitt, I.M. (2000). The immune system. First of two parts. *New England Journal of Medicine, 343,* 37–49. doi:10.1056/NEJM200007063430107

Dorner, T. (2006). Crossroads of B cell activation in autoimmunity: Rationale of targeting B cells. *Journal of Rheumatology, 77*(Suppl.), 3–11.

Harvey, R.A., Champe, P.C., Doan, T., Melvold, R., Viselli, S., & Waltenbaugh, C. (2008). Antigen and receptors. In R.A. Harvey, P.C. Champe, T. Doan, R. Melvold, S. Viselli, & C. Waltenbaugh (Eds.), *Lippincott's illustrated reviews: Immunology* (pp. 1–154). Philadelphia, PA: Lippincott Williams & Wilkins.

Hillman, R.S., Ault, K.A., & Rinder, H.M. (2005). Plasma cell disorders. In R.S. Hillman, K.A. Ault, & H.M. Rinder (Eds.), *Hematology in clinical practice* (4th ed., pp. 300–312). New York, NY: McGraw-Hill.

Sommer, C. (2005). The immune response. In C.M. Porth (Ed.), *Pathophysiology: Concepts of altered health states* (7th ed., pp. 365–502). Philadelphia, PA: Lippincott Williams & Wilkins.

CHAPTER 3

Pathophysiology

Kimberly Noonan, RN, ANP, AOCN®

INTRODUCTION

Multiple myeloma is an uncontrolled growth of cells with the phenotype of terminally differentiated plasma cells. The disease often appears in the bone marrow (BM) and is associated with skeletal pathology, which in most patients presents as multiple lytic bone lesions and osteoporosis. Monoclonal plasmacytosis, monoclonal protein, and osteolytic lesions are the classic triad of myeloma (Lokhorst, 2002). The development of myeloma is an interdependent multistep process beginning with the emergence of a limited number of monoclonal plasma cells. During the early phase of development, a small number (less than 10%) of these monoclonal plasma cells can be present without calcium elevation, renal insufficiency, anemia, or bone lytic lesions (known as CRAB symptoms), and less than 3 g/dl of a monoclonal spike (referred to as *M spike*). This condition is categorized as *monoclonal gammopathy of undetermined significance* (MGUS) (Jagannath, 2008). MGUS is a well-described precursor of multiple myeloma and has a conversion rate of 1% per year into malignant myeloma (Kyle et al., 2002).

THE ROLE OF GENETICS

Both MGUS and multiple myeloma have demonstrated a marked karyotypic complexity with gains and losses of whole chromosomes, nonrandom chromosomal translocations causing dysregulation of genes (Avet-Loiseau et al., 1998), and point mutations of genes, all leading to myeloma pathogenesis (Raab & Anderson, 2008). Other genetic changes include early-onset reciprocal chromosomal translocations involving the heavy-chain (IgH) locus or occasionally the IgL light-chain locus, chromosome 13 monosomy, loss of the short arm of chromosome 17, and gains and losses of chromosome 1 (Raab & Anderson, 2008).

Myeloma Cells and Bone Marrow Microenvironment Interplay

The concept of tumor-microenvironment interaction is closely linked to multiple myeloma, but it is also shared by a wide spectrum of other hematologic malignancies. A better understanding of the interplay between myeloma cells and the BM microenvironment has been the source of new molecular targets and therapeutic strategies, leading to several clinical trials (Raab & Anderson, 2008). Figure 3-1 illustrates the interaction of myeloma cells and their BM microenvironment, validating the current therapeutic targets for the disease.

The main pathophysiologic changes in multiple myeloma relate to the abnormalities within the BM microenvironment, BM stromal cells (BMSCs), and cytokine interactions that cause disease progression and resistance to chemotherapy. BMSCs, such as fibroblastic stromal cells, osteoblasts, osteoclasts, vascular endothelial cells, and lymphocytes, play a significant role in myeloma pathogenesis by contributing to the growth and proliferation of myeloma cells. In a collaborative fashion, cytokines also contribute to the growth, progression, and dissemination of the myeloma cells in conjunction with BMSCs (Lauta, 2003; Zdzisinska, Bojarska-Junak, Dmoszynska, & Kandefer-Szerszen, 2008). These pathophysiologic abnormalities are interdependent; therefore, some may be referred to repeatedly while explaining other difficult concepts.

The interaction of myeloma cells with the BM microenvironment involves the activation by cytokines, growth factors, and/or adhesion molecules of a cascade series that add to the proliferation and antiapoptosis of myeloma cells (Podar, Chauhan, & Anderson, 2009). Some of these pathways are listed and explained in Table 3-1, including phosphatidylinositol-3 kinase (PI3K)/Akt, inhibitor kappa-B (IκB) kinase, nuclear factor-kappa-B (NF-κB), Ras/Raf/mitogen-activated protein kinase (MAPK), mitogen-activated kinase (MEKK)/extracellular signal-regulated kinase (ERK), Janus kinase (JAK)-2/signal transducer and activator of transcription (STAT)-3, and Wingless type (Wnt, pronounced "wint") pathway (Hideshima & Raje, 2008). Figure 3-2 lists additional factors associated with the growth and proliferations of myeloma cells.

Bone Marrow Microenvironment

The BM microenvironment is composed of a variety of extracellular matrix (ECM) proteins, such as fibronectin, collagen, laminin, osteopontin, proteoglycans, and glycosaminoglycans, as well as cell components, including hematopoietic stem cells, progenitor and precursor cells, immune cells, erythrocytes, BM endothelial cells, and BMSCs (Podar, Ghobrial, Iseshima, Chauhan, & Anderson, 2008; Raab & Anderson, 2008). ECM cells provide a protective foundation for the microenvironment cellular components to

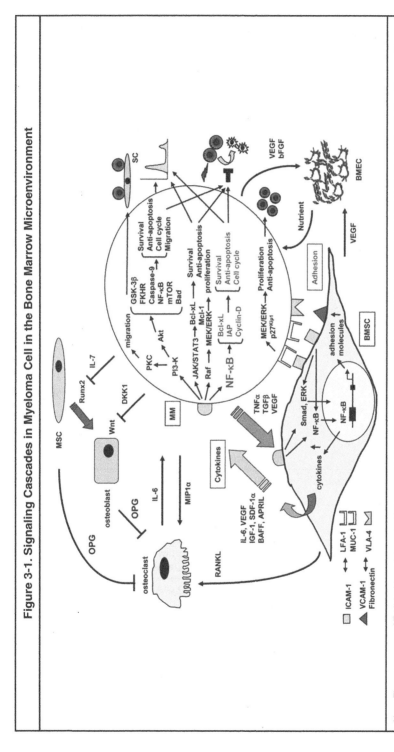

Figure 3-1. Signaling Cascades in Myeloma Cell in the Bone Marrow Microenvironment

Note. Figure courtesy of T. Hideshima. Adapted with permission from "Understanding Multiple Myeloma Pathogenesis in the Bone Marrow to Identify New Therapeutic Targets," by T. Hideshima, C. Mitsiades, G. Tonon, P.G. Richardson, and K.C. Anderson, 2007, *Nature Reviews Cancer, 7,* p. 588. Copyright 2007 by Macmillan Publishers Ltd; and "Advances in Biology of Multiple Myeloma: Clinical Applications," by T. Hideshima, P.L. Bergsagel, W.M. Kuehl, and K.C. Anderson, 2004, *Blood, 104,* p. 611. Copyright 2003 by American Society of Hematology.

| Table 3-1. Survival Pathways in Multiple Myeloma ||
Pathway	Function
Phosphatidylinositol-3 kinase (PI3K/Akt) Threonine protein kinase	• Activates downstream targets • Prevents the degradation of nuclear factor-kappa-B • Regulates cell proliferation by targeting the activity of glycogen synthase kinase β • Prevents cyclin D1 degradation • Targets mammalian target of rapamycin
Mitogen-activated protein kinases (MAPKs) Types: • Extracellular signal-regulated kinase (ERK) family • P 38 MAPK family • Jun amino-terminal kinases (JNK) family—c-Jun NH2 terminal kinase	• Regulate the production and secretion of cytokines • Regulate key cellular processes, such as cell cycle progression, growth, differentiation, and apoptosis
Janus kinase/signal transducer and activator of transcription 3 (JAK/STAT3)	• Upregulates gene transcription • Cytokine signaling by phosphorylating the intracellular domains of cytokine receptors • Activation associated with multiple myeloma cell survival
Wingless type (Wnt) pathway	• Regulates plasma and B-cell motility • Plays a key role in bone disease by prompting proliferation and survival of osteoblastic cells • DKK1 is elevated in patients with multiple myeloma, inhibits Wnt pathway, and blocks transcription factor Runx2/Cbfa1 necessary for osteoblast cell differentiation.

Note. Based on information from Esteve & Roodman, 2007; Hideshima et al., 2005; Leleu & Anderson, 2008; Podar et al., 2009.

Figure 3-2. Contributing Factors of Multiple Myeloma Growth and Proliferation

- Homing and adhesion of myeloma cells to the bone marrow via bone marrow stromal cells or extracellular matrix proteins
- Spread of tumor via the bloodstream from one site to another site within the bone marrow
- Paracrine factors involved in survival, differentiation, and proliferation of myeloma cells
- Angiogenesis
- Osteoclastogenesis and osteolysis
- Inhibition of osteogenesis
- Humoral and cellular immunodeficiency
- Anemia

Note. Based on information from Bergsagel, 2004; Hideshima & Raje, 2008.

perform the function they are assigned (Mitsiades et al., 2007). ECM cells also secrete growth and antiapoptotic cytokine factors known as interleukin-6 (IL-6), insulin-like growth factor-1 (IGF1), vascular endothelial growth factor (VEGF), and tumor necrosis factor alpha (TNF-α).

Nonhematopoietic and hematopoietic cells, as well as an extracellular and a liquid compartment of the BM microenvironment, are organized in a complex structure of sub-helminthic parasitic microenvironments or niches within protective mineralized bone. Within this well-orchestrated system, niches remain quiescent and preserved until there is an insult, such as the development of myeloma cells, creating a significant imbalance. In multiple myeloma, homeostasis between the cellular, extracellular, and liquid compartments within the BM is disrupted. The BM microenvironment provides signals that influence the behavior of myeloma cells and has a network of connective tissue containing immature blood cells (Mitsiades et al., 2007).

BM comprises three types of cells: self-renewing stem cells, differentiated progenitor cells, and functional mature blood cells. Erythrocytes, myelocytes, lymphocytes, and megakaryocytes are derived from a small population of primitive cells called the pluripotent stem cells. Several levels of differentiation lead to the development of progenitor cells for each blood cell type. These cells are referred to as *colony-forming units*, giving rise to precursor cells that develop into mature hematopoietic cells. During healthy conditions, or homeostasis, the number and total mass for each type of circulating blood cell remain relatively constant. Blood cells from each lineage are produced or destroyed according to health needs. Cytokines produced by BMSCs control the regulation of blood cells (Sommer, 2005). Figure 3-3 categorizes the cellular and noncellular elements found in the BM microenvironment of patients with multiple myeloma.

Bone Marrow Stromal Cells

BMSCs include fibroblastic stromal cells, osteoblasts, osteoclasts, vascular endothelial cells, and lymphocytes. They play a critical role of linking the myeloma cells to the BM microenvironment. BMSCs have shown to provide efficient support for the survival and proliferation of myeloma cells by producing high levels of cytokines, specifically IL-6, further promoting myeloma cell growth, survival, drug resistance, and migration (Raab & Anderson, 2008). The interactions of these cells with BMSCs enable the myeloma cells to stimulate the production of other cytokines that support osteoclastogenesis and angiogenesis (Mitsiades et al., 2007; Zdzisinska et al., 2008).

The interactions of myeloma cells with the BM microenvironment activates proliferative or antiapoptotic signaling cascades. Examples of cascades activated include PI3K/Akt, NF-κB, MEK/ERK, and JAK/STAT3. The signaling cascades also have the potential to mediate other interactions leading to my-

eloma proliferation. These interactions (Hideshima & Raje, 2008) include
- The cytoplasmic sequestration of many transcription factors
- Upregulation of cell cycle–regulating proteins such as cyclin D and anti-apoptotic proteins (Bcl2, Bcl-xL, Mcl1)
- More activation of telomerase of the BMSCs.

All of these molecular interactions are triggered either directly via cell adhesion molecule-mediated interactions of myeloma cells with BMSCs and ECM or indirectly by growth factors released by BMSCs or myeloma cells. Specifically, interaction of myeloma cells and BMSCs, as well as VEGF secreted by

---

Figure 3-3. Cellular and Noncellular Elements of the Bone Marrow

Cellular
- Hematopoietic cells
  - Hematopoietic stem cells
  - Progenitor/precursor cells
  - Natural killer cells
  - Macrophages
  - Platelets
  - Megakaryocytes
  - Erythrocytes
  - Lymphocytes
  - Dendritic cells
- Nonhematopoietic cells (bone marrow stromal cells)
  - Fibroblasts
  - Chondrocytes
  - Osteoclast
  - Osteoblast
  - Endothelial cell precursors

Noncellular
- Noncellular or extracellular matrix
  - Collagen
  - Fibronectin
  - Laminin
  - Proteoglycans
  - Glycosaminoglycans
- Liquid (cytokines)
  - IL-6, VEGF, IGF1, TNF-α
  - IGF2, IL-21, HGF, bFGF
  - IL-1, IL-10, IL-11, SDF1α
  - CD40, TNF, Wnt, MIP1α
  - TGF-β, IL-15

CD—cluster of differentiation; bFGF—basic fibroblast growth factor; HGF—hepatocyte growth factor; IGF—insulin-like growth factor; IL—interleukin; MIP—macrophage inflammatory protein; SDF—stromal-derived factor; TGF—tumor growth factor; TNF—tumor necrosis factor; VEGF—vascular endothelial growth factor; Wnt—"wingless"-type signaling pathway

Note. Based on information from Podar et al., 2009.

myeloma cells, triggers NF-κB-dependent transcription and the secretion of IL-6 in BMSCs, which enhances the production and secretion of VEGF, stimulating angiogenesis and proliferation of myeloma cells (Hideshima & Raje, 2008).

It is conceivable that BMSCs use similar molecular mediators such as cytokines, growth factors, and adhesion molecules to interact with normal hematopoietic cells, as well as myeloma cells. Growth factors can also modulate adhesion molecules profiles on myeloma cells and BMSCs. The relationship of growth factors, myeloma cells, and BMSCs in the BM milieu promotes the cellular growth, survival, and migration of myeloma cells. The combined interaction contributes to the progression and resistance to conventional therapies. In fact, BMSCs attenuate the response to conventional chemotherapy, such as corticosteroids and cytotoxic chemotherapy (Hideshima & Raje, 2008; Mitsiades et al., 2007; Podar et al., 2009).

BM endothelial cells are involved in the initial process of homing myeloma cells to the BM stromal compartment. Angiogenesis in active or symptomatic multiple myeloma is driven by paracrine (involving cytokines that act on adjacent cells) activation of BM endothelial cells by angiogenic cytokines such as VEGF and fibroblast growth factor, as well as proteases secreted by myeloma cells, fibroblasts, and osteoclasts. The adhesion, which occurs between myeloma cells and BMSCs, regulates many cytokines that have angiogenic activity. In myeloma cells, these angiogenic factors may be produced by genetic mutations. BM angiogenesis is sustained by VEGF and basic fibroblast growth factor, promoting myeloma cell growth in the BM milieu (Rajkumar & Kyle, 2001). Clearly, these autocrine (involving cytokines that act on the cells that produce them) and paracrine loops in the BM microenvironment mediate multiple myeloma proliferation. Angiogenesis promotes tumor cell growth by enhancing the delivery of oxygen and nutrients, removing catabolites, and secreting growth factors for tumor cells from endothelial cells.

Myeloma Cells' Interaction With Osteoclasts and Osteoblasts

Growth factors such as IL-6, IL-1, VEGF, stromal-derived factor-1α (SDF1α), and macrophage inflammatory protein-1α (known as MIP1α) also stimulate osteoclastogenesis. It is common for myeloma cells to migrate to bone structures in the body. Osteoclastic cells remove bone tissue as bone remodeling occurs, whereas osteoblastic cells build bone. Many stimuli, such as cytokines, hormones, calcium, phosphate, and mechanical stress, activate osteoclastic bone resorption and osteoblastic bone formation. A key question remains unanswered as to whether skeletal lesions are caused by the fertile "soil" provided by myeloma cells or if the BM microenvironment attracts myeloma cells more than other tissues do. No matter what the reason is, BMSCs play a critical role in bone destruction in patients with multiple myeloma. Skeletal involvement in this patient population is obviously related to the increased activity of osteoclasts but, arguably, is equally related to the lack of appropriate compensatory osteoblastic responses. Osteoclast activation and formation is involved in the development of osteolytic lesions that are characteristic in patients with multiple myeloma. Myeloma cells enhance the activity of osteoclasts and osteoclastogenesis, adjacent to myeloma cells, causing an enhanced bone resorption (Giuliani et al., 2002).

Osteoblastic cells regulate bone resorption by two processes. The first process is through osteoprotegerin (OPG, also called osteoclastogenesis inhibitory factor), a member of the TNF receptor family (Hideshima & Raje, 2008; Mitsiades et al., 2007). The second process is the receptor activator of the NF-κB ligand (RANKL), also a member of the TNF family. OPG binds to RANKL and inhibits bone resorption. RANKL stimulates osteoclast differentiation and activity, whereas OPG inhibits these processes. These two processes play a significant role in myeloma bone pathobiology. BMSCs secrete OPG, which prevents excessive activation of osteoclast by serving as a decoy receptor and competing with RANK for binding RANKL. The blockade of RANKL binding to RANK or the binding of OPG to RANKL inhibits osteoclast maturation and bone destruction. The important point is that myeloma cells affect the OPG/RANKL ratio in the BM microenvironment, which causes bone disease in patients with myeloma (Hideshima & Raje, 2008; Zdzisinska et al., 2008). Figure 3-4 explains the OPG/RANKL abnormality that occurs in patients with multiple myeloma.

In addition to activated osteoclastogenesis, a decrease in osteoblast activity may contribute to osteolytic lesions in patients with myeloma. The formation and differentiation of osteoblastic cells from mesenchymal stem cells require the help of a transcription factor, Runx2/Cbfa1 (Runt-related transcription factor 2/core binding factor alpha 1). When Runx2/Cbfa1 is blocked, osteoblastic progenitors are the result, increasing osteoclastogenesis (Giuliani, Rizzoli, & Roodman, 2006). Very late antigen-4 (VLA4) and cluster of differentiation-106 (CD106) or vascular cell adhesion molecule (VCAM1) can inhibit the effects of Runx2/Cbfa1, an important transcription factor for osteoblastic cell formation. Myeloma cells secrete soluble factors such as Dickkopf-1 (DKK1) and IL-7, which also inhibit Runx2/Cbfa1. The Wnt signaling pathway also plays an important role in osteoblast differentiation. Aside from its inhibitory effect on Runx2/Cbfa1, DKK1 is also a Wnt inhibitor (Tian et al., 2003). Studies have shown that elevated levels of DKK1 in BM plasma cells and in the peripheral blood of patients with myeloma are associated with a decrease in osteoblastic production that can lead to focal bone lytic lesions (Raab & Anderson, 2008).

CYTOKINES

The BM microenvironment consists of cytokines and growth factors. Myeloma cells and BMSCs trigger the paracrine and autocrine production and secretion of cytokines and growth factors into the BM microenvironment

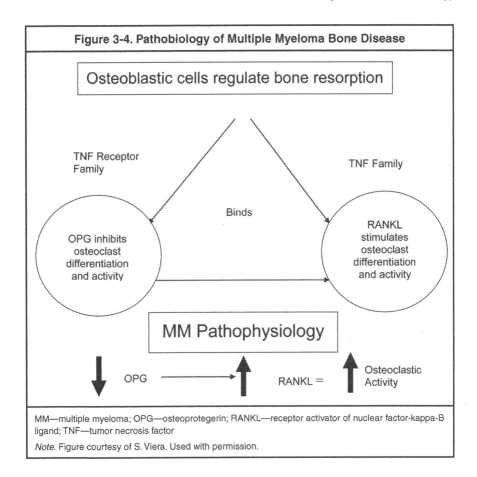

Figure 3-4. Pathobiology of Multiple Myeloma Bone Disease

Osteoblastic cells regulate bone resorption

TNF Receptor Family

TNF Family

Binds

OPG inhibits osteoclast differentiation and activity

RANKL stimulates osteoclast differentiation and activity

MM Pathophysiology

OPG ⟶ RANKL = Osteoclastic Activity

MM—multiple myeloma; OPG—osteoprotegerin; RANKL—receptor activator of nuclear factor-kappa-B ligand; TNF—tumor necrosis factor

Note. Figure courtesy of S. Viera. Used with permission.

(Podar, Richardson, Hideshima, Chauhan, & Anderson, 2007). Cytokines contribute to myeloma pathogenesis directly and indirectly. Cytokines directly affect multiple myeloma growth by triggering key tumor cell responses by adding to the growth, survival, migration, and drug resistance of myeloma cells. Indirectly, cytokines modify the tumor microenvironment by increasing tumor angiogenesis and bone resorption. Figure 3-5 lists cytokines that play a significant role in disease development (Hideshima, Bergsagel, Kuehl, & Anderson, 2004; Mitsiades et al., 2007; Podar et al., 2007).

Interleukin-6

IL-6 is an important cytokine in normal hematopoiesis as well as in the development of multiple myeloma. IL-6 promotes differentiation of normal B-cell lineage cells, which ultimately leads to an increased production of immunoglobulin by plasma cells. IL-6 stimulates the proliferation and drug resistance of malignant plasma cells in myeloma. If not the most essen-

Figure 3-5. Cytokines With a Role in Multiple Myeloma Development

- Interleukin (IL)-6
- Insulin-like growth factor-1 (IGF1)
- Vascular endothelial growth factor (VEGF)
- Tumor necrosis factor alpha (TNF-α)
- Stromal-derived factor-1 alpha (SDF1α)
- Tumor growth factor-beta (TGF-β)
- Basic fibroblast growth factor (bFGF)
- Macrophage inflammatory protein-1 alpha (MIP1α)
- Stem cell factor (SCF)
- Hepatocyte growth factor (HGF)
- IL-1β
- IL-3
- IL-10
- IL-15
- IL-21
- Ang-1
- B-cell activating factor (BAFF)
- Matrix metalloproteinases-2 (MMP2)
- Matrix metalloproteinases-9 (MMP9)
- A proliferation-inducing ligand (APRIL)

tial cytokine involved in myeloma production, it is a key growth and survival factor in the disease. IL-6 is produced and secreted by BMSCs and osteoblasts. IL-6 production increases in myeloma. As IL-6 production increases, tumor cell mass increases. IL-6 induces the expression of a transcription factor, Xbp-1, which is involved in plasma cell/myeloma differentiation (Podar et al., 2009). IL-6 triggers the activation of many myeloma pathways, including MEK/MAPK, JAK/STAT3, and PI3K/Akt.

Most IL-6 in the BM milieu is secreted by BMSCs. The transcription and secretion of IL-6 are augmented by the binding capacity of myeloma tumor cells and the secretion of other cytokines such as TNF-α, VEGF, and tumor growth factor beta. It is interesting to note that TNF-α-induced IL-6 in BMSCs is mediated via NF-κB activation. This is an important sequencing of events, as it displays and exemplifies the interconnection of several cytokines on one specific pathway (Hideshima & Raje, 2008; Mitsiades et al., 2007). Figure 3-6 depicts the interaction of IL-6 with other cytokines.

Vascular Endothelial Growth Factor

Both myeloma cells and BMSCs produce VEGF, which contributes to the increased angiogenesis in the BM of patients with multiple myeloma (Raab & Anderson, 2008). VEGF1 is expressed by myeloma cells in autocrine signaling pathways such as PI3K/protein kinase Ca-dependent cascade, MEK/ERK, and Mcl-1, leading to myeloma cell proliferation and survival. VEGF also affects osteoblasts, NK cells, monocytes, and endothelial progenitors (Podar et al., 2009).

Tumor Necrosis Factor Alpha

TNF-α is a combination cytokine known as the TNF-α superfamily. A superfamily is a large group of related proteins or molecules. The TNF-α superfamily includes SDF1α, CD40, B-cell activating factor (BAFF), and a proliferation-inducing ligand (APRIL). This superfamily-induced signaling

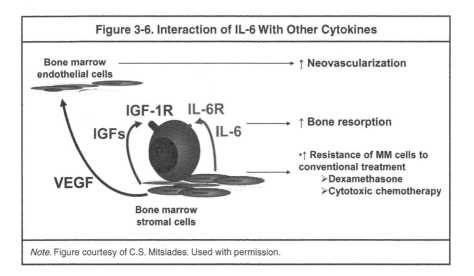

Figure 3-6. Interaction of IL-6 With Other Cytokines

Bone marrow endothelial cells ⟶ ↑ Neovascularization

IGF-1R IL-6R

IGFs

IL-6 ⟶ ↑ Bone resorption

VEGF

•↑ Resistance of MM cells to conventional treatment
➢Dexamethasone
➢Cytotoxic chemotherapy

Bone marrow stromal cells

Note. Figure courtesy of C.S. Mitsiades. Used with permission.

pathway in multiple myeloma is expressed by both myeloma cells and BMSCs. As a group, they are produced by macrophages, monocytes, dendritic cells, lymphocytes, myeloma cells, and BMSCs. Specifically, SDF1α promotes proliferation, induces migration, and protects against dexamethasone-induced apoptosis via the MAPK pathway, as well as the NF-κB and Akt pathways. SDF1α upregulates adhesion molecules, VLA4 and VCAM1, while SDF1α upregulates the secretion of IL-6 and VEGF in BMSCs, thereby stimulating angiogenesis and tumor proliferation (Raab & Anderson, 2008).

Cluster of Differentiation-40

CD40, a member of the TNF-α superfamily, is expressed by antigen-presenting cells (APCs) and T cells, as well as B-cell malignancies. This superfamily member mediates PI3K/Akt and NF-κB pathways, as well as increases the cellular growth in p53-dependent multiple myeloma and triggers VEGF secretions. BAFF and APRIL protect myeloma cells from apoptosis induced by IL-6 deprivation and dexamethasone. They promote cellular growth and adhesion to BMSCs. These processes are mediated through NF-κB, PI3K/Akt, and MAPK pathways (Podar et al., 2009).

Insulin Growth Factor-1

IGF1 is a multifunctional peptide that regulates cell proliferation, differentiation, and apoptosis. It is an important paracrine growth factor that induces proliferation, survival, migration, and drug resistance in myeloma cells (Raab & Anderson, 2008). In addition to an autocrine effect based on production of IGF by myeloma cells, activation of the IGF1 receptor results from the interaction between myeloma cells and BMSCs. IGF1 promotes proliferation and drug resistance in myeloma cells through the activation of MAPK and PI3K/ Akt signaling cascades. IGF1 induces cell migration and invasion via a PI3K-dependent pathway, through the Akt1-independent pathway, and through protein kinase D, RhoA, and β1-integrin. IGF1 appears to be a more potent inducer of Akt signaling than IL-6 (Podar et al., 2009).

CONCLUSION

The pathophysiology of multiple myeloma is a complicated but well-orchestrated and organized sequence of interactions. Many of these interactions are linked together and are interdependent. Understanding the interconnections involved in the development of myeloma, as well as the complicated pathways, is a critical step in treating and managing patients with this disease. As the knowledge of multiple myeloma grows and research progresses, the goal of finding a cure may not be a distant reality.

REFERENCES

Avet-Loiseau, H., Li, J.Y., Facon, T., Brigaudeau, C., Morineau, N., Maloisel, F., … Bataille, R. (1998). High incidence of translocations t(11;14) (q13;q32) and t(4;14) (p16;q32) in patients with plasma cell malignancies. *Cancer Research, 58*, 5640–5645.

Bergsagel, P.L. (2004). Epidemiology, etiology, and molecular pathogenesis In P. Richardson & K.C. Anderson (Eds.), *Multiple myeloma* (pp. 1–24). London, England: Remedica Publishing.

Esteve, F.R., & Roodman, G.D. (2007). Pathophysiology of myeloma bone disease. *Best Practice and Research: Clinical Haematology, 20*, 613–624. doi:10.1016/j.beha.2007.08.003

Giuliani, N., Colla, S., Sala, R., Moroni, M., Lazzaretti, M., La Monica, S., … Rizzoli, V. (2002). Human myeloma cells stimulate the receptor activator of nuclear factor-κB ligand (RANKL) in T lymphocytes: A potential role in multiple myeloma bone disease. *Blood, 100*, 4615–4621. doi:10.1182/blood-2002-04-1121

Giuliani, N., Rizzoli, V., & Roodman, G.D. (2006). Multiple myeloma bone disease: Pathophysiology of osteoblast inhibition. *Blood, 108*, 3992–3996. doi:10.1182/ blood-2006-05-026112

Hideshima, T., Bergsagel, P.L., Kuehl, W.M., & Anderson, K.C. (2004). Advances in biology of multiple myeloma: Clinical applications. *Blood, 104*, 607–618. doi:10.1182/ blood-2004-01-0037

Hideshima, T., Chauhan, D., Richardson, P., & Anderson, K.C. (2005). Identification and validation of novel therapeutic targets for multiple myeloma. *Journal of Clinical Oncology, 23*, 6345–6350. doi:10.1200/JCO.2005.05.024

Hideshima, T., & Raje, N. (2008). The role of bone marrow microenvironment in the pathogenesis of multiple myeloma. In K.C. Anderson & I.M. Ghobrial (Eds.), *Multiple myeloma: Translational and emerging therapies* (pp. 23–44). New York, NY: Informa Healthcare.

Jagannath, S. (2008). Pathophysiological underpinnings of multiple myeloma progression. *Journal of Managed Care Pharmacy, 14*(Suppl. 7), 7–11.

Kyle, R.A., Therneau, T.M., Rajkumar, S.V., Offord, J.R., Larson, D.R., Plevak, M.F., & Melton, L.J. (2002). A long-term study of prognosis in monoclonal gammopathy of undetermined significance. *New England Journal of Medicine, 346,* 564–569. doi:10.1056/NEJMoa01133202

Lauta, V.M. (2003). A review of the cytokine network in multiple myeloma: Diagnostic, prognostic, and therapeutic implications. *Cancer, 97,* 2440–2452. doi:10.1002/cncr.11072

Leleu, X., & Anderson, K.C. (2008). Promising new agents in phase I and II clinical trials in multiple myeloma. In K.C. Anderson & I.M. Ghobrial (Eds.), *Multiple myeloma: Translational and emerging therapies* (pp. 211–242). New York, NY: Informa Healthcare.

Lokhorst, H. (2002). Clinical features and diagnostic criteria. In J. Mehta & S. Singhal (Eds.), *Myeloma* (pp. 151–168). London, England: Martin Dunitz.

Mitsiades, C.S., McMillin, D.W., Klippel, S., Hideshima, T., Chauhan, D., Richardson, P.G., ... Anderson, K.C. (2007). The role of the bone marrow microenvironment in the pathophysiology of myeloma and its significance in the development of more effective therapies. *Hematology/Oncology Clinics of North America, 21,* 1007–1034, vii–viii. doi:10.1016/j.hoc.2007.08.007

Podar, K., Chauhan, D., & Anderson, K.C. (2009). Bone marrow microenvironment and the identification of new targets for myeloma therapy. *Leukemia, 23,* 10–24. doi:10.1038/leu.2008.259

Podar, K., Ghobrial, I., Iseshima, T., Chauhan, D., & Anderson, K.C. (2008). Niches within the multiple myeloma bone marrow microenvironment. In K.C. Anderson & I.M. Ghobrial (Eds.), *Multiple myeloma: Translational and emerging therapies* (pp. 61–74). New York, NY: Informa Healthcare.

Podar, K., Richardson, P.G., Hideshima, T., Chauhan, D., & Anderson, K.C. (2007). The malignant clone and the bone-marrow environment. *Best Practice and Research: Clinical Haematology, 20,* 597–612. doi:10.1016/j.beha.2007.08.002

Raab, M.S., & Anderson, K.C. (2008). Basic biology of plasma cell dyscrasias: Focus on the role of the tumor microenvironment. In S. Lonial (Ed.), *Myeloma therapy: Pursuing the plasma cell* (pp. 23–39). Totowa, NJ: Humana Press.

Rajkumar, S.V., & Kyle, R.A. (2001). Angiogenesis in multiple myeloma. *Seminars in Oncology, 28,* 560–564. doi:10.1016/S0093-7754(01)90024-7

Sommer, C. (2005). The immune response. In C.M. Porth (Ed.), *Pathophysiology: Concepts of altered health states* (7th ed., pp. 365–502). Philadelphia, PA: Lippincott Williams & Wilkins.

Tian, E., Zhan, F., Walker, R., Rasmussen, E., Ma, Y., Barlogie, B., & Shaughnessy, J.D. (2003). The role of the Wnt-signaling antagonist DKK1 in the development of osteolytic lesions in multiple myeloma. *New England Journal of Medicine, 349,* 2483–2494. doi:10.1056/NEJMoa030847

Zdzisinska, B., Bojarska-Junak, A., Dmoszynska, A., & Kandefer-Szerszen, M. (2008). Abnormal cytokine production by bone marrow stromal cells of multiple myeloma patients in response to RPMI8226 myeloma cells. *Archivum Immunologiae et Therapiae Experimentalis, 56,* 207–221. doi:10.1007/s00005-008-0022-5

CHAPTER 4

Epidemiology

Charise Gleason, MSN, NP-BC, AOCNP®

INTRODUCTION

Multiple myeloma is the second most common hematologic disorder in the United States, constituting approximately 1% of all cancer cases (Jemal et al., 2009; National Cancer Institute, 2009). The past 10 years have seen a wealth of new knowledge about the biology and therapeutics for myeloma. These advances are being applied to diagnosis and treatments and have resulted in improved overall survival for patients, yet little is known about the underlying causes. Multiple myeloma represents about 0.8% of all cancers worldwide, with more than 86,000 new cases occurring annually, and incidence varies from 0.4–5 per 100,000 people in various parts of the world (Parkin, Bray, Ferlay, & Pisani, 2005). The number of newly diagnosed cases is highest in North America, Australia and New Zealand, Northern Europe, and Western Europe when compared to Asian countries. A modest increase in incidence and mortality from the disease has occurred in most regions of the world over the past two decades without an obvious explanation (National Cancer Institute, 2009; Parkin et al., 2005).

ETIOLOGY

The exact etiology is unknown, and unlike other types of cancer that have documented risk factors, myeloma has few known predisposing factors for its development. The factors that contribute to the evolution and prevalence of monoclonal gammopathy of undetermined significance (MGUS) to multiple myeloma remain unclear (Gerkes, de Jong, Sijmons, & Vellenga, 2007; Lynch et al., 2008), although there is great interest in the role of genetic factors, race, environmental exposures, diet, immunologic function, and infection. Because MGUS is a well-known precursor, this chapter will provide a comprehensive review of the epidemiology of both MGUS and myeloma and the role of genetics, race, environmental factors, diet, immunology, and infection in the development of multiple myeloma.

INCIDENCE

Cancer is the number-two cause of death in the United States, with 562,340 deaths estimated to have occurred in 2009 (approximately 1,500 deaths per day), and 10,580 (5,640 in men and 4,940 in women) of those attributable to myeloma (American Cancer Society, 2009b; Jemal et al., 2009). Myeloma is the ninth most common cause of cancer death in women and the fourteenth cause of cancer death in men (Alexander et al., 2007). An estimated 20,580 new cases occurred in the United States in 2009, with 11,680 in men and 8,900 in women. Approximately 59,203 men and women were living with myeloma as of 2006 (Horner et al., 2006; Jemal et al., 2009). The disease most commonly affects older adults, with the median age at diagnosis being 70 years; incidence rises exponentially with age (Horner et al., 2006). In the United States, the lifetime risk of developing myeloma is 1 in 161 (0.62%), and it is rarely diagnosed before the age of 40 years.

Incidence rates of myeloma in North America, Australia and New Zealand, and Europe are similar, with an increased incidence in men compared to women and a higher incidence in African Americans (Parkin, Whelan, Ferlay, Teppo, & Thomas, 2002). Within the United States, the incidence is greater in men than in women (7.1 per 100,000 versus 4.6 per 100,000). Among African American men, the incidence rate is double that of Caucasians (14.3 per 100,000 versus 6.6 per 100,000), whereas people of Asian origin living in the United States have lower rates (Horner et al., 2006; Parkin et al., 2005). Higher incidence is also observed in the Caribbean and South and Central African countries, which is consistent with the increased risk seen in those of African descent (Parkin et al., 2005). Table 4-1 shows incidence by race per the National Cancer Institute Surveillance, Epidemiology, and End Results Program data. In large myeloma centers, half of the patients with monoclonal gammopathy have MGUS, whereas 15%–20% have multiple myeloma (Kyle et al., 2006).

RISK FACTORS

Risk factors for MGUS are similar to those for multiple myeloma, with age as a predominant factor. MGUS is present in more than 3% of the population older than age 50, with approximately 1% of patients with MGUS progressing to myeloma each year. Because the rate of conversion from MGUS to myeloma does not decrease with time, patients with MGUS will need to follow up with their healthcare provider indefinitely or refer to a myeloma center as needed (Kyle & Rajkumar, 2008; Kyle et al., 2002, 2006). In a large population-based study with 21,463 patients in Olmsted County, Minnesota, the prevalence of MGUS was 3.2% in people age 50 or older and 5.3% in residents age 70 or older (Kyle et al., 2002, 2006). It is not clear how many cases of myeloma are preceded by MGUS, as MGUS is not typically found on routine laboratory

Table 4-1. Incidence of Multiple Myeloma by Race		
Race/Ethnicity	Male	Female
All Races	7.1 per 100,000 men	4.6 per 100,000 women
White	6.6 per 100,000 men	4.1 per 100,000 women
Black	14.3 per 100,000 men	10.0 per 100,000 women
Asian/Pacific Islander	3.9 per 100,000 men	2.8 per 100,000 women
American Indian/Alaska Native	4.6 per 100,000 men	5.1 per 100,000 women
Hispanic	6.4 per 100,000 men	4.7 per 100,000 women

The age-adjusted incidence rate was 5.6 per 100,000 men and women per year. These rates are based on cases diagnosed in 2002–2006 from 17 SEER geographic areas.

Note. From SEER Stat Fact Sheets: Multiple Myeloma, by National Cancer Institute Surveillance, Epidemiology, and End Results Program, 2009. Retrieved from http://seer.cancer.gov/statfacts/html/mulmy.html.

analysis and patients are usually asymptomatic. The diagnosis of MGUS is frequently a coincidental finding and for the most part is underdiagnosed in the typical clinical setting (Kyle et al., 2006). A newer study by Weiss, Abadie, Verma, Howard, and Kuehl (2009) looked at the proportion of patients with newly diagnosed myeloma who had preexisting plasma cell disorders (PPCDs). The authors found that myeloma had evolved from PPCD in 27 out of 30 patients (90%), and the researchers suspected that PPCD incidence is even higher. They concluded that nearly all multiple myeloma is preceded by MGUS (Weiss et al., 2009). The main risk factors for progression to a malignant condition are the presence of an abnormal serum free light-chain ratio, a serum monoclonal protein of at least 1.5 g/dl, and a monoclonal immunoglobulin other than IgG (Kyle et al., 2006; Rajkumar et al., 2005). These risk factors help classify which patients with MGUS are at greatest risk for progressing to myeloma.

Family History and Genetics

Over the years, reports of myeloma occurring in the same family suggest a possible involvement of genetic factors in its development. Landgren et al. (2006) conducted a large population-based study comparing familial characteristics of autoimmune and hematologic disorders in patients with myeloma. The results showed a threefold increased risk among patients with a history of pernicious anemia and an increased risk in participants who had a history of systemic lupus erythematosus. The researchers reported no significant increased risk among individuals with a first-degree relative with MGUS and an elevated risk among those with a first-degree family history of myeloma. Ogmundsdottir et al. (2005) evaluated the occurrence of multiple myeloma in 218 Icelandic patients, noting that the risk for relatives of patients with myeloma developing MGUS was not increased, but there was a significant risk of developing myeloma for females separately and for males and females combined when looking at first-degree relatives of patients with myeloma.

Lynch et al. (2005) conducted a large observational study looking at 39 families with multiple cases of myeloma or related disorders. The conclusion noted that a diagnosis of myeloma *does* carry a risk of myeloma to other family members: the odds ratio for myeloma and a first-degree relative was 3.7. Their results reflected a lower age at diagnosis in successive generations. Interestingly, they reported on one family in which three siblings had the disease. A diagnosis of myeloma carries a familial risk for other types of cancers, particularly lymphoma and leukemia, as well as certain types of solid tumors (Bourguet, Grufferman, Delzell, Delong, & Cohen, 1985; Eriksson & Hallberg, 1992; Grosbois et al., 1999; Lynch et al., 2005, 2008).

A possible association exists between the human leukocyte antigens (HLAs) and incidence of myeloma. In an early study by Leech et al. (1983), researchers found an increased frequency of HLA-Cw5 and increased risk of myeloma among Black men. In a later population-based study by Pottern et al. (1992), researchers found an association between the HLA-Cw2 allele and the incidence of myeloma in both Black and White men. The associated risk was 5.7 for Blacks and 2.6 for Whites. These studies suggest a possible genetic component, but other factors also play a role, and further studies are needed.

Evidence has demonstrated an increased risk of myeloma in families with cases of breast cancer. *BRCA1* and *BRCA2* mutations among Ashkenazi Jewish patients and an increased risk of myeloma have been reported (Struewing et al., 1997). Sobol et al. (2002) noted that the *BRCA2* nonsense mutation, A10204T, might play a role in the development of a myeloma phenotype. In one family that has been prone to melanoma, a germ-line mutation of the *CDKN2A* (*p16*) gene was found in a family member who had myeloma. Additionally, researchers found that the wild-type *CDKN2A* allele was lost in malignant plasma cells, suggesting an increased susceptibility to multiple myeloma as well as a few other types of cancer (Dilworth et al., 2000).

Race

While hematopoietic neoplasms are more common in Caucasians, both MGUS and myeloma occur more frequently in African Americans, with the incidence of myeloma being twice as high in African American patients when compared to their Caucasian counterparts (Jain, Ascensao, & Schechter, 2009; Ries et al., 2003). Landgren et al. (2006) looked at the risk of MGUS and subsequent myeloma among African Americans and Caucasian veterans, noting a twofold higher incidence of myeloma and a threefold higher prevalence of MGUS in African Americans compared to Caucasians. The authors suggested that focus be shifted to studies examining risk factors for MGUS in order to better understand the etiology of myeloma. Although many accounts exist of familial history of myeloma, most of the studies have been done with Caucasian families. Lynch et al. (2008) reported on an African American family that had five cases of multiple myeloma, three cases of MGUS, and five cases of prostate cancer in two generations. In Ghana, the prevalence of MGUS in Black men was twice as high than in White men, supporting the hypothesis that race-related genetic susceptibility might explain the higher rates of MGUS among Blacks (Landgren et al., 2007).

Jain et al. (2009) reported on eight African American families with familial myeloma and MGUS over a 30-year period, which is one of the largest studies to date focusing on the African American population. The eight families were identified over three decades in a medical center whose clinic population was greater than 75% African American. They reported that out of eight families, 20 of 58 (35%) first-degree relatives had plasma cell dyscrasias, including 12 cases of myeloma, 8 cases of MGUS, and 1 case of amyloidosis. In this particular study, the median age at diagnosis for the patients with myeloma was 61 years. Some of the other factors thought to explain the increased risk of MGUS and myeloma in African American patients include environmental factors, diet, tobacco and alcohol use, and socioeconomic factors (Benjamin, Reddy, & Brawley, 2003).

Environmental Factors

It is not unusual for patients to ask what caused their myeloma and whether their occupation or lifestyle choices could be a factor. Known suspected risk factors include ionizing radiation and farming and agricultural exposures along with other occupational exposures, including exposure to organic solvents and pesticides. Alexander et al. (2007) performed an extensive epidemiologic literature review and noted the small numbers of cases in occupational cohort studies and a lack of statistical power and appearance of bias due to differential recall of exposures between the cases and controls. Although organic solvents, pesticides, and other exposures to chemicals have been studied, results continue to be varied and inconsistent (Alexander et al., 2007; Bergsagel et al., 1999).

Ionizing Radiation

Ichimaru, Ishimaru, Mikami, and Matsunaga (1982) evaluated the relationship between ionizing radiation from the atomic bomb and the incidence of myeloma in a fixed cohort of atomic bomb survivors for Hiroshima and Nagasaki and found an increased risk of myeloma. The analysis showed that the standardized relative risk adjusted for city, sex, and age at the time of the bombings increased with marrow-absorbed radiation dose. Furthermore, the researchers noted that the effect of radiation did not become apparent in individuals receiving 50 rad or more until 20 years or more after exposure. In a more recent study looking at the incidence of MGUS and myeloma in atomic bomb survivors, transformation from MGUS to myeloma occurred in 16% of unexposed patients, 17% in dose-unknown patients, and 26% in exposed patients, suggesting that exposure to the radiation accelerated the transformation of MGUS to myeloma (Alexander et al., 2007; Neriishi, Nakashima, & Suzuki, 2003). However, Preston et al. (1994) analyzed the incidence of myeloma after exposure to the atomic bomb through 1987 and found no increased risk.

Occupational Risk Factors

Farmers and agricultural workers have been exposed to potentially hazardous substances, including pesticides and other chemicals, for years, but they typically have a lower cancer mortality rate when compared to the general population. In a meta-analysis from various epidemiologic studies of agricultural workers published between 1977 and 1996 (Acquavella et al., 1998; Blair, Zahm, Pearce, Heineman, & Fraumeni, 1992; Khuder & Mutgi, 1997), results suggested that the risk of myeloma among farmers is similar to that of the general population. Because farmers and agricultural workers are exposed to so many chemicals and activities that could put them at risk, studies have failed to show consistent association to the risk of developing MGUS or myeloma.

Pesticides have also been widely examined to evaluate the risk of myeloma based on exposures by agricultural workers and licensed pesticide applicators. An extensive review of the literature by Alexander et al. (2007) revealed inconsistent results, with some studies suggesting a positive correlation and other studies finding no relationship (Blair, Sandler, et al., 2005; Freeman et al., 2005; Rusiecki et al., 2004; Semenciw et al., 1993). In one study, the risk of cancer was low overall, and researchers hypothesized that the cancer rates seemed to be a result of low smoking prevalence and other positive lifestyle factors (Lee et al., 2004). Exposure to organic solvents does not appear to be a risk factor for myeloma. Although exposure to high levels of benzene places a person at higher risk for developing acute myeloid leukemia, no evidence exists to support a high risk for developing myeloma (Bertazzi et al., 2001). A meta-analysis among workers who were exposed to solvents did not show an increased risk of developing myeloma and pointed out confounding factors of smoking and alcohol use (Chen & Seaton, 1996).

Approximately three million Americans in the military who were deployed to Vietnam in the 1960s and early 1970s were exposed to large amounts of defoliant mixtures known as Agent Orange (name given because of the orange stripe on the container). About 19 million gallons of a 50:50 mixture of two phenoxy herbicides were used on approximately 3.6 million acres in Vietnam and Laos (Frumkin, 2003). Many studies have been done on the relationship between Agent Orange and the development of hematologic malignancies, and the U.S. Department of Veterans Affairs has presumptively recognized the association of Agent Orange and myeloma as a service connection (U.S. Department of Veterans Affairs, 2008). The study results usually have yielded limited information on the link of Agent Orange to cancer. Moreover, results have been sparse and inconclusive, but myeloma has been labeled as a cancer with limited evidence of association to Agent Orange (American Cancer Society, 2009a; Frumkin, 2003).

Researchers also have studied the relationship between myeloma and personal or occupational exposure to hair coloring and dyes. An increase in the disease in a small fraction of hair dye users, particularly those using black dye, has been reported, but researchers found no significant exposure response based on the duration for all hair colors combined (Herrinton et al., 1994; Takkouche, Etminan, & Montes-Martinez, 2005; Thun et al., 1994). Using hair colors that do not contain carcinogens and that have appropriate labeling helps to reduce risk. In other environmental studies among rubber workers and people in wood-related occupations (Alder et al., 2006; Demers et al., 1995; Greenberg et al., 2001), results have been inconsistent. Occupational exposure to certain chemicals, solvents, or pesticides may contribute to the development of myeloma, but the evidence remains inconclusive.

Socioeconomic Status and Lifestyle Factors

Baris et al. (2000) evaluated the impact of socioeconomic status (SES) and the incidence of multiple myeloma and observed an inverse correlation between occupation-based SES and the risk for myeloma in both Black and White individuals. Their study found that low occupation-based SES accounted for 37% of myeloma cases in Blacks but only 17% in Whites because of the higher percentage of Black (62.9%) compared to White (34.7%) controls. It remains unclear whether low SES-related factors, such as poor housing, jobs with exposure to occupational carcinogens, unemployment, poor nutrition, and lack of health care, contribute to a higher incidence (Gorey & Vena, 1994). The authors noted no relationship to lifestyle factors such as tobacco or alcohol use, and further studies are warranted (Baris et al., 2000).

Epidemiologists have investigated the correlation between diet and multiple myeloma. Tavani et al. (2000) examined the relationship between red meat consumption and cancers. Although red meat intake has been associated with digestive track cancers, it seems to have no relationship to myeloma. In a very large case-control study by Fritschi, Ambrosini, Kliewer, and Johnson (2004), the authors reported that an increase in proportions of total energy and fat from fresh fish seems to protect against the development of hematologic malignancies, including myeloma. In contrast, the number of myeloma deaths was greater among Swedish fishermen on the Baltic Sea when they consumed more than twice as much fatty fish as the general Swedish population (Hagmar, Nilsson, Aakesson, Schuetz, & Moeller, 1992; Svensson, Mikoczy, Stromberg, & Hagmar, 1995; Svensson, Nilsson, et al., 1995). Other foods such as grains, meats, vegetables, and dairy products have shown mixed results with no significant increased risk of developing myeloma (Brown et al., 2001; Chatenoud et al., 1998; Negri, La Vecchia, Franceschi, D'Avanzo, & Parazzini, 1991; Tavani et al., 1997, 2000).

Researchers have studied the link between obesity and development of myeloma and have found an association. Brown et al. (2001) reported an association between increased obesity trends that may contribute to the incidence of myeloma in both Blacks and Whites. Blair, Cerhan, Folsom, and Ross (2005) noted that although obesity studies have been inconsistent, increased amounts of adipose tissue may elevate the risk of myeloma. A large Canadian study over eight provinces found an increased risk in both men and women who were obese, but smoking and alcohol use did not modify this association (Pan, Johnson, Ugnat, Wen, & Mao, 2004). The authors noted that the mechanism for the link was unclear and hypothesized that it could be related to a decreased immune response. In an earlier study by Friedman and Herrington (1994), researchers found the same association between myeloma and obesity, but only in White males.

Several studies have looked at the relationship of tobacco or alcohol use and multiple myeloma. Brown et al. (2001) did not find an association between smoking and myeloma; neither did Pan et al. (2004) with smoking or alcohol use. A large Swedish study of 333,000 male construction workers found that the use of cigarettes, pipes, snuff, or a mix of these was not linked to an increased risk of developing myeloma, and body mass index did not seem to modify the risk (Fernberg et al., 2007). A German case study showed a positive association between smoking and increased risk for myeloma (Nieters, Deeg, & Becker, 2006). However, overall, studies do not support an association between tobacco use and increased risk.

Immunologic Factors

There has been an interest in the relationship between chronic or recurrent infections and the development of myeloma. Case studies to identify the associations of infections and autoimmune disorders have failed to demonstrate consistent findings (Cohen, Bernstein, & Grufferman, 1987; Gramenzi et al., 1991; Koepsell et al., 1987). Research has not shown links between chronic or acute immune stimulation and myeloma, nor associations with certain immunizations such as those for influenza, polio, smallpox, and tetanus (Alexander et al., 2007; Gramenzi et al., 1991; Koepsell et al., 1987; Lewis et al., 1994). Koepsell et al. (1987) reported a link between rheumatoid arthritis and myeloma in one case-control study, whereas another large case-control study by Lewis et al. (1994) showed no correlation.

Several studies have linked AIDS with an increased incidence of myeloma, especially in the older adult population. Several studies have shown an increased risk in those living with AIDS (Biggar, Kirby, Atkinson, McNeel, & Engels, 2004; Frisch, Biggar, Engels, & Goedert, 2001; Grulich et al., 2002; Grulich, Wan, Law, Coates, & Kaldor, 1999). An Australian study found a significantly elevated risk of AIDS in an Australian cohort (Grulich et al., 1999), and a U.S. and Puerto Rican AIDS registry study reported an increased incidence following the diagnosis of AIDS (Goedert et al., 1998).

CONCLUSION

Approximately 20,000 new cases of myeloma were diagnosed in the United States in 2009, and one of the greatest known risk factors continues to be age. The incidence is higher in men and is twice as high in African Americans. Unlike for other cancers, few risk factors and predisposing factors are known. The etiology remains unknown; hence, no type of screening tool is available as with other cancers. There has been a positive link to ionizing radiation exposure at higher doses and questionable links to environmental factors such as pesticide exposure and occupational hazards. Vietnam veterans who were exposed to Agent Orange have a suggestive association, and per the Veterans Administration, a presumptive service connection.

The role of genetics is still undefined in myeloma, but several studies have reported an increased risk of developing myeloma when there is a positive family history. Known cases exist of myeloma occurring in the same family over several generations. Race plays a factor in the incidence of MGUS and multiple myeloma, with higher rates occurring in African Americans. MGUS is linked to the subsequent development of myeloma, with higher risk factors including the association of an abnormal free light-chain ratio and a higher level of monoclonal protein at the time of MGUS diagnosis.

Obesity, diet, and exercise may be contributing factors, as well as poor SES, but studies are inconclusive, and these are more likely related to a factor that has yet to be discovered. An increased risk among people with AIDS has been noted, especially as this population ages. As the general population ages, the risk of developing myeloma will continue to rise. Although a wealth of progress has taken place in the past 10 years regarding both the biology and treatment of multiple myeloma, continued studies are needed to further understand the disease and associated risk factors.

REFERENCES

Acquavella, J., Olsen, G., Cole, P., Ireland, B., Kaneene, J., Schuman, S., & Holden, L. (1998). Cancer among farmers: A meta-analysis. *Annals of Epidemiology, 8,* 64–74. doi:10.1016/S1047-2797(97)00120-8

Alder, N., Fenty, J., Warren, F., Sutton, A.J., Rushton, L., Jones, D.R., & Abrams, K.R. (2006). Meta-analysis of mortality and cancer incidence among workers in the synthetic rubber-producing industry. *American Journal of Epidemiology, 164,* 405–420. doi:10.1093/aje/kwj252

Alexander, D.D., Mink, P.J., Adami, H.O., Cole, P., Mandel, J.S., Oken, M.M., & Trichopoulos, D. (2007). Multiple myeloma: A review of the epidemiologic literature. *International Journal of Cancer, 120*(Suppl. 12), 40–61. doi:10.1002/ijc.22718

American Cancer Society. (2009a). *Agent orange and cancer*. Retrieved from http://www.cancer.org/docroot/PED/content/PED_1_3x_Agent_Orange_and_Cancer.asp?sitearea=PED

American Cancer Society. (2009b). *Cancer facts and figures 2009*. Retrieved from http://www.cancer.org/downloads/STT/500809web.pdf

Baris, D., Brown, L.M., Silverman, D.T., Hayes, R., Hoover, R.N., Swanson, G.M., ... Fraumeni, J.F., Jr. (2000). Socioeconomic status and multiple myeloma among US blacks and whites. *American Journal of Public Health, 90,* 1277–1281. doi:10.2105/AJPH.90.8.1277

Benjamin, M., Reddy, S., & Brawley, O.W. (2003). Myeloma and race: A review of the literature. *Cancer and Metastasis Reviews, 22,* 87–93. doi:10.1023/A:1022268103136

Bergsagel, D.E., Wong, O., Bergsagel, P.L., Alexanian, R., Anderson, K., Kyle, R.A., & Raabe, G.K. (1999). Benzene and multiple myeloma: Appraisal of the scientific evidence. *Blood, 94,* 1174–1182.

Bertazzi, P.A., Consonni, D., Bachetti, S., Rubagotti, M., Baccarelli, A., Zocchetti, C., & Pesatori, A.C. (2001). Health effects of dioxin exposure: A 20-year mortality study. *American Journal of Epidemiology, 153,* 1031–1044. doi:10.1093/aje/153.11.1031

Biggar, R.J., Kirby, K.A., Atkinson, J., McNeel, T.S., & Engels, E. (2004). Cancer risk in elderly persons with HIV/AIDS. *Journal of Acquired Immune Deficiency Syndromes, 36,* 861–868. doi:10.1097/00126334-200407010-00014

Blair, A., Sandler, D.P., Tarone, R., Lubin, J., Thomas, K., Hoppin, J.A., Samanic, C., ... Alavanja, M.C.R. (2005). Mortality among participants in the Agricultural Health Study. *Annals of Epidemiology, 15,* 279–285. doi:10.1016/j.annepidem.2004.08.008

Blair, A., Zahm, S.H., Pearce, N.E., Heineman, E.F., & Fraumeni, J.F., Jr. (1992). Clues to cancer etiology from studies of farmers. *Scandinavian Journal of Work, Environment and Health, 18,* 209–215.

Blair, C.K., Cerhan, J.R., Folsom, A.R., & Ross, J.A. (2005). Anthropometric characteristics and risk of multiple myeloma. *Epidemiology, 16,* 691–694. doi:10.1097/01.ede.0000172135.61188.2d

Bourguet, C.C., Grufferman, S., Delzell, E., Delong, E.R., & Cohen, H.J. (1985). Multiple myeloma and family history of cancer: A case-control study. *Cancer, 56,* 2133–2139. doi:10.1002/1097-0142(19851015)56:8<2133::AID-CNCR2820560842>3.0.CO;2-F

Brown, L.M., Gridley, G., Pottern, L.M., Baris, D., Swanson, C.A., Silverman, D.T., ... Fraumeni, J.F. (2001). Diet and nutrition as risk factors for multiple myeloma among blacks and whites in the United States. *Cancer Causes and Control, 12,* 117–125. doi:10.1023/A:1008937901586

Chatenoud, L., Tavani, A., La Vecchia, C., Jacobs, D.R., Jr., Negri, E., Levi, F., & Franceschi, S. (1998). Whole grain food intake and cancer risk. *International Journal of Cancer, 77,* 24–28. doi:10.1002/(SICI)1097-0215(19980703)77:1<24::AID-IJC5>3.0.CO;2-1

Chen, R., & Seaton, A. (1996). A meta-analysis of mortality among workers exposed to organic solvents. *Occupational Medicine, 46,* 337–344.

Cohen, H.J., Bernstein, R., & Grufferman S. (1987). Role of immune stimulation in the etiology of multiple myeloma. *American Journal of Hematology, 24,* 119–126. doi:10.1002/ajh.2830240202

Demers, P.A., Boffetta, P., Kogevinas, M., Blair, A., Miller, B.A., Robinson, C.F., ... Vainio, H. (1995). Pooled re-analysis of cancer mortality among five cohorts of workers in wood-related industries. *Scandinavian Journal of Work, Environment and Health, 21,* 179–190.

Dilworth, D., Liu, L., Stewart, A.K., Berenson, J.R., Lassam, N., & Hogg, D. (2000). Germline CDKN2A mutation implicated in predisposition to multiple myeloma. *Blood, 95,* 1869–1871.

Eriksson, M., & Hallberg, B. (1992). Familial occurrence of hematologic malignancies and other diseases in multiple myeloma: A case-control study. *Cancer Causes and Control, 3,* 63–67. doi:10.1007/BF00051914

Fernberg, P., Odenbro, A., Bellocco, R., Boffetta, P., Pawitan, Y., Zendehdel, K., & Adami, J. (2007). Tobacco use, body mass index, and the risk of leukemia and multiple myeloma:

A nationwide cohort study in Sweden. *Cancer Research, 67,* 5983–5986. doi:10.1158/0008-5472.CAN-07-0274

Freeman, L.E.B., Bonner, M.R., Blair, A., Hoppin, J.A., Sandler, D.P., Lubin, J.H., … Alavanja, M.C.R. (2005). Cancer incidence among male pesticide applicators in the Agricultural Health Study cohort exposed to diazinon. *American Journal of Epidemiology, 162,* 1070–1079. doi:10.1093/aje/kwi321

Friedman, G.D., & Herrington, H.L. (1994). Obesity and multiple myeloma. *Cancer Causes and Control, 5,* 479–483. doi:10.1007/BF01694762

Frisch, M., Biggar, R.J., Engels, E.A., & Goedert, J.J. (2001). Association of cancer with AIDS-related immunosuppression in adults. *JAMA, 285,* 1736–1745. doi:10.1001/jama.285.13.1736

Fritschi, L., Ambrosini, G.L., Kliewer, E.V., & Johnson, K.C. (2004). Dietary fish intake and risk of leukaemia, multiple myeloma, and non-Hodgkin lymphoma. *Cancer Epidemiology, Biomarkers and Prevention, 13,* 532–537.

Frumkin, H. (2003). Agent orange and cancer: An overview for clinicians. *CA: A Cancer Journal for Clinicians, 53,* 245–255. doi:10.3322/canjclin.53.4.245

Gerkes, E.H., de Jong, M.M., Sijmons, R.H., & Vellenga, E. (2007). Familial multiple myeloma: Report on two families and discussion of screening options. *Hereditary Cancer in Clinical Practice, 5,* 72–78. doi:10.1186/1897-4287-5-2-72

Goedert, J.J., Cote, T.R., Virgo, P., Scoppa, S.M., Kingma, D.W., Gail, M.H., … Biggar, R.J. (1998). Spectrum of AIDS-associated malignant disorders. *Lancet, 351,* 1833–1839. doi:10.1016/S0140-6736(97)09028-4

Gorey, K.M., & Vena, J.E. (1994). Cancer differentials among US blacks and whites: Quantitative estimates of socioeconomic-related risks. *Journal of the National Medical Association, 86,* 209–215.

Gramenzi, A., Buttino, I., D'Avanzo, B., Negri, E., Franceschi, S., & La Vecchia, C. (1991). Medical history and the risk of multiple myeloma. *British Journal of Haematology, 63,* 769–772.

Greenberg, R.S., Mandel, J.S., Pastides, H., Britton, N.L., Rudenko, L., & Starr, T.B. (2001). A meta-analysis of cohort studies describing mortality and cancer incidence among chemical workers in the United States and Western Europe. *Epidemiology, 12,* 727–740. doi:10.1097/00001648-200111000-00023

Grosbois, B., Jego, P., Attal, M., Payen, C., Rapp, M.J., Fuzibet, J.G., … Bataille, R. (1999). Familial multiple myeloma: Report of fifteen families. *British Journal of Haematology, 105,* 768–770. doi:10.1046/j.1365-2141.1999.01415.x

Grulich, A.E., Li, Y., McDonald, A., Correll, P.K.L., Law, M.G., & Kaldor, J.M. (2002). Rates of non-AIDS-defining cancers in people with HIV infection before and after AIDS diagnosis. *AIDS, 16,* 1155–1161. doi:10.1097/00002030-200205240-00009

Grulich, A.E., Wan, X., Law, M.G., Coates, M., & Kaldor, J.M. (1999). Risk of cancer in people with AIDS. *AIDS, 13,* 839–843. doi:10.1097/00002030-199905070-00014

Hagmar, L.L.K., Nilsson, A., Aakesson, B., Schuetz, A., & Moeller, T. (1992). Cancer incidence and mortality among Swedish Baltic sea fishermen. *Scandinavian Journal of Work, Environment and Health, 18,* 217–224.

Herrinton, L.J., Weiss, N.S., Koepsell, T.D., Daling, J.R., Taylor, J.W., Lyon, J.L., … Greenberg, R.S. (1994). Exposure to hair-coloring products and the risk of multiple myeloma. *American Journal of Public Health, 84,* 1142–1144. doi:10.2105/AJPH.84.7.1142

Horner, M.J., Ries, L.A.G., Krapcho, M., Neyman, N., Aminou, R., Howlader, N., … Edwards, B.K. (2006). *SEER cancer statistics review, 1975–2006.* Retrieved from http://SEER.cancer.gov/csr/1975_2006

Ichimaru, M., Ishimaru, T., Mikami, M., & Matsunaga, M. (1982). Multiple myeloma among atomic bomb survivors in Hiroshima and Nagasaki, 1950–1976: Relationship to radiation dose absorbed by marrow. *Journal of the National Cancer Institute, 69,* 323–328.

Jain, M., Ascensao, J., & Schechter, G.P. (2009). Familial myeloma and monoclonal gammopathy: A report of eight African American families. *American Journal of Hematology, 84,* 34–38. doi:10.1002/ajh.21325

Jemal, A., Siegel, R., Ward, E., Hao, Y., Xu, J., & Thun, M.J. (2009). Cancer statistics, 2009. *CA: A Cancer Journal for Clinicians, 59,* 225–249. doi:10.3322/caac.20006

Khuder, S.A., & Mutgi, A.B. (1997). Meta-analyses of multiple myeloma and farming. *American Journal of Industrial Medicine, 32,* 510–516. doi:10.1002/(SICI)1097-0274(199711)32:5<510::AID-AJIM11>3.0.CO;2-5

Koepsell, T.D., Daling, J.R., Weiss, N.S., Taylor, J.W., Olshan, A.F., Lyon, J.L., ... Child, M. (1987). Antigenic stimulation and the occurrence of multiple myeloma. *American Journal of Epidemiology, 126,* 1051–1062.

Kyle, R.A., & Rajkumar, S.V. (2008). Multiple myeloma. *Blood, 111,* 2962–2972. doi:10.1182/blood-2007-10-078022

Kyle, R.A., Therneau, T.M., Rajkumar, S.V., Larson, D.R., Plevak, M.F., Offord, J.R., ... Melton, J. (2006). Prevalence of monoclonal gammopathy of undetermined significance. *New England Journal of Medicine, 354,* 1362–1369. doi:10.1056/NEJMoa054494

Kyle, R.A., Therneau, T.M., Rajkumar, S.V., Offord, J.R., Larson, D.R., Plevak, M.F., & Melton, L.J., 3rd. (2002). A long-term study of prognosis in monoclonal gammopathy of undetermined significance. *New England Journal of Medicine, 346,* 564–569. doi:10.1056/NEJMoa01133202

Landgren, O., Gridley, G., Turesson, I., Caporaso, N.E., Goldin, L.R., Baris, D., ... Linet, M.S. (2006). Risk of monoclonal gammopathy of undetermined significance (MGUS) and subsequent multiple myeloma among African American and white veterans in the United States. *Blood, 107,* 904–906. doi:10.1182/blood-2005-08-3449

Landgren, O., Katzmann, J.A., Hsing, A.W., Pfeiffer, R.M., Kyle, R.A., Yeboah, E.D., ... Rajkumar, S.V. (2007). Prevalence of monoclonal gammopathy of undetermined significance among men in Ghana. *Mayo Clinic Proceedings, 82,* 1468–1473. doi:10.4065/82.12.1468

Lee, W.J., Hoppin, J.A., Blair, A., Lubin, J.H., Dosemeci, M., Sandler, D.P., & Alavanja, M.C.R. (2004). Cancer incidence among pesticide applicators exposed to alachlor in the agricultural health study. *American Journal of Epidemiology, 159,* 373–380. doi:10.1093/aje/kwh040

Leech, S.H., Bryan, C.F., Elston, R.C., Rainey, J., Bickers, J.N., & Pelias, M.Z. (1983). Genetic studies in multiple myeloma: Association with HLA-Cw5. *Cancer, 51,* 1408–1411. doi:10.1002/1097-0142(19830415)51:8<1408::AID-CNCR2820510814>3.0.CO;2-7

Lewis, D.R., Pottern, L.M., Brown, L.L.M., Silverman, D.T., Haves, R.B., Schoenberg, J.B., ... Hoover, R.N. (1994). Multiple myeloma among blacks and whites in the United States: The role of chronic antigenic stimulation. *Cancer Causes and Control, 5,* 529–539. doi:10.1007/BF01831381

Lynch, H.T., Ferrara, K., Barlogie, B., Coleman, E.A., Lynch, J.F., Weisenburger, D., ... Thome, S. (2008). Familial myeloma. *New England Journal of Medicine, 359,* 152–157. doi:10.1056/NEJMoa0708704

Lynch, H.T., Watson, P., Tarantolo, S., Wiernik, P.H., Quinn-Laquer, B., Bergsagel, K.I., ... Weisenburger, D. (2005). Phenotypic heterogeneity in multiple myeloma families. *Journal of Clinical Oncology, 23,* 685–693. doi:10.1200/JCO.2005.10.126

National Cancer Institute. (2009). *A snapshot of multiple myeloma.* Retrieved from http://planning.cancer.gov/disease/Myeloma-Snapshot.pdf

Negri, E., La Vecchia, C., Franceschi, S., D'Avanzo, B., & Parazzini, F. (1991). Vegetable and fruit consumption and cancer risk. *International Journal of Cancer, 48,* 350–354. doi:10.1002/ijc.2910480307

Neriishi, K., Nakashima, E., & Suzuki, G. (2003). Monoclonal gammopathy of undetermined significance in atomic bomb survivors: Incidence and transformation to multiple myeloma. *British Journal of Haematology, 121,* 405–410. doi:10.1046/j.1365-2141.2003.04287.x

Nieters, A., Deeg, E., & Becker, N. (2006). Tobacco and alcohol consumption and risk of lymphoma: Results of a population-based case-control study in Germany. *International Journal of Cancer, 118,* 422–430. doi:10.1002/ijc.21306

Ogmundsdottir, H.M., Haraldsdottirm, V., Johannesson, G.M., Olafsdottir, G., Bjarnadottir, K., Sigvaldason, H., & Tulinius, H. (2005). Familiality of benign and malignant paraproteinemias. A population-based cancer-registry study of multiple myeloma families. *Haematologica, 90,* 66–71.

Pan, S.Y., Johnson, K.C., Ugnat, A.M., Wen, S.W., & Mao, Y. (2004). Association of obesity and cancer risk in Canada. *American Journal of Epidemiology, 159,* 259–268. doi:10.1093/ aje/kwh041

Parkin, D.M., Bray, F., Ferlay, J., & Pisani, P. (2005). Global cancer statistics, 2002. *CA: A Cancer Journal for Clinicians, 55,* 74–108. doi:10.3322/canjclin.55.2.74

Parkin, D.M., Whelan, S.L., Ferlay, J., Teppo, L., & Thomas, D.B. (2002). Cancer in five continents. *IARC Scientific Publications, VIII*(155), 1–781.

Pottern, L.M., Gart, J.J., Nam, J.M., Dunston, G., Wilson, J., Greenberg, R., ... Hoover, R.N. (1992). HLA and multiple myeloma among black and white men: Evidence of a genetic association. *Cancer Epidemiology, Biomarkers and Prevention, 1,* 177–182.

Preston, D.L., Kusumi, S., Tomonaga, M., Izumi, S., Ron, E., Kuramoto, A., ... Mabuchi, K. (1994). Cancer incidence in atomic bomb survivors. Part III. Leukemia, lymphoma, and multiple myeloma, 1950–1987. *Radiation Research, 137*(Suppl. 2), S68–S97.

Rajkumar, S.V., Kyle, R.A., Therneau, T.M., Melton, L.J., III, Bradwell, A.R., Clark, R.J., ... Katzmann, J.A. (2005). Serum free light chain ratio is an independent risk factor for progression in monoclonal gammopathy of undetermined significance. *Blood, 106,* 812–817. doi:10.1182/blood-2005-03-1038

Ries, L.A.G., Harkins, D., Krapcho, M., Mariotto, A., Miller, B.A., Feuer, E.J., ... Edwards, B.K. (Eds.). (2003). *SEER cancer statistics review, 1975–2003.* Retrieved from http://seer .cancer.gov/csr/1975_2003/

Rusiecki, J.A., De Roos, A., Lee, W.J., Dosemeci, M., Lubin, J.H., Hoppin, J.A., ... Alavanja, M.C. (2004). Cancer incidence among pesticide applicators exposed to atrazine in the agricultural health study. *Journal of the National Cancer Institute, 96,* 1375–1382.

Semenciw, R.M., Morrison, H.I., Riedel, D., Wilkins, K., Ritter, L., & Mao, Y. (1993). Multiple myeloma mortality and agricultural practices in the prairie provinces of Canada. *Journal of Occupational Medicine, 36,* 557–561. doi:10.1097/00043764-199306000-00010

Sobol, H., Vey, N., Sauvan, R., Philip, N., Noguchi, T., & Eisinger, F. (2002). Familial multiple myeloma: A family study and review of the literature. *Journal of the National Cancer Institute, 94,* 461–462.

Struewing, J.P., Hartge, P., Wacholder, S., Baker, S.M., Berlin, M., McAdams, M., ... Tucker, M.A. (1997). The risk of cancer associated with specific mutations of BRCA1 and BRCA2 among Ashkenazi Jews. *New England Journal of Medicine, 336,* 1401–1408. doi:10.1056/ NEJM199705153362001

Svensson, B.G., Mikoczy, Z., Stromberg, U., & Hagmar, L. (1995). Mortality and cancer incidence among Swedish fishermen with a high dietary intake of persistent organochlorine compounds. *Scandinavian Journal of Work, Environment and Health, 21,* 106–115.

Svensson, B.G., Nilsson, A., Jonsson, E., Schutz, A., Akesson, B., & Hagmar, L. (1995). Fish consumption and exposure to persistent organochlorine compounds, mercury, selenium and methylamines among Swedish fishermen. *Scandinavian Journal of Work, Environment and Health, 21,* 96–105.

Takkouche, B., Etminan, M., & Montes-Martinez, A. (2005). Personal use of hair dyes and risk of cancer: A meta-analysis. *JAMA, 293,* 2516–2525. doi:10.1001/jama.293.20.2516

Tavani, A., La Vecchia, C., Gallus, S., Lagiou, P., Trichopoulos, D., Levi, F., & Negri. E. (2000). Red meat intake and cancer risk: A study in Italy. *International Journal of Cancer, 86,* 425–428. doi:10.1002/(SICI)1097-0215(20000501)86:3<425::AID-IJC19>3.0.CO;2-S

Tavani, A., Pregnolato, A., Negri, E., Franceschi, S., Serraino, D., Carbone A., & La Vecchia, C. (1997). Diet and risk of lymphoid neoplasms and soft tissue sarcomas. *Nutrition and Cancer, 27,* 256–260. doi:10.1080/01635589709514535

Thun, M.J., Altekruse, S.F., Namboodiri, M.M., Calle, E.E., Myers, D.G., & Heath, C.W., Jr. (1994). Hair dye use and risk of fatal cancers in U.S. women. *Journal of the National Cancer Institute, 86,* 210–215. doi:10.1093/jnci/86.3.210

U.S. Department of Veterans Affairs. (2008). *Information for veterans, their families and others about VA health care programs related to Agent Orange.* Retrieved from http://www1.va.gov/agentorange

Weiss, B.M., Abadie, J., Verma, P., Howard, R.S., & Kuehl, W.M. (2009). A monoclonal gammopathy precedes multiple myeloma in most patients. *Blood, 113,* 5418–5422. doi:10.1182/blood-2008-12-195008

CHAPTER 5

Patient Assessment

Patricia A. Mangan, MSN, APRN-BC

INTRODUCTION

One of the most rewarding and yet difficult aspects of the care of patients with multiple myeloma is analyzing the unique constellation of clinical manifestations for each individual. Myeloma can present completely asymptomatically upon routine blood testing but at times presents with life-threatening symptoms requiring immediate attention. Proper identification of symptomatic clues to the diagnosis through a comprehensive workup that includes extensive laboratory and radiologic evaluation can lead to better decisions concerning disease management (Mangan, 2005).

Over the past decade, much has been learned concerning the interaction of malignant plasma cells with the bone marrow microenvironment. Biologic factors such as cytogenetics, myeloma cell proliferation rates, biophysical properties of the abnormal monoclonal protein (known as *M protein*), and cytokine activities lead to a varying range of symptoms, dysfunctional organs, and survival potentials that can range from days or weeks to decades.

It is critical that clinicians have adequate knowledge of myeloma's clinical manifestations, diagnostic criteria, and diagnostic tests and procedures to make an accurate diagnosis and manage it appropriately. Finally, an excellent comprehension of the factors relating to tumor burden or staging and prognosis is a vital component of evidence-based treatment decision making.

CLINICAL MANIFESTATIONS OF MULTIPLE MYELOMA

The classic presentation of multiple myeloma is a man in his seventh decade of life or later, with a pathologic fracture and bone pain, x-rays positive for lytic bone lesions, anemia, monoclonal protein in his blood, and bone marrow plasmacytosis. Because of the increased awareness of myeloma by primary healthcare providers, diagnostic testing is initiated for patients who exhibit myeloma-associated symptoms or laboratory abnormalities. The ease and availability of diagnostic testing, including blood tests for quantitative immunoglobulins and serum protein electrophoresis or urine tests for albuminuria and light-chain proteinuria using electrophoresis, have made the consideration of this disease relatively straightforward and inexpensive.

Currently, approximately 20% of all patients are diagnosed while they are completely asymptomatic (Katzel, Hari, & Vesole, 2007). An elevated serum total protein, increased creatinine, elevated calcium, and anemia are among the numerous myeloma-related abnormalities that will be identified by routine serum chemistries and complete blood counts during annual physical examinations. Checking for these abnormal laboratory findings may lead to the diagnosis of myeloma well before signs and symptoms develop.

Clinical features of symptomatic or active disease include bone pain, fatigue, weight loss, and paresthesias. The most common clinical features at presentation are anemia, lytic bone lesions, renal insufficiency, hypercalcemia, and infection (Rajkumar & Kyle, 2005). The presence of one or more of these symptoms or laboratory abnormalities often is the first clue of myeloma.

Myeloma Bone Disease

Bone pain is the most common presenting symptom and can occur any time during the course of the disease. The bone pain, related to bone destruction associated with myeloma, often dominates the clinical presentation. Skeletal involvement, particularly the spine, affects nearly 70% of patients during the course of the disease, and in fact, one-third of patients are diagnosed following a pathologic fracture (Roodman, 2008). Ultimately, lytic bone lesions occur in up to 90% of patients during the course of their disease (Dimopoulos et al., 2009). Typically, movement exacerbates the pain, which is different than with pain seen in other metastatic carcinomas that often worsens at night without activity (Kyle et al., 2003; Longo & Anderson, 2005). The pain is often experienced in the weight-bearing areas, such as the back and the ribs, and pain need not be associated with fracture (Caers et al., 2008). Fractures may occur because of a plasmacytoma or a large lytic lesion or as a result of a relatively minor trauma in an area of osteoporosis.

Reasons for myeloma bone disease include myeloma tumors expanding to the point that mass lesions cause vertebral collapse and spinal cord compression. A common reason is the malignant plasma cells' production of osteoclast-activating factors (OAFs) that stimulate normal osteoclasts, causing extensive bone resorption, whereas other cytokines inhibit osteoblast bone formation. Interleukin-6 is one of the more important OAFs inducing the differentiation and maturation of osteoclast progenitors (Esteve & Roodman, 2007; Giuliani, Rizzoli, & Roodman, 2006). Because of the exhausted osteoblast function and reduced bone formation, bony lesions seldom heal, even when patients are in remission of myeloma (Sezer, 2009). The lack of osteoblastic activity is also why bone scans are often negative in patients with myeloma despite extensive lytic lesions. Therefore, radioisotopic bone scanning is less useful in diagnosis and monitoring than plain radiography, which can reveal the lytic lesions (Dimopoulos et al., 2009; Longo & Anderson, 2005; Roodman, 2008).

Bone findings can range from diffuse osteopenia to lytic bone lesions and myeloma tumors originating from the bones (bony plasmacytomas). The bone x-rays frequently show a punched-out effect with hypo-intense appearance. Bony plasmacytomas may expand to the point that the tumors will involve more than 50% of a vertebral column, placing patients at a higher risk for a vertebral collapse, spinal cord compression, or other compression symptomatology. Compression fractures can occur in up to 50% of patients with myeloma bony disease, and certainly the diagnosis of myeloma should be considered in all patients with nontraumatic vertebral compression fractures (Angtuaco, Fassas, Walker, Sethi, & Barlogie, 2004; Katzel et al., 2007; Longo & Anderson, 2005).

Severe osteopenia and lytic lesions confer a high fracture potential. Even minor movements, such as turning in bed or lifting a grocery bag, can lead to a pathologic fracture. Bone lysis also results in substantial mobilization of calcium from bone, and hypercalcemia may dominate the clinical picture (Dimopoulos et al., 2009). It is crucial that oncology nurses check not only the number and sites of lytic lesions but also the sizes of these lesions to determine whether a patient is at risk for a spontaneous or pathologic fracture.

Anemia

At the time of diagnosis, up to 70% of patients will have anemia, defined as a hemoglobin level below the lower limit of normal (usually less than 10 g/dl). A moderate anemia is seen in the majority of patients with myeloma, but severe anemia with a hemoglobin less than 8 g/dl can be seen in up to 20% of patients (Fonseca & San Miguel, 2007; Rajkumar & Buadi, 2007). The anemia tends to be of a normocytic, normochromic nature and generally is multifactorial. Marrow infiltration with plasma cells can replace erythrocyte precursors and inhibit normal hematopoiesis and decrease red cell production (Blade & Rosinol, 2005). Renal insufficiency can lead to a decreased level of the red blood cell growth hormone, erythropoietin, also reducing production (Silvestris, Tucci, Quatraro, & Dammacco, 2003). There can be a component of anemia of chronic disease, as well as iron deficiency from microscopic blood loss, if the patient also has thrombocytopenia (Blade, Rosinol, & Cibeira, 2008). Additionally, treatment of the disease can result in anemia. A blunted erythropoietin response to anemia may be caused by cytokines that are being produced by the myeloma cells and an abnormal marrow microenvironment. Cytokines such as interleukin-6, interleukin-1, and tumor necrosis factor beta are most likely involved (Silvestris et al., 2003). Anemia of any sort, but certainly once the hemoglobin drops below 8–9 g/dl, can result in significant clinical symptoms of fatigue, weakness, and dyspnea on exertion. Improving anemia by virtue of treatment of the underlying disease, use of exogenous erythropoietin products, resolution of renal insufficiency, and, if needed, transfusion, can substantially improve these symptoms.

Other cytopenias, including neutropenia and thrombocytopenia, are less common at diagnosis but can occur. Usually an alteration of neutrophil and platelet counts suggests a more advanced disease. Thrombocytopenia occurs in less than 15% of patients, and neutropenia is even far less common (Fonseca & San Miguel, 2007).

An increased risk of bleeding occurs in myeloma and is multifactorial. Thrombocytopenia, a quantitative decrease in platelet numbers, can certainly increase the risk of bleeding, particularly with the use of aspirin or nonsteroidal anti-inflammatory medications, which may alter platelet function (Pedersen-Bjergaard, Andersen, & Hansen, 1998). The monoclonal immunoglobulin can occasionally interfere with platelet function and result in an increased risk of bleeding, potentially interfering with red cell clearance and increasing destruction of both red cells and platelets. Finally, clotting factors can be dysfunctional or decreased in amount in patients with myeloma. In particular, fibrinogen, factor V, factor VII, and factor VIII have been implicated in an increased risk for bleeding (Longo & Anderson, 2005).

Renal Insufficiency

Renal insufficiency and failure occurs in up to 25% of patients with myeloma. In fact, an elevated serum creatinine is found in up to one-half of patients, with 20% of patients having a creatinine level greater than 2 g/dl (Fonseca & San Miguel, 2007; Longo & Anderson, 2005). Renal insufficiency is a poor prognostic factor in this disease. Renal failure is second only to infection as the leading cause of death for individuals with myeloma.

Renal dysfunction is multifactorial. Its causes include poor hydration and volume depletion, urinary tract infection and sepsis, nephrotoxins such as certain antibiotics, nonsteroidal anti-inflammatory medications, IV contrast dyes and bisphosphonates, hypercalcemia and nephrocalcinosis, hyperuricemia and urate nephropathy, and even infiltration of the kidney by plasma cells (Ailawadhi & Chanan-Khan, 2008; Choudhury & Ahmed, 2006; Coleman, 2008; Gertz, 2005; Perazella & Markowitz, 2008; Taber & Mueller, 2006). Deposition in the kidney by monoclonal light chains, also known as *myeloma kidney*, may result in renal insufficiency or failure. Proximal tubular damage or interstitial nephritis usually is caused by the free light chain (Leung et al., 2008). Whole immunoglobulins do not pass through the glomeruli and are less commonly involved (Longo & Anderson, 2005). Part of the reason for tubular damage is the overloading of the normal process of light-chain metabolism. Normally, serum light chains are filtered in the kidneys, reabsorbed in the tubules, and metabolized. The increased amount of light chains present in myeloma overloads the tubular cells, thus resulting in tubular damage (Leung et al., 2008).

Hypercalcemia

As noted previously, up to 25% of patients with myeloma will have hypercalcemia (Angtuaco et al., 2004; Rajkumar & Kyle, 2005). When the serum calcium level rises slowly, the patient can remain relatively asymptomatic for a long period of time. Early symptoms can include fatigue, nausea, vomiting, anorexia, polydipsia, dry mucous membranes, or constipation (Kaplan, 2006). If the rise is sudden, a hypercalcemic crisis can occur and result in coma, renal failure, or cardiac arrest. As the imbalance worsens, dehydration, confusion, loss of deep tendon reflexes, electrocardiogram changes, and orthostatic hypotension can occur (Kaplan, 2006).

Normally, 99% of the body's total calcium supply is in the bone, while the other 1% circulates in the blood and exists in two forms, ionized or free calcium that is primarily attached to serum albumin (Mangan, 2005). It therefore is important to note that if the albumin level is decreased, the fraction of ionized or free calcium is greater than the fraction of total calcium level, and the relative severity of the hypercalcemia may be underestimated. Thus, it is important to correct the serum calcium level for hypoalbuminemia to obtain a true total serum calcium level.

A calcium level greater than 10.5 mg/L indicates active myeloma, and patients require immediate treatment (Durie et al., 2003). Patients experiencing hypercalcemia attributable to uncontrolled disease must receive aggressive hydration with diuretics, bisphosphonates, and calcitonin to correct the high calcium level and prevent acute renal failure secondary to hypercalcemia and dehydration (Kaplan, 2006; Terpos, Cibeira, Blade, & Ludwig, 2009). Myeloma treatment must be initiated immediately to treat the cause of hypercalcemia.

Infection

Up to 10% of patients will be diagnosed with myeloma after presenting with infection to their primary care clinicians (Lokhorst, 2002). Up to two-thirds of patients will have a serious infection at some time during their life (Longo & Anderson, 2005). The immune deficiencies in this patient population account for the recurrent infections resulting because of a depression of normal immunoglobulin production or immune paresis (Katzel et al., 2007). Additionally, the ability to mount a humoral immune response, such as those on bacterial cell walls, is impaired. Therefore, bacterial infections, especially in the respiratory and urinary tracts, are the most common sites of infection (Blade & Rosinol, 2007).

The most common infection early in the course of the disease is *Streptococcus pneumoniae* infection and pyelonephritis. Gram-negative infections become more common with treatment, particularly with the use of corticosteroids. Infection is the leading cause of death in patients with myeloma (Ludwig & Zojer, 2007). Anti-infectious vaccinations, such as the Pneumovax® (Merck &

Co., Inc.) and influenza vaccines, should be administered, but they are less effective in this patient population.

Viral reactivation, such as herpes simplex and herpes zoster, which are related to decreased humoral and cellular immunities caused by myeloma, occur more frequently during the course of this disease.

Neurologic Symptoms

Specific neurologic symptoms, such as weakness and pain from spinal cord compression by direct mass effect on the bone or tumor, occur frequently in patients with multiple myeloma. The second most common is peripheral neuropathy, with up to 80% of patients having some form of compensatory or motor paresthesias (Richardson et al., 2006). The most troubling of these is related to demyelinating polyneuropathy, associated with monoclonal antibody interference in which the myelin sheath and nerve conduction are altered in some affected patients. Aside from myeloma, other monoclonal disorders associated with peripheral neuropathy include Waldenström macroglobuline-mia, solitary plasmacytoma, systemic immunoglobulin light-chain amyloido-sis, POEMS (polyneuropathy, organomegaly, endocrinopathy, monoclonal gammopathy, and skin changes), and cryoglobulinemia (Hoffman-Snyder & Smith, 2008). The clinician must rule out these other monoclonal disorders during the diagnostic workup.

The spectrum of neurologic complications of multiple myeloma and related conditions is diverse, with complications ranging from direct compression of bone on nerves (radiculopathy, spinal cord compression, base-of-the-skull tumor) to nerve infiltration by the monoclonal protein (amyloids, peripheral neuropathies, and in rare cases, a change in sensation known as numb chin syndrome of myeloma), metabolic (slowed mentation from hyperviscosity, hypercalcemia, or uremia), and autoimmune or cytokine-mediated compli-cations such as peripheral neuropathy (Dispenzieri & Kyle, 2005). Oncology nurses must perform a careful assessment of the signs and symptoms of seri-ous neurologic complications and initiate immediate interventions to prevent fatal complications.

Hyperviscosity

Up to 5% of patients can have a substantial increase in blood viscosity lead-ing to symptoms of hyperviscosity. Hyperviscosity syndrome occurs most com-monly with the IgM subclass of myeloma, as IgM antibodies tend to circulate as pentamers (Lokhorst, 2002). Up to 50% of patients with IgM paraprotein can have hyperviscosity signs and symptoms. For IgG and IgA subclasses, hy-perviscosity is related more directly to the quantity of M protein in the blood. Normal blood viscosity is 1.8 cP (almost twice as much as the viscosity of water, which is 1.0). Symptomatic hyperviscosity can occur at any elevated viscosity but usually not until levels greater than 4.0 are reached. Patients with levels above 4.0 should undergo viscosity-lowering treatment urgently, as should those who have lower levels but are symptomatic. Usually, high viscosity levels are not reached until monoclonal immunoglobulin levels are greater than 5 g/dl (Longo & Anderson, 2005).

Most of the symptoms of hyperviscosity result from impediment of blood circulation leading to cerebral, pulmonary, and renal dysfunction. Patients can experience bleeding, blurred vision, headache, drowsiness, confusion, or irritability. Patients with hypertension and diabetes are at higher risk for organ damage from hyperviscosity. Symptomatic hyperviscosity is an oncologic emergency, and urgent plasmapheresis should be initiated.

DIAGNOSIS OF MYELOMA

The classic diagnosis is the infiltration of bone marrow with 10% or greater malignant plasma cells with the presence of M protein in the serum or urine (Durie et al., 2003; Longo & Anderson, 2005). M protein in the serum or urine is not sufficient to make the diagnosis of myeloma. Patients with no other evidence of disease except M protein have monoclonal gammopathy of undetermined significance (MGUS). In 2003, the scientific advisers of the International Myeloma Foundation established broadly accepted diagnostic criteria for both asymptomatic, or smoldering, myeloma and symptomatic, or active, myeloma. These criteria are widely used today. The diagnosis system requires evidence of myeloma-related organ dysfunction as the defining element for the diagnosis of symptomatic or active disease. Four major areas of dysfunction are considered: elevated calcium, renal insufficiency, anemia, and bony abnormalities, and are represented by the acronym CRAB (Durie et al., 2003). Figure 5-1 outlines the diagnostic criteria. A classic patient has a triad of findings including marrow plasmacytosis (10% or greater), lytic bone lesions, and serum or urine M protein (Longo & Anderson, 2005). Using these criteria, a patient with M protein in the serum or urine can be classified as either having MGUS, smoldering myeloma, or active myeloma.

Up to 1% of the population older than age 50 have M protein in the blood or urine and have no other manifestations of multiple myeloma (Longo & Anderson, 2005). These patients with MGUS actually have less than 3 g/dl of M protein in the serum, less than 10% plasma cells in the bone marrow, at most a small amount of M protein in the urine, and no lytic bone lesions, anemia, hypercalcemia, or renal insufficiency (Durie et al., 2003; Kyle et al., 2002). Figure 5-2 outlines the diagnostic criteria for MGUS. The diagnosis should not be made until the patient has been observed for 12 months, has demonstrated very stable levels of M protein, and has had no development of the CRAB criteria. Long-term follow-up of patients with MGUS showed that the vast majority of these patients will never develop myeloma or any lymphoid malignancy (Longo & Anderson, 2005). However, in 30 years of follow-up, up to 30% of these patients will develop myeloma; therefore, blood monitoring of these patients is warranted.

Asymptomatic or smoldering disease is defined with the diagnosis of myeloma with at least 10% bone marrow involvement with malignant plasma cells

---

Figure 5-1. Multiple Myeloma Diagnostic Criteria

Multiple myeloma diagnostic criteria: all three required
1. Monoclonal plasma cells in the bone marrow ≥ 10% and/or presence of a biopsy-proven plasmacytoma
2. Monoclonal protein present in the serum and/or urine*
3. Myeloma-related organ dysfunction (1 or more)**
   - [C] Calcium elevation in the blood (serum calcium > 10.5 mg/L or upper limit of normal)
   - [R] Renal insufficiency (serum creatinine > 2 mg/dl)
   - [A] Anemia (hemoglobin < 10 g/dl or 2 g < normal)
   - [B] Lytic bone lesions or osteoporosis***

Note: These criteria identify stage IB and stages II and III A/B myeloma by Durie-Salmon stage. Stage IA becomes smoldering or indolent myeloma.

* If no monoclonal protein is detected (nonsecretory disease), then ≥ 30% monoclonal bone marrow plasma cells and/or a biopsy-proven plasmacytoma required.

** A variety of other types of end organ dysfunctions can occasionally occur and lead to a need for therapy. Such dysfunction is sufficient to support classification as myeloma if proven to be myeloma related.

*** If a solitary (biopsy-proven) plasmacytoma or osteoporosis alone (without fractures) are the sole defining criteria, then ≥ 30% plasma cells are required in the bone marrow.

Note. From "Myeloma Management Guidelines: A Consensus Report from the Scientific Advisors of the International Myeloma Foundation," by B.G.M. Durie, R. Kyle, A. Belch, W. Bensinger, J. Blade, M. Boccadoro, ... B. Van Ness, 2003, *Hematology Journal, 4,* p. 380. Copyright 2003 by European Hematology Association. Open access article distributed under the terms of the Bethesda Statement on Open Access Publishing (http://www.earlham.edu/~peters/fos/bethesda.htm). Retrieved from http://online .haematologica.org/thj/2003/6200312a.pdf.

Figure 5-2. Monoclonal Gammopathy of Undetermined Significance (MGUS) Diagnostic Criteria

MGUS diagnostic criteria: all three required
1. Serum monoclonal protein and/or urine monoclonal protein level low*
2. Monoclonal bone marrow plasma cells < 10%
3. Normal serum calcium, hemoglobin level and serum creatinine
   No bone lesions on full skeletal x-ray survey and/or other imaging if performed
   No clinical or laboratory features of amyloidosis or light-chain deposition disease

* Low is defined as: Serum IgG < 3.0 g/dl; serum IgA < 2.0 g/dl; urine monoclonal kappa or lambda < 1.0 g/24 h.

Note. Reprinted from "Myeloma Management Guidelines: A Consensus Report from the Scientific Advisors of the International Myeloma Foundation," by B.G.M. Durie, R. Kyle, A. Belch, W. Bensinger, J. Blade, M. Boccadoro, ... B. Van Ness, 2003, *Hematology Journal, 4,* p. 380. Copyright 2003 by European Hematology Association. Open access article distributed under the terms of the Bethesda Statement on Open Access Publishing (http://www.earlham.edu/~peters/fos/bethesda.htm). Retrieved from http://online.haematologica.org/thj/2003/6200312a.pdf.

or multiple plasmacytomas and measurable M protein in the blood or urine. These patients, however, do not have any of the CRAB criteria (Durie et al., 2003). Figure 5-3 outlines the diagnostic criteria of asymptomatic or smoldering disease. These patients generally are monitored without therapy until showing evidence of progressive disease. Although many of these patients will develop overt myeloma within a short period of time, many can be observed for years, if not decades, before needing therapy. Symptomatic or active disease requires at least 10% bone marrow involvement with malignant plasma cells or a biopsy-proven plasmacytoma, as well as M protein in the serum or urine, but requires evidence of end-organ damage associated with the CRAB criteria. These patients require immediate therapy to prevent serious and irreversible organ damage (Rajkumar & Kyle, 2005).

Figure 5-3. Smoldering or Indolent Myeloma Diagnostic Criteria

Smoldering or indolent myeloma diagnostic criteria*: all three required
1. Monoclonal protein present in the serum and/or urine
2. Monoclonal plasma cells present in the bone marrow and/or a tissue biopsy
3. Not meeting criteria for monoclonal gammopathy of undetermined significance, multiple myeloma, or solitary plasmacytoma of bone or soft tissue

*These criteria identify stage IA myeloma by Durie-Salmon stage.

Note. Reprinted from "Myeloma Management Guidelines: A Consensus Report From the Scientific Advisors of the International Myeloma Foundation," by B.G.M. Durie, R. Kyle, A. Belch, W. Bensinger, J. Blade, M. Boccadoro, ... B. Van Ness, 2003, *Hematology Journal, 4,* p. 380. Copyright 2003 by European Hematology Association. Open access article distributed under the terms of the Bethesda Statement on Open Access Publishing (http://www.earlham.edu/~peters/fos/bethesda.htm). Retrieved from http://online.haematologica.org/thj/2003/6200312a.pdf.

STAGING

The median survival for patients with multiple myeloma is approximately 3–4 years, with some patients living longer than 10 years. Survival is related to disease stage (Rajkumar & Buadi, 2007). Staging is an important component of the diagnostic workup because it guides clinicians and patients with treatment decisions based on known median survival associated with each disease stage. For example, the Durie-Salmon staging system, developed in 1975, is a clinical staging system to help estimate suspected tumor burden and predict patient outcome (Durie & Salmon, 1975). It is one of the most used classification systems of myeloma (Blade et al., 2008). This system is based on a combination of clinical factors: amount of M protein, serum hemoglobin level, serum calcium level, number of lytic bone lesions on a skeletal radiographic survey, and renal function (Durie & Salmon, 1975). Despite the general use of the Durie-Salmon staging system, the complexity of the criteria made its implementation difficult (Caers et al., 2008). Clinicians argue that the measurement of the tumor mass or bulk of disease is cumbersome, with no universal agreement on its prognostic value. Table 5-1 illustrates the Durie-Salmon staging system.

In 2004, the International Myeloma Working Group (IMWG) identified the need for a universally reliable and simple staging system for consistent classification and stratification of disease and developed the International Staging System (ISS). The ISS is based on two laboratory measurements, serum β_2-microglobulin (β_2M) and albumin, which are known as markers of disease activity in myeloma (Greipp et al., 2005). It nicely defines three risk groups (stage I, II, III) with the median survival of 62, 44, and 29 months, respectively. Table 5-2 demonstrates the ISS. It is a validated alternative to the Durie-Salmon staging system for predicting survival duration at diagnosis (Hari et al., 2009; Katzel et al., 2007).

β_2M is a well-recognized prognostic marker; Longo and Anderson (2005) posited that it is the single most powerful predictor of survival. Patients with β_2M levels less than 3.5 mg/L and albumin levels greater than or equal to 3.5 g/dl have stage I disease by the ISS criteria and have a favorable prognosis with a median survival of 62 months. Patients with β_2M levels greater than 5.5 mg/L are assigned stage III by the ISS and have a poor prognosis with a median survival of approximately 29 months. Stage II disease meets neither stage I nor III ISS criteria and is considered an intermediate stage with a median survival of 44 months (Caers et al., 2008; Greipp et al., 2005).

Both the Durie-Salmon and the ISS staging systems are important in predicting survival but are not useful for therapeutic risk stratification (Kyle & Rajkumar, 2009). Because myeloma is a biologically heterogeneous disease, it is unlikely that any one clinical staging system can fully accommodate the factors that affect outcome. Efforts are under way to develop improved staging criteria that will include other prognostic features, such as cytogenetics and gene expression profiling markers, to predict outcomes (Chng & Bergsagel, 2008). Staging systems have been developed based on cytogenetic and gene expression profiling to uniformly stage myeloma; however, these sophisticated tests are limited by availability and cost.

DIAGNOSTIC TESTS AND PROCEDURES

Complete Physical Assessment and Past Medical and Surgical History

Patients suspected of having myeloma should undergo an initial diagnostic evaluation to ensure the accuracy of the diagnosis and investigate for any manifestation of the disease. As with all medical conditions, a careful physical assessment and a complete past medical and surgical history—including recent infections, fatigue, unintentional weight loss, and pain—should be undertaken. During a complete physical examination, clinicians must pay particular attention in noting masses or point tenderness.

Table 5-1. Durie-Salmon Staging System		
Stage	**Criteria**	**Measured Myeloma Mass (cells × 10^{12}/m^2)***

I	*All* of the following:
	1. Hemoglobin value > 10 g/100 ml
	2. Serum calcium value normal (≤ 12 mg/100 ml)
	3. On roentgenogram, normal bone structure (scale 0) or solitary bone plasmacytoma only
	4. Low M-component production rates
	  a. IgG value < 5 g/100 ml
	  b. IgA value < 3 g/100 ml
	  c. Urine light chain M-component on electrophoresis < 4 g/24 hours
		< 0.6 (Low)

II	Fitting neither stage I nor stage III	0.6–1.20 (Intermediate)

III	*One or more* of the following:
	1. Hemoglobin value < 8.5 g/100 ml
	2. Serum calcium value > 12 mg/100 ml
	3. Advanced lytic bone lesions (scale 3)
	4. High M-component production rates
	  a. IgG value > 7 g/100 ml
	  b. IgA value > 5 g/100 ml
	  c. Urine light chain M-component on electrophoresis > 12 g/24 hours
		> 1.20 (High)

Subclassification
A = Relatively normal renal function (serum creatinine value < 2.0 mg/100 ml)**
B = Abnormal renal function (serum creatinine value ≥ 2.0 mg/100 ml)

Examples
Stage IA = low cell mass with normal renal function
Stage IIIB = high cell mass with abnormal renal function

IgA—immunoglobulin A; IgG—immunoglobulin G

* 10^{12} cells = approximately 1 kg or 2.2 lbs; m^2 = square meter of body surface area.

** If the serum creatinine value is not available, the blood urea nitrogen (BUN) value may be used as an indicator of renal function. (A BUN value of 30 mg/100 ml is roughly equal to a serum creatinine value of 2 mg/100 ml.)

Note. From "A Clinical Staging System for Multiple Myeloma Correlation of Measured Myeloma Cell Mass With Presenting Clinical Feature, Response to Treatment, and Survival," by B. Durie and S. Salmon, 1975, *Cancer, 36,* p. 852. Copyright 1975 by American Cancer Society. Reprinted with permission of Wiley-Liss, Inc., a subsidiary of John Wiley & Sons, Inc.

Laboratory Tests

Laboratory evaluation should include a complete blood count (CBC) with differential, which may reveal cytopenias. Additionally, the presence of circulating plasma cells in the CBC, although rare, occurs in up to 2% of patients with multiple myeloma (Longo & Anderson, 2005).

Table 5-2. International Staging System for Multiple Myeloma		
Stage	Criteria	Median Survival
Stage I	Serum β_2-microglobulin less than 3.5 mg/L Serum albumin greater than or equal to 3.5 g/dl	62 months

Stage II	Not stage I or stage III
	Two possibilities:
	Serum β2-microglobulin less than 3.5 mg/L but serum
	   albumin less than 3.5 g/dl
	Serum β_2-microglobulin 3.5–5.5 mg/L irrespective of
	   serum albumin level
		44 months

Stage III	Serum β_2-microglobulin greater than or equal to 5.5 mg/L	29 months
Note. Based on information from Greipp et al., 2005.		

Evaluation of serum chemistries should include blood urea nitrogen and creatinine to assess renal function and electrolytes, calcium, albumin, and lactate dehydrogenase to evaluate for electrolyte imbalances, hypercalcemia, and other abnormalities. A quantitative measurement of serum immunoglobulin (IgG, IgA, and IgM) levels should be made to detect an abnormal elevation of a particular immunoglobulin or to seek immune paresis (low levels of immunoglobulins).

Protein electrophoresis is the most important test for identifying and characterizing M protein directly produced by myeloma cells. Of myeloma cells, 97% produce and secrete a monoclonal heavy-chain or light-chain protein, and less than 3% are nonsecretory. This M protein in the blood or urine is most commonly intact IgG paraprotein (60%) or IgA (25%). Nonsecretory myelomas and myelomas that secrete IgM, IgD, or IgE M protein are very rare. Up to 20% of cases will secrete just a kappa or lambda light-chain M protein (Longo & Anderson, 2005). Thus, it is important to perform a 24-hour urine protein electrophoresis (UPEP) and urine immunofixation electrophoresis (UIFE) to detect light-chain-type disease. M protein in the blood can be detected by serum protein electrophoresis (SPEP) in approximately 80% of patients and by serum immunofixation electrophoresis (SIFE) 93% of the time (Caers et al., 2008; Katzel et al., 2007; Rajkumar & Kyle, 2005). Therefore, SPEP and SIFE should always be conducted as part of the initial diagnostic evaluation. Table 5-3 shows the different types of myeloma and their corresponding tests.

All patients with suspected myeloma should undergo a 24-hour UPEP and UIFE to determine the presence of urinary M protein (also called *Bence-Jones proteinuria*). Up to 20% of patients will lack serum M protein but have the presence of urinary M protein (Kyle et al., 2003). Other myeloma centers have reported approximately 15% of cases presenting with light-chain disease only, detectable in the urine by performing UPEP and UIFE (Pratt, 2008) or in the serum by performing a serum free light-chain assay (Bradwell, 2005; Bradwell, Carr-Smith, Mead, Harvey, & Drayson, 2003).

Up to 5% of patients have no detectable M protein in the serum or urine by SPEP, UPEP, SIFE, or UIFE, but the majority of these patients will have detectable free light chains in the serum, if serum free light-chain assay is performed (Kyle et al., 2003; Rajkumar & Kyle, 2005; Shaw, 2006). Serum free light-chain assay measures the level of free or unbound kappa and lambda light chains in the serum and can detect M protein in more than two-thirds of these patients. Normally the ratio of kappa light chains to lambda light chains is near equal. An abnormal kappa to lambda ratio indicates an excess of one light-chain type and suggests a clonal plasma cell disorder. A normal concentration of free light chain, however, also may result from nonmalignant conditions; therefore, other laboratory testing is necessary (Dispenzieri et al., 2008, 2009).

Table 5-3. Types of Multiple Myeloma and Diagnostic Tests		
Type	Diagnostic Tests	Findings
Heavy-chain (immunoglobulins IgG or IgA)	Quantitative immuno-globulins	One of immunoglobulins will be elevated (IgG or IgA). IgM, IgD, or IgE elevation is rare.
	Serum protein electrophoresis (SPEP)	Presence of a serum M-spike in the beta or gamma region of the electrophoresis
	Serum immunofixation electrophoresis (SIFE)	Presence of a specific monoclonal protein (e.g., IgG kappa or lambda, IgA kappa or lambda)
Light-chain (kappa or lambda light chain)	24-hour urine protein electrophoresis (UPEP)	One of the light-chain proteins will be elevated (kappa or lambda light chain).
	Urine immunofixation electrophoresis (UIFE)	Presence of a monoclonal kappa or lambda light-chain protein
	Serum free light-chain assay	One of the light chain proteins will be elevated (kappa or lambda light chain). Kappa/lambda ratio will be abnormal.
Nonsecretory	Serum free light chain assay	One of the light-chain proteins will be elevated (kappa or lambda light chain). Kappa/lambda ratio will be abnormal.
	SPEP/SIFE and UPEP/UIFE	No measurable serum or urine M protein. SIFE or UIFE may or may not detect the specific monoclonal protein.

Note. Based on information from Bradwell, 2005; Bradwell et al., 2003; Kyle et al., 2003.

Procedures

A bone marrow aspirate and biopsy or biopsy of a plasmacytoma is necessary for the diagnosis of multiple myeloma. Routine histology and immunohistochemistry stains are performed, as well as flow cytometry for B-cell markers and clonality. Clinicians also should perform cytogenetic evaluation, including conventional cytogenetics as well as fluorescent in situ hybridization (FISH), for the presence of myeloma-related gene translocations or deletions, in conjunction with bone marrow biopsy and aspirate (Fonseca & San Miguel, 2007).

Radiographic evaluation of the bones is necessary to complete the evaluation. Metastatic skeletal surveys (head-to-toe x-rays of axial bones) remain the standard method for screening for lytic lesions, osteopenia, or osteoporosis (Winterbottom & Shaw, 2009). In addition, symptomatic areas should be specifically visualized.

Subtle bone changes can occur well before changes are visible on skeletal radiography. A more sensitive whole body magnetic resonance imaging (MRI), including the skull, spine, and pelvis, and computed tomography (CT) scans of suspected body areas should be considered to give complementary information to skeletal surveys, particularly for patients with normal conventional radiography but with bony symptoms (Roodman, 2008). MRI can detect involvement in vertebral marrow in 50% of patients with indolent (asymptomatic or smoldering) disease, and CT scans can detect early signs of bone-destructive lesions (Dimopoulos et al., 2009). MRI is the standard procedure for patients with pain syndromes or neurologic signs and symptoms to identify soft tissue involvement and early epidural or spinal cord compression.

Nuclear bone scans are less valuable in detecting lesions in myeloma and have no role in routine staging. Bone scans reflect osteoblastic activity and thus underestimate the extent of osteolytic lesions characteristic of myeloma bone disease. Fluoro-2-deoxy-D-glucose (FDG) and positron-emission tomography (PET) imaging, however, may be useful in detecting myeloma, particularly in patients with nonsecretory disease or patients who have symptoms but without clear findings by other diagnostic methods.

Limited data are available regarding the prognostic information of imaging studies such as MRI or PET following treatment, but abnormal medullary or extramedullary FDG activity on PET imaging following high-dose therapy stem cell transplantation carries a particularly poor prognosis (Katzel et al., 2007). MRI and CT scan results can be helpful for determining appropriate biopsy sites and diagnosis when the diagnosis is still in question. Table 5-4 summarizes the diagnostic tests and procedures when multiple myeloma is suspected.

PROGNOSTICATION

Once the diagnosis of multiple myeloma has been made, an assessment of prognosis, or more importantly, the anticipated aggressiveness of the disease,

Table 5-4. Diagnostic Evaluation for Multiple Myeloma	
Test	**Findings Associated With Myeloma**
Complete blood count/platelets/ differential	Decreased hemoglobin; decreased white blood cell count; decreased platelets
Chemistry panel	Increased creatinine; increased calcium; increased uric acid; decreased albumin; increased lactate dehydrogenase
Serum protein electrophoresis	Presence of monoclonal protein
Quantitative immunoglobulins	May be hypogammuloglobulinemic with immuno-electrophoresis
β_2-microglobulin	Elevated level indicates poorer prognosis.
C-reactive protein	Elevated level indicates poorer prognosis.
Kappa/lambda light-chain analysis	Abnormal ratio
Plasma cell labeling index	Elevated level indicates poorer prognosis.
24-hour urine protein electrophoresis	Presence of monoclonal protein/Bence-Jones protein
Bone marrow biopsy/aspirate with cytogenetics/fluorescence in situ hybridization evaluation	Greater than 10% involvement with plasma cells Presence of del 13 indicates poorer prognosis. Presence of del 17p indicates poorer prognosis. Presence of t(4;14) indicates poorer prognosis. Presence of t(14;16) indicates poorer prognosis.
Skeletal survey	Presence of osteolytic lesions Presence of osteoporosis
Magnetic resonance imaging*	Possible cord compression, plasmacytoma, and marrow infiltration
* If symptoms indicate	

can be helpful to determine treatment. The median survival for patients ranges widely from months to decades depending on the disease characteristics. In general, the median survival is approximately five years (Kyle et al., 2003; Rajkumar & Kyle, 2005). Attempts have been made to categorize patients' disease as low risk or high risk, but more research is needed to establish a risk-stratified approach to treatment.

Stage of Myeloma

A number of clinical and laboratory parameters are dependent predictors of survival. Traditionally, the Durie-Salmon staging system classified patients as indolent and not requiring therapy (stage I) versus those with a low tumor burden (stage II) or a high tumor burden (stage III). More recently, a simpler system (the ISS) uses the albumin and serum β_2M levels to determine prognosis. The β_2M is a small protein that forms the light chain of the human leukocyte antigen. β_2M is the single most important prognostic factor in myeloma, and the level is a measure of tumor burden (Blade et al., 2008; Garewal et al., 1984). β_2M, however, is normally excreted by the kidneys, and its serum concentration increases in patients with renal failure. Therefore, it also is a measure of renal function. In the absence of renal problems, a clear correlation exists between serum β_2M levels and myeloma tumor burden. A high β_2M is a predictor of poor survival. The variability of this test, however, makes it a poor measure of tumor burden throughout treatment and is therefore not used for disease monitoring (Blade et al., 2008; San Miguel & Garcia-Sanz, 2005).

Recent multivariable meta-analysis of clinical laboratory data obtained from numerous clinical trials has identified serum albumin as another dominant prognostic factor (Decaux et al., 2008; Kyrtsonis, Maltezas, Tzenou, Koulieris, & Bradwell, 2009). Along with β_2M, these two measurements make up the ISS. It is important to note that all patients analyzed to develop this system had active disease and were undergoing active therapy. Therefore, the ISS cannot be easily related to the Durie-Salmon staging system. Patients with normal albumin and low β_2M levels had the best prognosis. Patients with either elevated β_2M or low albumin levels had intermediate prognosis, and those with high β_2M levels had the highest-risk disease (Greipp et al., 2005).

C-Reactive Protein

A number of studies have linked C-reactive protein to prognosis. It is a surrogate marker for interleukin-6, which is an osteoclast-activating factor, and elevated levels have been associated with poor prognosis (San Miguel & Garcia-Sanz, 2005).

Plasma Cell Labeling Index

Similarly, the plasma cell labeling index (PCLI), popularized by the Mayo Clinic as a marker of rapid tumor cell division, has been shown to be a marker of prognosis (Rajkumar & Kyle, 2005). The higher the PCLI level (1% or higher), the poorer the patient's prognosis. The limited availability of this test, however, has limited its use.

Performance Status

Patient performance status is a powerful predictor of survival in multiple myeloma. Various performance status scales, such as the Eastern Cooperative Oncology Group and the Karnofsky performance scales, measure patients' ability to ambulate and conduct activities of daily living. Patients with good performance status have a substantially better and improved median survival (36 months) when compared to those with poor performance status (11 months) (Rajkumar & Buadi, 2007). Similarly, younger patients tend to have a better prognosis than those who are older (Blade et al., 2008; Kyrtsonis et al., 2009). Older patients generally have a poor performance status and other comorbidities that may preclude aggressive therapy and increase the incidence of infection and thrombosis, contributing to poor survival.

Organ Dysfunction

One particular organ dysfunction associated with a poor prognosis is renal insufficiency. Patients with irreversible renal failure have a median survival of less than one year. Patients with reversible renal failure, on the other hand, have a survival that is similar to those with initial normal renal function (Blade et al., 2008).

Lambda Light Chain–Type Myeloma

Some investigators have suggested that the type of light chain produced may affect survival. Lambda light chain–secreting disease has demonstrated a shorter survival than kappa light chain–secreting disease in some studies (Longo & Anderson, 2005). If this observation is confirmed, it may be because of increased renal dysfunction caused by lambda light chains.

Abnormal Cytogenetics

Cytogenetic abnormalities are emerging as a powerful predictor of prognosis. Because of the low proliferative rates of myeloma cells, karyotypic abnormalities are detected in less than 30% of patients by routine testing (Kyle & Rajkumar, 2009). The detection of abnormal metaphases, especially on chromosome 13, by conventional cytogenetic evaluation has been reported to result in poor survival, but newer therapies such as the immunomodulatory agents and proteasome inhibitors may have altered this prognostication (Dewald et al., 2005). Cytogenetic studies using FISH have been more sensitive in identifying chromosomal translocations. Up to 90% of patients with multiple myeloma have an abnormality detected by FISH (Kyle & Rajkumar). The prognostic significance of these abnormalities is less clear, however. Patients with chromosome 13 abnormalities detected by FISH, for instance, have a similar outcome as those with normal cytogenetics determined by conventional methods. However, abnormalities such as t(4;14), t(14;16), or del(17) are associated with a poor survival (Dewald et al., 2005; Rajkumar & Kyle, 2005; San Miguel & Garcia-Sanz, 2005; Stewart et al., 2007).

The number and type of chromosomal abnormalities identified by karyotype are associated with a shortened survival. Patients with mostly numerical gains of chromosomes (hyperdiploidy) have a good or neutral prognosis. Patients who have deletions or loss of chromosomes (hypodiploidy) have been identified by some investigators to have more aggressive disease with shorter survival (Fonseca et al., 2004; Kyle & Rajkumar, 2009).

Gene Expression Profile

Most recently, microarray technology has allowed for the assessment of gene expression in hundreds of thousands of genes in a particular tumor at one time. Researchers are now assessing the patterns of gene expression, or gene expression profiling, for correlation with survival and various treatments. Likely over the next decade, the understanding of gene expression patterns will allow for personalized therapy for multiple myeloma and an increased predictability of outcome.

CONCLUSION

The assessment and monitoring of patients with multiple myeloma have been marked with extensive advancement in diagnostics and imaging. The ISS is gaining popularity in clinical practice and is now used in major clinical trials. More advances are expected in biologic classification, staging, and molecular-based risk stratification. Continued progress in these areas will undoubtedly improve the management of patients with myeloma and eventually lead to better overall survival.

REFERENCES

Ailawadhi, S., & Chanan-Khan, A. (2008). Management of multiple myeloma patients with renal dysfunction. In S. Lonial (Ed.), *Myeloma therapy: Pursuing the plasma cell* (pp. 499–516). Totowa, NJ: Humana Press.

Angtuaco, E.J., Fassas, A.B., Walker, R., Sethi, R., & Barlogie, B. (2004). Multiple myeloma: Clinical review and diagnostic imaging. *Radiology, 231*, 11–23. doi:10.1148/radiol.2311020452

Blade, J., & Rosinol, L. (2005). Renal, hematologic and infectious complications in multiple myeloma. *Best Practice and Research in Clinical Haematology, 18*, 635–652. doi:10.1016/j.beha.2005.01.013

Blade, J., & Rosinol, L. (2007). Complications of multiple myeloma. *Hematology/Oncology Clinics of North America, 21*, 1231–1246. doi:10.1016/j.hoc.2007.08.006

Blade, J., Rosinol, L., & Cibeira, M.T. (2008). Prognostic factors for multiple myeloma in the era of novel agents. *Annals of Oncology, 19*, vii117–vii120. doi:10.1093/annonc/mdn437

Bradwell, A.R. (2005). Serum free light chain measurements move to center stage. *Clinical Chemistry, 51*, 805–807. doi:10.1373/clinchem.2005.048017

Bradwell, A.R., Carr-Smith, H.D., Mead, G.P., Harvey, T.C., & Drayson, M.T. (2003). Serum test for assessment of patients with Bence Jones myeloma. *Lancet, 361*, 489–491. doi:10.1016/S0140-6736(03)12457-9

Caers, J., Vande broek, I., De Raeve, H., Michaux, L., Trullemans, F., Schots, R., ... Vanderkerken, K. (2008). Multiple myeloma—An update on diagnosis and treatment. *European Journal of Haematology, 81,* 329–343. doi:10.1111/j.1600-0609.2008.01127.x

Chng, W.J., & Bergsagel, P.L. (2008). Biologically-based classification and staging of multiple myeloma. In S. Lonial (Ed.), *Myeloma therapy: Pursuing the plasma cell* (pp. 41–56). Totowa, NJ: Humana Press.

Choudhury, D., & Ahmed, Z. (2006). Drug-associated renal dysfunction and injury. *Nature Clinical Practice in Nephrology, 2,* 80–91. doi:10.1038/ncpneph0076

Coleman, R.E. (2008). Risks and benefits of bisphosphonates. *British Journal of Cancer, 98,* 1736–1740. doi:10.1038/sj.bjc.6604382

Decaux, O., Lode, L., Magrangeas, F., Charbonnel, C., Gouraud, W., Jezequel, P., ... Minvielle, S. (2008). Prediction of survival in multiple myeloma based on gene expression profiles reveals cell cycle and chromosomal instability signatures in high-risk patients and hyperdiploid signatures in low-risk patients: A study of the Intergroupe Francophone du Myélome. *Journal of Clinical Oncology, 26,* 4798–4805. doi:10.1200/JCO.2007.13.8545

Dewald, G.W., Therneau, T., Larson, D., Lee, Y.K., Fink, S., Smoley, S., ... Kyle, R. (2005). Relationship of patient survival and chromosome anomalies detected in metaphase and/or interphase cells at diagnosis of myeloma. *Blood, 106,* 3553–3558. doi:10.1182/blood-2005-05-1981

Dimopoulos, M., Terpos, E., Comenzo, R. L., Tosi, P., Beksac, M., Sezer, O., ... Durie, B.G.M. (2009). International Myeloma Working Group consensus statement and guidelines regarding the current role of imaging techniques in the diagnosis and monitoring of multiple myeloma. *Leukemia.* Advance online publication. doi:10.1038/leu.2009 .89

Dispenzieri, A., & Kyle, R.A. (2005). Neurological aspects of multiple myeloma and related disorders. *Best Practice and Research in Clinical Haematology, 18,* 673–688. doi:10.1016/j. beha.2005.01.024

Dispenzieri, A., Kyle, R.A., Katzmann, J.A., Therneau, T.M., Larson, D., Benson, J., ... Rajkumar, S.V. (2008). Immunoglobulin free light chain ratio is an independent risk factor for progression of smoldering (asymptomatic) multiple myeloma. *Blood, 111,* 785–789. doi:10.1182/blood-2007-08-108357

Dispenzieri, A., Kyle, R., Merlini, G., Miguel, J.S., Ludwig, H., Hajek, R., ... Durie, B.G.M. (2009). International Myeloma Working Group guidelines for serum-free light chain analysis in multiple myeloma and related disorders. *Leukemia, 23,* 215–224. doi:10.1038/ leu.2008.307

Durie, B.G., Kyle, R.A., Belch, A., Bensinger, W., Blade, J., Boccadoro, M., ... Van Ness, B. (2003). Myeloma management guidelines: A consensus report from the Scientific Advisors of the International Myeloma Foundation. *Hematology Journal, 4,* 379–398. doi:10.1038/sj.thj.6200312

Durie, B.G., & Salmon, S.E. (1975). A clinical staging system for multiple myeloma. Correlation of measured myeloma cell mass with presenting clinical features, response to treatment, and survival. *Cancer, 36,* 842–854. doi:10.1002/1097-0142(197509)36:3<842:: AID-CNCR2820360303>3.0.CO;2-U

Esteve, F.R., & Roodman, G.D. (2007). Pathophysiology of myeloma bone disease. *Best Practice in Research and Clinical Haematology, 20,* 613–624. doi:10.1016/j.beha.2007.08.003

Fonseca, R., Barlogie, B., Bataille, R., Bastard, C., Bergsagel, P.L., Chesi, M., ... Avet-Loiseau, H. (2004). Genetics and cytogenetics of multiple myeloma: A workshop report. *Cancer Research, 64,* 1546–1558. doi:10.1158/0008-5472.CAN-03-2876

Fonseca, R., & San Miguel, J. (2007). Prognostic factors and staging in multiple myeloma. *Hematology/Oncology Clinics of North America, 21,* 1115–1140, ix. doi:10.1016/ j.hoc.2007.08.010

Garewal, H., Durie, B.G., Kyle, R.A., Finley, P., Bower, B., & Serokman, R. (1984). Serum beta 2-microglobulin in the initial staging and subsequent monitoring of monoclonal plasma cell disorders. *Journal of Clinical Oncology, 2,* 51–57.

Gertz, M.A. (2005). Managing myeloma kidney. *Annals of Internal Medicine, 143*(11), 835–837.

Giuliani, N., Rizzoli, V., & Roodman, G.D. (2006). Multiple myeloma bone disease: Pathophysiology of osteoblast inhibition. *Blood, 108,* 3992–3996. doi:10.1182/blood-2006-05-026112

Greipp, P.R., San Miguel, J., Durie, B.G., Crowley, J.J., Barlogie, B., Blade, J., ... Westin, J. (2005). International staging system for multiple myeloma. *Journal of Clinical Oncology, 23,* 3412–3420. doi:10.1200/JCO.2005.04.242

Hari, P.N., Zhang, M.J., Roy, V., Perez, W.S., Bashey, A., To, L.B., ... Vesole, D. (2009). Is the international staging system superior to the Durie-Salmon staging system? A comparison in multiple myeloma patients undergoing autologous transplant. *Leukemia, 23,* 1528–1534. doi:10.1038/leu.2009.61

Hoffman-Snyder, C., & Smith, B.E. (2008). Neuromuscular disorders associated with paraproteinemia. *Physical Medicine and Rehabilitation Clinics of North America, 19,* 61–79. doi:10.1016/j.pmr.2007.10.005

Kaplan, M. (2006). Hypercalcemia of malignancy. In M. Kaplan (Ed.), *Understanding and managing oncologic emergencies* (pp. 51–97). Pittsburgh, PA: Oncology Nursing Society.

Katzel, J.A., Hari, P., & Vesole, D.H. (2007). Multiple myeloma: Charging toward a bright future. *CA: A Cancer Journal for Clinicians, 57,* 301–318. doi:10.3322/CA.57.5.301

Kyle, R.A., Gertz, M.A., Witzig, T.E., Lust, J.A., Lacy, M.Q., Dispenzieri, A., ... Greipp, P.R. (2003). Review of 1027 patients with newly diagnosed multiple myeloma. *Mayo Clinic Proceedings, 78,* 21–33. doi:10.4065/78.1.21

Kyle, R.A., & Rajkumar, S.V. (2009). Criteria for diagnosis, staging, risk stratification and response assessment of multiple myeloma. *Leukemia, 23,* 3–9. doi:10.1038/leu.2008.291

Kyle, R.A., Therneau, T.M., Rajkumar, S.V., Offord, J.R., Larson, D.R., Plevak, M.F., & Melton, L.J. (2002). A long-term study of prognosis in monoclonal gammopathy of undetermined significance. *New England Journal of Medicine, 346,* 564–569. doi:10.1056/NEJMoa01133202

Kyrtsonis, M.C., Maltezas, D., Tzenou, T., Koulieris, E., & Bradwell, A.R. (2009). Staging systems and prognostic factors as a guide to therapeutic decisions in multiple myeloma. *Seminars in Hematology, 46,* 110–117. doi:10.1053/j.seminhematol.2009.02.004

Leung, N., Gertz, M.A., Zeldenrust, S.R., Rajkumar, S.V., Dispenzieri, A., Fervenza, F.C., ... Winters, J.L. (2008). Improvement of cast nephropathy with plasma exchange depends on the diagnosis and on reduction of serum free light chains. *Kidney International, 73,* 1282–1288. doi:10.1038/ki.2008.108

Lokhorst, H. (2002). Clinical features and diagnostic criteria. In J. Mehta & S. Singhal (Eds.), *Myeloma* (pp. 151–168). London, England: Martin Dunitz Ltd.

Longo, D., & Anderson, K. (2005). Plasma cell disorders. In D.L. Kasper, E. Braunwald, A.S. Fauci, S.L. Hauser, D.L. Longo, & J.L. Jameson (Eds.), *Harrison's principle of internal medicine* (16th ed., pp. 656–662). New York, NY: McGraw-Hill.

Ludwig, H., & Zojer, N. (2007). Supportive care in multiple myeloma. *Best Practice and Research in Clinical Haematology, 20,* 817–835. doi:10.1016/j.beha.2007.10.001

Mangan, P. (2005). Recognizing multiple myeloma. *Nurse Practitioner, 30*(3), 14–27. doi:10.1097/00006205-200503000-00003

Pedersen-Bjergaard, U., Andersen, M., & Hansen, P.B. (1998). Drug-specific characteristics of thrombocytopenia caused by non-cytotoxic drugs. *European Journal of Clinical Pharmacology, 54,* 701–706. doi:10.1007/s002280050538

Perazella, M.A., & Markowitz, G.S. (2008). Bisphosphonate nephrotoxicity. *Kidney International, 74,* 1385–1393. doi:10.1038/ki.2008.356

Pratt, G. (2008). The evolving use of serum free light chain assays in haematology. *British Journal of Haematology, 141,* 413–422. doi:10.1111/j.1365-2141.2008.07079.x

Rajkumar, S.V., & Buadi, F. (2007). Multiple myeloma: New staging systems for diagnosis, prognosis and response evaluation. *Best Practice and Research in Clinical Haematology, 20,* 665–680. doi:10.1016/j.beha.2007.10.002

Rajkumar, S.V., & Kyle, R.A. (2005). Multiple myeloma: Diagnosis and treatment. *Mayo Clinic Proceedings, 80,* 1371–1382. doi:10.4065/80.10.1371

Richardson, P.G., Briemberg, H., Jagannath, S., Wen, P.Y., Barlogie, B., Berenson, J., ... Amato, A.A. (2006). Frequency, characteristics, and reversibility of peripheral neuropathy during treatment of advanced multiple myeloma with bortezomib. *Journal of Clinical Oncology, 24,* 3113–3120. doi:10.1200/JCO.2005.04.7779

Roodman, G.D. (2008). Skeletal imaging and management of bone disease. *Hematology: American Society of Hematology Education Program Book, 2008,* 313–319. doi:10.1182/asheducation-2008.1.313

San Miguel, J.F., & Garcia-Sanz, R. (2005). Prognostic features of multiple myeloma. *Best Practice and Research in Clinical Haematology, 18,* 569–583. doi:10.1016/j.beha.2005.01.012

Sezer, O. (2009). Myeloma bone disease: Recent advances in biology, diagnosis, and treatment. *Oncologist, 14,* 276–283. doi:10.1634/theoncologist.2009-0003

Shaw, G.R. (2006). Nonsecretory plasma cell myeloma—Becoming even more rare with serum free light-chain assay: A brief review. *Archives of Pathology and Laboratory Medicine, 130,* 1212–1215.

Silvestris, F., Tucci, M., Quatraro, C., & Dammacco, F. (2003). Recent advances in understanding the pathogenesis of anemia in multiple myeloma. *International Journal of Hematology, 78,* 121–125. doi:10.1007/BF02983379

Stewart, A.K., Bergsagel, P.L., Greipp, P.R., Dispenzieri, A., Gertz, M.A., Hayman, S.R., ... Fonseca, R. (2007). A practical guide to defining high-risk myeloma for clinical trials, patient counseling and choice of therapy. *Leukemia, 21,* 529–534. doi:10.1038/sj.leu.2404516

Taber, S.S., & Mueller, B.A. (2006). Drug-associated renal dysfunction. *Critical Care Clinics, 22,* 357–374, viii. doi:10.1016/j.ccc.2006.02.003

Terpos, E., Cibeira, M.T., Blade, J., & Ludwig, H. (2009). Management of complications in multiple myeloma. *Seminars in Hematology, 46,* 176–189. doi:10.1053/j.seminhematol.2009.01.005

Winterbottom, A.P., & Shaw, A.S. (2009). Imaging patients with myeloma. *Clinical Radiology, 64,* 1–11. doi:10.1016/j.crad.2008.07.006

CHAPTER 6

Treatment of Newly Diagnosed, Transplant-Ineligible Patients

Beth Faiman, RN, MSN, APRN-BC, AOCN®

INTRODUCTION

Multiple myeloma is an incurable plasma cell malignancy that can affect adults at nearly any age. It is estimated that 63% of cases will occur in people older than age 65, and at least half of all patients with myeloma are older than 70 years of age (Horner et al., 2009; Hulin et al., 2009). The standard treatment for newly diagnosed, transplant-ineligible patients with myeloma was relatively unchanged for 30 years as evidenced in a study from the Myeloma Trialists' Collaborative Group (1998). Data were evaluated on 4,930 patients and an additional 1,703 patients from seven clinical trials to determine whether melphalan and prednisone (MP), the standard treatment for myeloma since the 1960s, was superior to any other available therapy. Although many patients were able to achieve remission from various combination chemotherapy regimens introduced during the decades prior to this analysis, the group noted no difference in overall survival (OS) when comparing MP to other available therapies (Myeloma Trialists' Group, 1998). This pivotal analysis demonstrated there was clearly room for improvement in the treatment of patients who are ineligible for stem cell transplantation.

A NEW ERA

An era of hope emerged shortly after the Myeloma Trialists' Group publication as thalidomide, an older drug with a notorious history, returned. This time, thalidomide shined brightly as the first in a new class of drugs and led the way for novel therapies. Thalidomide successfully renewed optimism and hope for better treatment options among patients with relapsed disease as initial case reports described a new mechanism of action and improved efficacy compared to existing chemotherapy agents (Faiman, 2007; Orlowski et al., 1998; Singhal et al., 1999). This led the way for drug discovery, finding new pathways and newer antimyeloma agents that demonstrated improved response rates and, in many instances, less toxicity than the regimens that preceded the novel agents. The landscape of multiple myeloma management has dramatically changed for the better. Clinicians once had few treatment options and saw little improvement in survival. Cure has not yet been identified, but with the advances of the past decade, the outlook is infinitely more optimistic, as myeloma has successfully transitioned from a short, life-threatening disease course to a chronic disease.

Multiple factors have played a role in improving outcomes that are seen with myeloma therapy today. Better diagnostic strategies, improved supportive care techniques, and a heightened awareness of myeloma incidence are a few factors that may have contributed to improved survival (Kumar et al., 2008). A study by the Mayo Clinic Group evaluated 2,981 patients with newly diagnosed disease in several patient groups from January 1971 to December 2006. The data showed that individuals who were diagnosed in the 1990s had an OS of 44.8 months versus 29.9 months for people diagnosed in the 1980s. Older individuals benefited from new technology, as patients who were diagnosed after age 65 had an increased survival of 32 months versus 26 months. These data suggest an improvement in the outcome of patients with myeloma in the past decade regardless of age (Kumar et al., 2008).

Patients typically are diagnosed at an older age, yet the approach to treatment is essentially the same for older and younger individuals alike. Initial therapy for nearly all patients historically consisted of oral MP, which was considered to be the standard of care well into the 1990s. Autologous stem cell transplant (ASCT) became a recognized treatment option in the 1980s, but it was not until the mid-1990s that treatment options were more closely examined based on data from the Intergroupe Francophone du Myélome. A landmark study suggested that tandem ASCTs would successfully improve survival and was superior to a single transplant; therefore, all individuals younger than age 65 should be considered for ASCT (Attal et al., 2003). Based on results of this and other trials, attention increased as to whether patients were eligible for ASCT (Barlogie, Kyle, et al., 2006; Palumbo et al., 2004).

STANDARD AUTOLOGOUS STEM CELL TRANSPLANT

Patients must be evaluated for ASCT eligibility for two main reasons. First, intensive therapy with high-dose chemotherapy not only provides an additional therapeutic option to patients but also has been shown to prolong remissions in a majority of patients (Attal et al., 1996, 2003; Barlogie, Tricot, et al., 2006;

Child et al., 2003). Furthermore, ASCT eligibility must be established prior to therapy that involves preservation of the pluripotent bone marrow stem cell. Stem cells of patients who are considered candidates for ASCT must be used or harvested and stored for future use prior to receiving therapies such as alkylating agents. Melphalan is a widely used alkylating agent and can interfere with adequate stem cell mobilization, regardless of whether an early or delayed transplant is contemplated (Kyle & Rajkumar, 2004). Some data suggest that although adequate stem cell harvest can be achieved with patients who have received lenalidomide, granulocyte–colony-stimulating factor (G-CSF) alone may be inadequate for harvesting of stem cells for reasons that are unclear. Therefore, patients receiving lenalidomide may require cyclophosphamide and G-CSF in order to harvest adequate number of stem cells (Cook et al., 2008).

A PHILOSOPHICAL DIVIDE

Two principal, but different, philosophical approaches exist to the treatment of patients with newly diagnosed multiple myeloma, and these are centered on transplant eligibility. General criteria exist for determining whether patients are transplant eligible. Patients are deemed eligible for transplant based on multiple factors, which include physiologic health status, chronologic age, and other comorbid medical conditions that would put them at higher risk for transplant-related mortality (Kyle & Rajkumar, 2008). In addition, patients must be willing to undergo this type of intensive procedure, and not all eligible patients are willing to do so (Kyle & Rajkumar, 2008). Multiple myeloma has been traditionally viewed as an incurable disease, and although most will achieve remission status from ASCT, only a small subset of patients who undergo aggressive therapies may enjoy the benefits of a prolonged remission until the malignant clone reemerges. For individuals who meet the criteria for diagnosis of symptomatic myeloma and are considered ineligible for transplant, many therapies can be administered to control disease. This was not the case even a few years ago.

Patients with multiple myeloma face the challenge of determining the best treatment for them among the available options. The number of antimyeloma therapies has increased dramatically in the past decade, and selecting the appropriate therapy may be quite overwhelming to patients. Transplant-ineligible patients once had a limited number of treatment options, and most drugs, such as oral MP, had a response rate of up to 50% in earlier studies (Alexanian et al., 1969). Furthermore, lower response rates with MP have been noted in modern clinical trials with more stringent response criteria when compared to newer therapies (Kyle & Rajkumar, 2008). Only rarely will patients achieve a complete remission with oral MP.

Improved OS is a goal that most clinical trials attempt to achieve as an end point, and several have successfully identified treatment options better than the previous standard of care regimens (e.g., MP) for patients with myeloma (Facon et al., 2006; Hernandez et al., 2004; San Miguel et al., 2008). ASCT is an effective treatment modality for some, but not all, patients. While several international groups are establishing the role of transplant in younger patients (Attal et al., 1996; Barlogie, Tricot, et al., 2006; Child et al., 2003; Palumbo et al., 1999), the role of transplant in patients who are ineligible for traditional high-dose therapy or in older adults has yet to be clearly defined.

REDUCED-INTENSITY AUTOLOGOUS STEM CELL TRANSPLANT

Reduced-intensity ASCT is a viable treatment option for transplant-ineligible patients. Advanced age has been a poor prognostic factor in several conventional chemotherapy trials in patients with myeloma, characterized by a median survival of less than three years, even after adjusting for major variables such as concurrent illnesses and general health status (Badros et al., 2001). Some researchers hypothesized that by reducing the dose of melphalan chemotherapy, which is the most common chemotherapy regimen used in ASCT, patients who were once deemed ineligible for transplant would now have another treatment option available to them.

The Italian Myeloma Group investigated the role of reduced-intensity IV melphalan in patients who were not candidates for traditional high-dose chemotherapy. The researchers found it was not well tolerated and that patients did not demonstrate improved response or survival rates as compared to conventional therapy (Palumbo et al., 1999). Investigators from the University of Arkansas evaluated 159 patients with myeloma who were older than age 70 from 1992 to 1999. Lower transplant-related doses of IV melphalan were better tolerated than what was received in the higher-dose group, and the transplant-related mortality was less in the lower-dose group (Badros et al., 2001). The Italian Study Group also found response was better with reduced-dose melphalan than the previous standard of care, oral melphalan (Palumbo et al., 1999).

In a study comparing melphalan, prednisone, and thalidomide (MPT) versus MP and ASCT in patients who were not eligible for standard transplant-related doses of melphalan, patients were randomized to MP, MPT, or melphalan 100 mg/m^2 IV as part of ASCT. Patients receiving the MPT regimen had fewer adverse events and improved OS versus the transplant group and showed improved progression-free survival, suggesting that the MPT regimen is superior to ASCT or MP alone when administered to newly diagnosed, transplant-ineligible patients with myeloma (Facon et al., 2006).

Newer agents that are now widely available tend to be more attractive in transplant-ineligible patients than reduced or standard doses of chemotherapy. Several studies have discussed the role of reduced doses of melphalan chemotherapy in patients not considered eligible for standard doses of melphalan, but considerable toxicity is associated with even a reduced-dose regimen (Palumbo et al., 2004). Based on the data, ASCT appears to lead to significant morbidity and mortality regardless of dose and does not improve OS. Because transplant in older adults can cause significant toxicity, caution must be exercised when selecting this as a treatment option. Novel therapies may provide patients a better survival advantage than undergoing transplantation even when reduced doses of melphalan are used. Balancing the risks and benefits of the treatment and quality of life is imperative. Table 6-1 outlines the alternative treatment options for patients who are not candidates for reduced or standard dose intensity transplant.

CONVENTIONAL THERAPIES

Melphalan and Prednisone

The oral MP regimen has been considered the standard induction regimen for patients with newly diagnosed multiple myeloma since the 1960s (Bergsagel, Sprague, Austin, & Griffith, 1962; Bergsagel & Stewart, 2004). Melphalan is administered via both oral and IV routes and belongs to the alkylating group of antineoplastic agents. Various clinical trials have studied this combination therapy, and as a result, dosing schedules may vary depending on which regimens were used in a particular trial. A common dosing schedule of MP is 12 six-week cycles of melphalan 0.25 mg/kg and prednisone 2 mg/kg given orally for four days (Facon et al., 2006). Alternative dosing of this regimen includes melphalan 9 mg/m²/day on days 1–4 every four weeks with prednisone 60 mg/m² PO daily on days 1–4 (San Miguel et al., 2008). Common side effects of melphalan that occur in at least 15% of patients include leukopenia, thrombocytopenia, and anemia. Gastrointestinal side effects (which include nausea, diarrhea, constipation, and vomiting), infections, and alopecia are rare (Alexanian et al., 1969; San Miguel et al., 2008).

Nursing care and monitoring of patients who are receiving melphalan include evaluation of laboratory parameters prior to each cycle. A complete blood count (CBC) and a renal function panel that includes serum blood urea nitrogen and creatinine are required to assess hematologic status and kidney function, respectively. These laboratory values should be checked before each cycle of MP. Although renal excretion of melphalan is low, caution must be exercised when administering melphalan to patients with decreased renal function; dose reduction should be considered to prevent myelosuppression and an increased risk of infection. One study suggested that a 50% reduction in the dose of melphalan decreased the incidence of myelosuppression in patients with compromised kidney function (Cornwell, Pajak, McIntyre, Kochwa, & Dosik, 1982). Melphalan is excreted renally; therefore, nurses must assess kidney function at baseline in any patient receiving melphalan because of the decreased renal clearance of melphalan.

Table 6-1. Comparison of Agents Available for Newly Diagnosed Transplant-Ineligible Patients With Multiple Myeloma

Regimen	Treatment Schema	Response Rate	Overall Survival (OS)	Side Effects
Melphalan and prednisone (MP) (Palumbo et al., 2006)	Six four-week cycles of melphalan 4 mg/m² PO days 1–7 and prednisone 40 mg/m² PO days 1–7	48%	47.6 months	Myelosuppression, fatigue
Dexamethasone (Alexanian et al., 1992)	Dexamethasone 40 mg PO days 1–4, 9–12, and 17–21 of a 28-day cycle	43%	24 months	Fatigue, asthenia, hyperglycemia, mood swings, increased risk of infection
MP plus bortezomib (San Miguel et al., 2008)	MP: Melphalan 9 mg/m² plus prednisone 60 mg/m² days 1–4 Bortezomib 1.3 mg/m² days 1, 4, 8, 11, 22, 25, 29, and 32 for cycles 1–4 and days 1, 8, 22, and 29 during cycles 5–9 (for maintenance) of a 42-day cycle	71%	At 26 months the median OS had not been reached; the projected three-year OS was 85%.	Myelosuppression, gastrointestinal events, infections; peripheral sensory neuropathy, neuralgias, and dizziness may occur.
MP plus thalidomide (MPT) (Palumbo et al., 2006)	Melphalan 4 mg/m² PO days 1–7 Prednisone 40 mg/m² PO days 1–7 Thalidomide 100 mg PO each day Given every four weeks for six months	76%	53.6 months	Myelosuppression, constipation, increased infection risk; peripheral neuropathy, rash (rare)
Thalidomide maintenance (Facon et al., 2006)	Thalidomide maintenance was offered until disease progression. Standard doses of MP for 12 courses at 6-week intervals with thalidomide up to 100 mg PO daily (no maintenance)	76%	51.5 months	—

(Continued on next page)

Table 6-1. Comparison of Agents Available for Newly Diagnosed Transplant-Ineligible Patients With Multiple Myeloma (Continued)

Regimen	Treatment Schema	Response Rate	Overall Survival (OS)	Side Effects
MP plus lenalidomide (Palumbo et al., 2007)	Melphalan 0.18 mg/kg PO days 1–4, prednisone 2 mg/kg PO days 1–4, and lenalidomide 10 mg PO days 1–28, repeated every 4–6 weeks for 9 cycles with aspirin 100 mg PO daily for deep vein thrombosis prophylaxis	81%	1-year OS 100%	Myelosuppression, rash, increased risk of venous thromboembolism (VTE)
Thalidomide plus dexamethasone (Gay et al., 2009; Rajkumar, Blood, et al., 2006)	Thalidomide 200 mg PO days 1–28 plus dexamethasone 40 mg PO days 1, 8, 15, and 22 every 28 days	58%–70%	OS not reported in thalidomide/dexamethasone trial (survival was not an end point for the study, and the study was not powered to compare differences in survival between arms). OS 57.2 months when compared to lenalidomide/dexamethasone	Sedation, somnolence, fatigue, constipation, rash, increased risk of VTE
Lenalidomide plus dexamethasone (Rajkumar et al., 2008)	Lenalidomide 25 mg PO days 1–21 every 28 days Dexamethasone 40 mg PO days 1, 8, 15, and 22 every 28 days	Not reported	2-year survival 91% with weekly dexamethasone 3-year survival 74% in patients receiving weekly dexamethasone	Myelosuppression, rash, change in bowel habits; fatigue, increased risk of VTE, hyperglycemia
Vincristine, doxorubicin, and dexamethasone (VAD) (Alexanian et al., 1990; Cavo et al., 2005; Harousseau et al., 2008)	Vincristine 0.4 mg/day IV and doxorubicin 9 mg/m²/day IV days 1–4 with standard doses of dexamethasone (40 mg PO or IV days 1–4, 9–12, and 17–20 of a 28-day cycle) Vincristine and doxorubicin are administered by continuous infusion.	59%	Data from Alexanian et al. (1990) and Cavo et al. (2005) do not report OS to exceed 30 months. OS at 18 months was 89.3% for VAD (Harousseau et al., 2008).	Granulocytopenia, neuropathy, increased risk of infection

Corticosteroids

Dexamethasone and prednisone are therapeutic agents that belong to a class of drugs called corticosteroids, which are the backbone of antimyeloma therapy. These drugs lead to the inhibition or expression of cytokines such as interleukin-6 (IL-6). IL-6 is a major cytokine growth factor for myeloma cells. Steroids exert their antimyeloma properties by effectively reducing the activity of nuclear factor-kappa-B (NF-κB), which leads to apoptosis or programmed cell death (Alexanian, Dimopoulos, Delasalle, & Barlogie, 1992; Berenson et al., 2002).

Although steroids are effective treatment for myeloma, steroid-related side effects affect nearly every organ system (see Table 6-2) (Faiman, Bilotti, Mangan, & Rogers, 2008). Patients may commonly experience side effects such as mood swings and personality changes as a result of steroids. Patients also have reported insomnia and sleeplessness. Weight gain, edema, and shortness of breath, especially in patients with known cardiac disease, should be assessed at each visit. Blurred vision and vision changes usually are transient and resolve once steroid therapy is completed, but early cataract formation may be a consequence that cannot be avoided. Eye examinations at least every six months are recommended for patients receiving steroid therapy to assess for side effects that may warrant intervention.

Leukocytosis and an increased risk of infection, such as pneumonia, can occur with short-term and long-term steroid use. Nurses should educate patients regarding the following concepts: increased risk of infection, signs and symptoms that should elicit prompt intervention, and the importance of hand washing. Avascular necrosis of the hip or other joints is a serious side effect of prolonged steroid use. Clinicians should encourage patients to notify their healthcare provider or nurse if symptoms of hip or joint pain present and do not improve within one week (Faiman et al., 2008).

Endocrinopathies are common when steroids are used alone or in combination with other therapies for the treatment of multiple myeloma. Steroid-induced hyperglycemia is one of the greatest concerns, as it places patients at risk for negative short-term and long-term consequences on various organ systems. In some patients, mild postprandial blood glucose levels of less than 200 mg/dl can be managed with a low-carbohydrate and low-sugar diet in combination with exercise. If serum glucose is higher than 300 mg/dl, the short-term effects of electrolyte imbalance and dehydration may occur, as well as potential long-term negative effects of microvascular changes. It is critical that nurses assess for a prior history of elevated blood sugar readings, as patients and family members must be made aware of the risk of developing high blood sugar. Clinicians should discuss the signs and symptoms of hyperglycemia and hypoglycemia and review a baseline assessment of risk (Faiman et al., 2008; Pogach et al., 2004). A primary care practitioner or endocrinologist may be helpful in identifying and managing hyperglycemia if medication intervention and home glucose monitoring are warranted.

Table 6-2. Side Effects of Steroids in Patients With Multiple Myeloma

System Affected	Side Effect	Nursing and Patient Intervention
Cardiovascular	Edema	Diuretics; avoid excess dietary sodium; compression stockings
Constitutional	Fatigue	Manage activities; timing of medication (dose steroids in early morning or late at night), dose reduction if affecting quality of life
	Insomnia	Good sleep hygiene
	"Let down" effect after discontinuing steroids	Steroid taper or dose reductions (if severe)
Dermatologic	Acneform rash	Good hygiene with nonirritating soaps; topical or oral antibiotics
	Thinning of skin	Good skin hygiene if skin tears develop
Endocrine	Hyperglycemia	Dietary modifications and avoidance of carbohydrates and sugars; oral hypoglycemic or subcutaneous insulin may be needed in some cases
	Adrenal insufficiency	Steroid taper if long-term steroids used
	Hypogonadism	Refer to primary care provider or an endocrinologist.
Gastrointestinal	Dyspepsia	H_2 receptor inhibitors and proton pump inhibitors
	Taste changes	Good oral hygiene; lozenges
	Hiccoughs	Hold breath while drinking water; drink from the other side of the water glass; if severe, may need chlorpromazine or dose reduction of steroids
Immune	Leukocytosis	Surveillance for infection
	Increased risk of infection	Instruct patient to promptly report signs and symptoms of infection to nurse or healthcare provider.

(Continued on next page)

System Affected	Side Effect	Nursing and Patient Intervention
Table 6-2. Side Effects of Steroids in Patients With Multiple Myeloma _(Continued)_		
Musculoskeletal	Bone thinning or osteoporosis	Monitor bone mineral density; calcium and vitamin D supplements; bisphosphonate therapy for patients with osteoporosis related to steroids or multiple myeloma
	Avascular necrosis	Prompt reporting of pain symptoms; refer to orthopedist if present
	Proximal myopathy	Regular exercise; dose reduce steroids if severe
	Muscle cramping	L-glutamine, quinine water; rule out restless leg syndrome if occurs only at nighttime
Ophthalmic	Vision changes (blurred)	Routine ophthalmic evaluation
	Early cataract formation	Follow with optometry; avoid changing eyeglass prescriptions; may need to be corrected
Psychiatric	Mood swings, personality changes	Screen for history of depression or mania before initiating steroids; educate patient regarding this potential side effect; antidepressants or pharmacologic therapy may be warranted.
	Weight gain, "moon face" or cushingoid appearance	Screen for hyperglycemia or insulin resistance with weight gain; screen for depression; provide support and education.
Sexual dysfunction	Decreased libido	Estrogen or testosterone may be indicated, but complete evaluation by primary care provider or urologist is the first step if pharmacologic interventions are warranted.

Note. Based on information from Faiman et al., 2008.

Nurses should be aware that adrenal insufficiency, which is characterized by dehydration, hypotension, hypoglycemia, or altered mental status, may occur from rapid cessation of long-term steroid use. Although tapering steroids over a long period of weeks is not necessary in patients who do not receive steroids on a daily basis, some degree of fatigue may result from steroid withdrawal (Faiman et al., 2008). Patients who are taking steroids more frequently are at risk for adrenal insufficiency, a potentially life-threatening side effect. Tapering steroids after long-term use in these patients is suggested (Arlt & Allolio, 2003; Wilson & Speiser, 2009).

Steroids are an effective antimyeloma therapy and are used in nearly every regimen, as they have been proved to enhance the effects of various novel and chemotherapy agents in nearly every therapeutic clinical trial in which they have been studied. It is critical to communicate to patients the importance of using steroids in combination with other treatments, such as melphalan; to reinforce side effects; and to implement best management strategies in order to strive for safe and effective delivery of these drugs.

Melphalan, Prednisone, and Bortezomib

Many of the newer agents have variable side effect profiles that allow patients to receive combination therapies that produce an improved remission rate with less toxicity. As mentioned, the combination of MP is associated with a median survival of 29–37 months, but for lack of a better treatment options, this had been the preferred therapy for treatment of newly diagnosed myeloma for many years (Kyle & Rajkumar, 2004). Preclinical studies suggested that adding bortezomib to MP would improve response rates, and a clinical trial was designed to evaluate this combination.

In a phase III clinical trial known as the VISTA (Velcade as Initial Standard Therapy in Multiple Myeloma: Assessment With Melphalan and Prednisone) trial, 682 patients were randomly assigned to receive nine 6-week cycles of melphalan (9 mg/m^2 of body surface area) and prednisone (60 mg/m^2) on days 1–4 of a 28-day cycle. MP was given to patients either by itself or in combination with bortezomib (1.3 mg/m^2) on days 1, 4, 8, 11, 22, 25, 29, and 32 of a 42-day cycle. Following the initial treatment phase, the bortezomib plus MP regimen was given to patients during cycles 1–4 and on days 1, 8, 22, and 29 of a 42-day cycle during cycles 5–9, which was considered to be the maintenance phase of therapy. The results of this randomized, controlled trial showed that the combination of bortezomib plus MP was superior to MP alone, as 71% of patients had at least a partial response to therapy compared to 35% of patients receiving MP. This was one of the first combinations to improve survival in patients with myeloma, and at 26 months, the median OS had not been reached. The projected three-year OS may reach 85% (San Miguel et al., 2008).

Side effects in patients receiving bortezomib plus MP were more prevalent than in those who received MP alone, yet no significant increase occurred in treatment-related deaths (1% and 2%, respectively). Key side effects that were noted in more than 15% of patients receiving bortezomib plus MP included myelosuppression, gastrointestinal events (i.e., nausea, diarrhea, constipation, and vomiting), and infections (pneumonia and herpes zoster) (San Miguel et al., 2008). Nervous system disorders also were common, as peripheral sensory neuropathy, neuralgias, and dizziness occurred.

Nursing implications are focused on patient education and monitoring of treatment-related side effects. Appropriate laboratory monitoring for patients receiving this three-drug regimen is critical. A CBC should be obtained prior to each dose of bortezomib to assess for myelosuppression and hematologic status. Dose reductions according to the package insert should be considered for moderate to severe leukopenia, anemia, or thrombocytopenia, or any other significant side effects that may be related to bortezomib and affect function or quality of life (Millennium Pharmaceuticals, Inc., 2007). Clinicians should evaluate patients' renal function prior to each cycle, as a dose reduction in melphalan may be warranted. It is important to note that patients with renal insufficiency can safely receive the standard dosing schedule of bortezomib (San Miguel et al., 2008).

Two studies have evaluated the safety and efficacy of bortezomib in patients with renal failure. Data from a National Cancer Institute–sponsored trial demonstrated safety in patients with impaired kidney function, as bortezomib is not primarily cleared through the kidneys but through hepatic cytochrome P450 enzymes (Mulkerin et al., 2006). A second subset analysis of patients receiving bortezomib in a phase III clinical trial also was performed. Patients who had impaired renal function with a calculated creatinine clearance less than 30 ml/min demonstrated a response rate of 30%. Of the patients with moderate renal impairment, 25% responded to therapy (Jagannath et al., 2005). The overall frequency of discontinuation of bortezomib was similar regardless of renal function at baseline.

Gastrointestinal side effects of bortezomib are fairly common. Nausea can be prevented by premedication with a $5-HT_3$ antagonist, such as ondansetron or granisetron, which may decrease the risk of nausea and vomiting associated with bortezomib (Colson, Doss, Swift, Tariman, & Thomas, 2004). Increased dietary fiber may help decrease diarrhea as it reabsorbs water in the colon and acts as a bulking agent. Some patients with predictable diarrhea following meals or bortezomib administration may take loperamide before meals or after each diarrhea stool but not to exceed eight tablets per day. Caution must be exercised when using loperamide and other potent antidiarrheal agents, as watery diarrhea accompanied by abdominal cramping may be a sign of a serious infection. Intermittent laboratory evaluation for *Clostridium difficile* or other serious gastrointestinal infections should be performed by assessing stools for *C. difficile* and cultures (Smith, Bertolotti, Curran, & Jenkins, 2008).

Neuropathy or neurotoxicity is a phenomenon that may occur in several different types of patients with cancer and non-cancer diagnoses such as peripheral vascular disease and diabetes but may be present in patients with untreated multiple myeloma as well. Oftentimes nurses and healthcare professionals will identify neuropathy in myeloma when patients have subjective sensory alteration characterized by burning, numbness, tingling, or a decrease in sensation (Tariman, Love, McCullagh, & Sandifer, 2008). These phenomena can be objectively measured with sensitive neurologic procedures such as electrophysiologic studies (EPS), but less expensive techniques may note the presence of neuropathy, such as the clinical examination of the practitioner (Mileshkin et al., 2006).

Nurses play an ongoing and critical role as educators regarding neuropathy, and this begins by raising patient awareness that peripheral neuropathy may occur. In most instances, the nurse administers the drug and interviews patients just prior to the scheduled treatment and, thus, may have more contact with patients than providers. Ongoing surveillance, recognition of symptoms, and intervention are critical to alleviating side effects that may impair the delivery of a drug or the patient's ability to stay on the recommended course of treatment (Richardson, Sonneveld, et al., 2009).

Neuropathy in patients receiving bortezomib should be evaluated before each dose and is one of the most serious side effects of bortezomib. Peripheral sensory neuropathy developed in nearly half of patients receiving bortezomib in the VISTA trial, and serious grade 3 toxicity was present in 13% of patients and warranted discontinuation of therapy (Colson et al., 2004; Tariman et al., 2008). Nurses should educate patients about the increased risk, which includes grade 3 dizziness that will occur in approximately 16% of patients. Prompt identification of side effects and dosage reduction of bortezomib are critical (Colson et al., 2004; Tariman et al., 2008).

In a study evaluating the benefits of dosage reduction in patients with myeloma who were receiving bortezomib therapy, the dose of bortezomib was held, reduced, or discontinued depending on the severity of peripheral neuropathy as reported by the patient and graded by the nurse or clinician. Overall, 124 of 331 patients (37%) had treatment-emergent peripheral neuropathy, which was lower than in a previous phase II trial that did not include dose reduction guidelines. Efficacy of the bortezomib was not affected by dose reduction in patients who reported painful neuropathy, and the neuropathy was noted in this study to be reversible in the majority of patients (Richardson, Sonneveld, et al., 2009). Based on these findings, close monitoring for neuropathy symptoms and dose reduction of bortezomib in patients with even mildly painful peripheral neuropathy are recommended.

Two types of infections were noted in patients receiving the combination of bortezomib and MP: pneumonia and herpes zoster. Nurses should alert patients to the increased risk of developing respiratory illness and implement intervention strategies such as ambulation, coughing and deep breathing, and prompt reporting of signs or symptoms of infection (Miceli, Colson, Gavino, & Lilleby, 2008). Screening patients to see if they are candidates for the pneumonia vaccine is also important. The Pneumovax® 23 (pneumococcal vaccine polyvalent) (Merck & Co., Inc.) is a sterile, liquid vaccine for intramuscular or subcutaneous injection that includes the 23 most prevalent or invasive pneumococcal types of Streptococcus pneumoniae and also includes the six serotypes that most frequently cause invasive drug-resistant pneumococcal infections among children and adults in the United States. The Centers for

Disease Control and Prevention (CDC) recommends the 23-valent Pneumovax, which may help decrease the incidence of pneumococcal infection, a life-threatening condition, for patients with myeloma. Although vaccines against pneumococcus are less effective in older adults than in younger adults, the CDC recommends that the vaccine be administered once after the age of 60 years (CDC, 2008).

Bortezomib has been attributed to an increased risk of herpes zoster or shingles activation in patients with myeloma. The incidence of herpes zoster activation when patients received bortezomib plus MP was 13%, and increased risk was also noted in the APEX (Assessment of Proteasome Inhibition for Extending Remissions) trial (Chanan-Khan et al., 2006; San Miguel et al., 2008). Prophylactic doses of antiviral therapy such as acyclovir or valacylovir should be given to patients receiving bortezomib, which may prevent the development of shingles or lesions.

Patient education is targeted toward awareness and prompt reporting of symptoms. Signs of a herpetic infection may include a prodrome of a tingling sensation followed by the eruption of a rash that may be described as itchy and painful. An erythematous, vesicular rash typically follows a dermatome, or nerve root, and will become evident. If the virus travels to the nerve root, the resulting pain can be particularly debilitating (Kim et al., 2008). It is especially important to note that although a herpes zoster vaccine called Zostavax® (Merck & Co., Inc.) is available, it is contraindicated in immunosuppressed individuals and those with hematologic malignancies. Zostavax is a live, attenuated vaccine and may reactivate a dormant viral infection in patients who lack an intact immune system (Merck & Co., Inc., 2007).

Melphalan, Prednisone, and Thalidomide

The addition of oral MP to oral thalidomide (MPT) has been studied and reported in three major randomized, controlled clinical trials that have accrued mainly transplant-ineligible patients and those older than the age of 65 (Facon et al., 2006; Hulin et al., 2009; Palumbo et al., 2006). One trial randomized patients to receive one of two oral regimens to include MP or MPT. The dose of MP in either arm was the same, and each of the two regimens was administered every month for 12 months. The result of this trial demonstrated that 47% of patients receiving MPT achieved a partial response to therapy versus 7% in the MP group. Researchers also noted a median OS of 51.6 months in the MPT group versus 33.2 months in the MP-alone group, which suggested the MPT regimen was superior to MP alone (Facon et al., 2006). Another trial by Palumbo et al. (2006) randomized patients either to standard-dose MP for six months or to MPT for six months followed by maintenance therapy with thalidomide. The results of this trial showed a trend toward an improved three-year survival with the combination of MPT followed by maintenance thalidomide. The third trial by the Intergroupe Francophone du Myélome demonstrated the safety and efficacy of MPT in patients older than age 75 and that the combination of MPT was superior to MP with a survival advantage in the MPT group (Hulin et al., 2009).

Despite the higher response rate and improved survival benefit of MPT as compared to MP, side effects with MPT therapy are more frequent than with the two-drug combination therapy, as expected. Incidence of grade 3–4 adverse events occurred in approximately 50% of patients who were treated with MPT compared to 25% of patients receiving MP (Hulin et al., 2009). Common side effects of MPT reported in each of the trials include fatigue, myelosuppression, increased risk of infection, deep vein thrombosis (DVT), and nervous system disorders.

The history of thalidomide is an interesting one and is not commonly reported. Chemie Grunenthal was a German pharmaceutical company that introduced thalidomide into the market as a sedative in October 1957. By 1960, the drug had been distributed in more than 409 countries and was commonly given to pregnant women to prevent nausea and emesis. The first report of fetal malformations came shortly thereafter and was thought to occur when the drug was taken in the first trimester between days 35 and 49 after the last menstrual period. By the end of 1961, thalidomide was taken off the market in most countries, but almost 10,000 infants had already been affected. The drug was not used in the United States, as the U.S. Food and Drug Administration (FDA) had denied approval of its use because of the lack of safety data (Kyle & Rajkumar, 2008). Discussion among the medical community regarding the potential antitumor effects of thalidomide had begun, but given its teratogenic effects, the drug had little use until the mid to late 1990s. At that time, thalidomide was studied in relapsed myeloma and quickly regained notoriety. Several key clinical studies have subsequently focused on the use of thalidomide alone and in combination with other therapies (Singhal et al., 1999). Similar to bortezomib, dose modifications are not necessary when thalidomide is administered to patients with renal disease.

Because of the teratogenic effects of thalidomide, the FDA has granted approval for its use in patients through a restrictive program designed to monitor the drug's distribution. Celgene Corp. instituted the S.T.E.P.S.® (System for Thalidomide Education and Prescribing Safety) program to educate patients, pharmacists, and providers about the side effects of thalidomide and to restrict its use to the population of patients who can benefit from the drug (Zeldis, Williams, Thomas, & Elsayed, 1999). Education and awareness of black box warnings, the risk of birth defects, and safe use must be ongoing. Patients must refill thalidomide on a monthly basis and can receive thalidomide only from a registered S.T.E.P.S. prescriber. Pharmacists must be specially trained and registered with Celgene to dispense thalidomide in accordance with FDA regulations. Unused drug must be returned to the company. The goal of this program is to eliminate the possibility of fetal exposure to thalidomide while allowing access to individuals who may benefit (Celgene Corp., 2006b).

Nursing interventions for patients receiving thalidomide include patient and family education about common side effects and strategies to alleviate these effects. Constipation is common in patients who are taking thalidomide for the treatment of multiple myeloma, and higher doses of thalidomide may lead to increased constipation. Patients who are concurrently taking other medicines that have constipation as a side effect, such as pain medications, may have a greater chance of developing constipation. It is important to initiate a bowel regimen and instruct patients to increase fiber in their diet when starting thalidomide therapy. Stool softeners and laxatives may be indicated and are effective as a preventive strategy. Increasing fluid intake will help decrease the risk of dehydration and constipation (Smith et al., 2008).

Many patients who are taking thalidomide complain of sleepiness and daytime or early-morning fatigue. Nurses must instruct patients that if they are taking thalidomide, they should start slowly with one pill a day taken at bedtime and then titrate the dose in weekly increments to achieve target dosing. To address early-morning fatigue and combat daytime sleepiness and sedation, patients may benefit from taking thalidomide early in the evening. Dose reductions of thalidomide may be warranted if the sleepiness and sedation interfere with daily activities (Faiman, 2007).

Peripheral neuropathy is a side effect of thalidomide that rarely occurs early in the treatment phase but more often develops late in the course of therapy. Thalidomide-induced neurotoxicity may be noted earlier in the treatment phase in patients with other health problems, such as diabetes or long-standing high blood pressure, that lead to microvascular changes and venous insufficiency. Although EPS monitoring provides quantitative data to verify the presence or absence of neuropathy, a clinical neurologic examination provides important information also. In a trial by Mileshkin et al. (2006), clinical examination was as effective as EPS monitoring in patients with neuropathy. Patients should be instructed to watch for numbness and tingling in their hands and feet and to promptly report these symptoms to their nurse or healthcare provider. Difficulty with tasks such as buttoning a shirt or opening a jar may be a sign of peripheral neuropathy, but other sensory changes may be present on clinical examination. Dizziness, shakiness, or unsteadiness while walking or standing may be other signs of motor neuropathy that should be reported, and the dose of thalidomide should be decreased (Colson et al., 2004; Faiman, 2007).

Myeloma is intrinsically a hypercoagulable disease, and certain antimyeloma regimens that contain thalidomide and lenalidomide may further increase the risk of venous thromboembolism (VTE). Therefore, patient education about the signs and symptoms of VTE is critical (Rome, Doss, Miller, & Westphal, 2008). For example, when thalidomide was given in combination with MP, the risk of DVT was approximately 20% in the absence of thromboprophylaxis. When patients received enoxaparin, the rate of DVT dropped to approximately 3% (Palumbo et al., 2006). Although VTE can occur with thalidomide and lenalidomide, the risk is low unless given in combination with dexamethasone, doxorubicin, multiagent chemotherapy, or erythropoiesis-stimulating factors, where the risk can be significantly increased up to 75%.

Additional risk factors for VTE exist and must be evaluated before initiation of antimyeloma therapy. Nurses should assess for signs and symptoms of DVT or VTE, including unilateral swelling or cyanosis of the extremity at baseline and at subsequent outpatient or hospital visits. Shortness of breath and anxiety may suggest pulmonary embolism and warrant prompt intervention (Rome et al., 2008; Wiley, 2007). Figure 6-1 lists risk factors and interventions for VTE.

Bortezomib and Dexamethasone

Bortezomib is approved by the FDA for use in combination with MP in patients with newly diagnosed myeloma, but it also can be given with dexamethasone. Aside from use in patients with relapsed or refractory disease, the combination of bortezomib and dexamethasone has been studied in patients with newly diagnosed myeloma and does not impair stem cell harvest in patients who may pursue future transplantation. Therefore, this regimen can be used in all types of patients to include transplant-ineligible patients, older adults, and those who are unsure if they wish to pursue stem cell transplantation at a later date (Harousseau et al., 2006; Jagannath et al., 2006). Long-term follow-up of patients receiving bortezomib 1.3 mg/m^2 on days 1, 4, 8, and 11 of a three-week cycle for up to six cycles, given with oral dexamethasone 40 mg by mouth on the day of and day after bortezomib, showed that while patients responded to single-agent bortezomib, their response was improved by the addition of dexamethasone to the regimen. Dexamethasone generally is administered at a dose of 40 mg by mouth the day of and the day after bortezomib (Harousseau et al., 2006; Jagannath et al., 2006; Richardson et al., 2007) but is generally not well tolerated in older adult patients (Ludwig et al., 2007). Caution must be exercised, and nurses should watch for side effects of dexamethasone when administered to older adults, as its use is discouraged in this population.

The side effects of bortezomib in combination with dexamethasone were similar to those seen in combination with melphalan, with the exception of myelosuppression. The most common blood count abnormality is the presence of a cyclic and predictable thrombocytopenia that in clinical trials was worse on day 11 of a 21-day cycle. A CBC should be obtained before each dose of bortezomib to evaluate blood counts. Dose reductions for thrombocytopenia are rarely needed with bortezomib and dexamethasone, but reduced dosing is indicated if platelets fall to less than 30,000 k/L. Peripheral sensory neuropathy, increased risk of infection, and gastrointestinal side effects such as diarrhea, nausea, and constipation have all been noted in clinical trials. These adverse affects are milder than what is seen when bortezomib is given in combination with MP and generally are predictable and manageable in most patients (Jagannath et al., 2006).

Figure 6-1. Selected Risk Factors for Development of Venous Thromboembolism in Multiple Myeloma

Risk Factors
- Independent risk factors
  - Age
  - Obesity (body mass index greater than 30 k/m^2)
  - History of venous thromboembolism
  - Central venous catheter
- Comorbidities
  - Diabetes
  - Active infections
  - Cardiac disease
  - Renal disease
  - Surgical procedures (including vertebroplasty and kyphoplasty)
  - Inherited thrombophilia or hereditary coagulopathies
  - Other concomitant malignancy
- Medications: Lenalidomide or thalidomide in combination with
  - Erythropoietin
  - Estrogens or hormone therapies
  - Pegylated liposomal doxorubicin or doxorubicin
  - High-dose steroids

Interventions
- Education regarding signs and symptoms
  - Slight fever
  - Tachycardia
  - Unilateral swelling
  - Shortness of breath
  - Cyanosis of extremity
  - Pain in extremity
  - Dull ache in one extremity
  - Venous distention
- Prevention
  - Avoid dehydration
  - Ambulation
  - Sequential compression devices
  - Prophylactic anticoagulation prior to surgical procedures (enoxaparin, heparin)
  - Risk assessment intervention (see below)

Low Risk
- 0–1 risk factors
- Aspirin 81–100 mg PO daily

Intermediate Risk
- 1–2 risk factors
- Aspirin 81–325 mg PO daily and watch closely for signs of venous thromboembolism

High Risk
- More than 2 risk factors
- Therapeutic anticoagulation with warfarin, low-molecular-weight heparin, or full-dose heparin for patients with two or more risk factors

Note. Based on information from Palumbo et al., 2008; Rome et al., 2008; Wiley, 2007.

Thalidomide and Dexamethasone

Thalidomide is a first drug in the class of drugs called *immunomodulatory agents* approved by the FDA for the treatment of newly diagnosed multiple myeloma. In addition, thalidomide is considered an effective treatment regimen in transplant-ineligible patients based on three key studies. In one multicenter, randomized, double-blind, placebo-controlled study, patients were randomized to thalidomide plus dexamethasone (TD) versus dexamethasone alone as initial therapy for newly diagnosed disease. Patients randomized to one arm received thalidomide 50–200 mg PO on days 1–28 and dexamethasone 40 mg on days 1–4, 9–12, and 17–20 of a 28-day cycle. The other group of patients received the same dose of dexamethasone alone. Patients who received TD had a median time to progression of 22.4 months versus 6.5 months in the dexamethasone-only group. OS rates have not been met yet, but many patients in the TD arm remain in remission (Rajkumar, Hussein, et al., 2006). A second Eastern Cooperative Oncology Group (ECOG) trial that was similar in study design randomized patients to receive TD versus dexamethasone alone. Patients who received the combination of TD had better response rates and longer time to progression than patients receiving glucocorticoids alone (Rajkumar, Blood, Vesole, Fonseca, & Greipp, 2006).

A third trial conducted by Ludwig et al. (2007) randomized older adult patients to receive oral MP or oral TD for treatment of newly diagnosed myeloma. Patients received thalidomide 50–200 mg PO daily and dexamethasone 40 mg PO on days 1–4, 9–12, and 17–20 of a 28-day regimen. MP was given on a standard dosing schedule. The combination of TD was shown to be superior to MP, with more patients responding to treatment and for a longer duration of time. Despite a higher response to therapy, the results of this trial showed that patients receiving TD had more neuropathy, a higher incidence of DVT, psychological toxicity, and a higher rate of early treatment discontinuation than patients receiving MP. The data also showed that patients receiving TD had a shorter OS than patients receiving MP therapy even though more hematologic toxicity occurred in those who had received MP (Ludwig et al., 2007). This suggests that high doses of dexamethasone in combination with other therapies such as thalidomide may not be well tolerated in older adults and should be avoided.

Major side effects of TD include increased risk of VTE, constipation, fatigue or sleepiness, and nervous system disorders such as neuropathy. Myelosuppression occurs in combination with melphalan but is not a side effect of thalidomide. Rash may occur in a small percentage of patients and usually resolves, but in rare cases (less than 1%), Stevens-Johnson syndrome may occur, which produces a widespread rash from head to toe that could be severe (Celgene Corp., 2006b).

Nursing considerations for patients receiving thalidomide in combination with dexamethasone or other agents focus mainly on education regarding drug safety and monitoring for side effects. Patients receiving thalidomide have an increased risk of developing VTE. The nurse's role is to educate patients regarding the increased risk of blood clots, to determine if they are candidates for aspirin or other therapeutic anticoagulation, and to educate patients regarding preventive strategies. Other important nursing interventions and management strategies for constipation, fatigue or sleepiness, and neuropathy also warrant special attention.

Lenalidomide and Dexamethasone

Lenalidomide is an analog of thalidomide and an oral immunomodulatory agent that has demonstrated efficacy in patients with newly diagnosed as well as relapsed disease. Despite its similarity to the first-in-class immunomodulatory agent for myeloma, lenalidomide carries a much different dosing schedule and side effect profile. The mechanism of action is not well known in lenalidomide (Doss, 2006; Faiman, 2007), but it clearly works in the bone marrow stroma to inhibit proliferation of the plasma cells. It is primarily excreted through the kidneys and does not undergo cytochrome P450 metabolism, meaning the risk for drug-drug interactions is low (Celgene Corp., 2006a).

Lenalidomide has been studied extensively in patients with relapsed myeloma and in several newly diagnosed myeloma trials, but the most convincing data for its use in transplant-ineligible patients have resulted from a randomized, controlled, phase III clinical trial sponsored by ECOG. In this trial, patients were randomized to lenalidomide 25 mg PO daily for 21 days with either high-dose dexamethasone (40 mg/day on days 1–4, 9–12, and 17–20 of a 28-day cycle) or low-dose dexamethasone (40 mg/day on days 1, 8, 15, and 22 of a 28-day cycle). The trial was halted early because of the increased one-year survival rate observed in the low-dose dexamethasone arm (96%) compared to the high-dose dexamethasone arm (87%), as the patients receiving high-dose dexamethasone had increased risk of infections and VTE. Differences in OS favored the low-dose dexamethasone arm in subgroup analysis of patients younger than age 65 and in those age 65 or older, which suggests that all patients with newly diagnosed disease, regardless of age, should receive the lower doses of steroids as opposed to higher doses of steroids, which traditionally was the standard of care (Rajkumar et al., 2008).

An important nursing consideration when caring for patients who are receiving lenalidomide is to counsel patients about the risk of birth defects. Preclinical studies suggest that lenalidomide does not appear to cause the same teratogenic effects seen with thalidomide. Despite this finding, no data support its safety in humans, and the potential increased risk for fetal birth defects is not worth taking. The chemical structure closely resembles thalidomide, which warrants caution (Kumar & Rajkumar, 2006). The RevAssist® program of Celgene Corp. is similar to the company's S.T.E.P.S. program and was developed to address the need for safety and education when prescribing lenalidomide. Female patients of child-bearing potential must be counseled before the start of lenalidomide therapy and on a monthly basis to avoid becoming pregnant;

men receiving the drug must not cause a woman to become pregnant. Two forms of birth control are required at all times, and patients must not donate blood or sperm. Counseling against fetal exposure to lenalidomide should be ongoing and performed at least on a monthly basis prior to prescription refills (Celgene Corp., 2006a).

A second important consideration for patients who are receiving lenalido- mide and dexamethasone would be education on the increased risk of VTE. Patients in the ECOG trial had an increased risk of VTE in the high-dose dexamethasone group as compared to the low-dose dexamethasone group. Intervention and management of these side effects are the same as with pa- tients receiving thalidomide and should be routinely discussed with patients. Guidelines have been established for the prevention, diagnosis, and manage- ment of VTE associated with lenalidomide and thalidomide (Palumbo et al., 2007; Rome et al., 2008).

The proper dosing and schedule of lenalidomide in patients with renal failure and compromised renal function has been described. Little was known about the effects of lenalidomide and renal function until recently, as only patients with serum creatinine levels less than 2.5 mg/dl were allowed to participate in the randomized clinical trials that described its efficacy. As of 2009, the FDA has approved changes to the product package insert to reflect renal dosing parameters (Celgene Corp., 2006a). Like many drugs that are excreted through the kidneys, dosing of lenalidomide for patients with my- eloma must be done on the basis of creatinine clearance. It is recommended that nurses and healthcare providers calculate serum creatinine clearance so that the correct starting dose of lenalidomide is ordered.

The most common consequence of inappropriate dosing of lenalidomide in patients with renal insufficiency or renal failure is myelosuppression. First reported by Niesvizky et al. (2007), this group observed that patients who received the oral combination of clarithromycin, lenalidomide, and dexam- ethasone and had concurrent renal dysfunction with a creatinine clearance of less than 40 ml/min experienced more significant myelosuppression than those with normal renal function (Niesvizky et al., 2007). Lenalidomide is safe in patients with renal dysfunction and in patients on dialysis, but it is important to initiate the appropriate dose and implement routine monitor- ing of serum creatinine clearance. Dosage reductions based on decreased renal function should be considered in all patients with myeloma. A CBC and differential should be obtained at least every two weeks at the beginning of therapy; serum creatinine should be monitored at the time of each blood draw (Celgene Corp., 2006a).

Melphalan, Prednisone, and Lenalidomide

In prior clinical trials, researchers have added either thalidomide or bort- ezomib to MP in an attempt to find the best standard of care regimen for older adult or transplant-ineligible patients. Palumbo et al. (2007) studied the combination of MP plus lenalidomide (MPR) in 54 newly diagnosed patients older than 65 years. In this trial, the dose of melphalan was 0.18 mg/kg PO on days 1–4, prednisone 2 mg/kg PO on days 1–4, and lenalidomide 5–10 mg PO on days 1–21 repeated every four to six weeks for nine cycles. The overall response rate in this trial was 81%, and 48% of patients achieved at least very good partial response to therapy, which suggests this is an effective regimen in patients with myeloma (Palumbo et al., 2007).

Side effects of MPR are similar to previous trials that used lenalidomide or MP. Neutropenia, thrombocytopenia, and anemia were the most common. Rash and gastrointestinal side effects were noted infrequently. All patients received prophylactic aspirin, and the incidence of VTE in the MPR trial was low and occurred in only three of the patients, and two patients actually developed DVT after aspirin discontinuation. MPR seems to be fairly well tolerated on the basis of this clinical trial, but clearly more studies are warranted (Palumbo et al., 2007).

High-Dose Dexamethasone

Corticosteroids such as prednisone and dexamethasone have been administered to patients with multiple myeloma for many decades and have been shown to induce remissions (Alexanian et al., 1992; Facon et al., 2006) and prolong remission as maintenance therapy (Berenson et al., 2002). The mechanism of action for steroids in myeloma includes several pathways. The antitumor effects of steroids have been documented, but the mechanism of action remains unclear. One hypothesis is that steroids induce apoptosis and promote myeloma cell death by inhibiting IL-6 activity, a growth factor for myeloma cells (Alexanian et al., 1969). Dosing schedules of steroids vary, but as a single agent, dexamethasone has been most widely administered in a pulse-like fashion given 40 mg PO days 1–4, 9–12, and 17–21 of a 28-day cycle. The toxicity of single-agent dexamethasone has been established and is no longer recommended for frontline management of myeloma (Ludwig et al., 2007).

Two recent studies suggest that the toxicities associated with high-dose steroids alone or in combination with other agents may outweigh the benefits to myeloma cell death when given to older adult patients with the disease. One study evaluated the effectiveness of different steroid combinations with oral melphalan in older adult patients. Facon et al. (2006) randomized 488 patients ages 65–75 to three different treatments including MP, melphalan and dexamethasone (MD), or dexamethasone alone. The treatment groups showed no difference in OS. Although the initial response to therapy appeared to be higher in patients receiving MD than in those receiving other treatments, the morbidity associated with the older adult patients receiving the dexamethasone-based regimen was significantly higher than in patients receiving MP. Patients experienced many side effects in the MD and dexamethasone arms, including febrile infections, bleeding, uncontrolled diabetes, and gastrointestinal and psychiatric complications (Facon et al., 2006).

Another study of MP versus MD in the treatment of older adult patients (N = 201) showed that they tolerated MP better than MD, and higher doses of dexamethasone did not improve OS and resulted in more side effects. Based on the results of these studies, oral MP appears to be safer than MD for older adult patients (Hernandez et al., 2004). Several key clinical trials have been designed to address the effectiveness of certain treatment regimens and reduce toxicity associated with high doses of steroids in combination with chemotherapy or novel agents (Hussein et al., 2006; Rajkumar et al., 2008). Side effects must be closely monitored to optimize treatment outcomes (see Figure 6-1). Nurses play a key role in educating patients about the side effects of steroids and providing interventions.

Vincristine, Doxorubicin, and Dexamethasone

The regimen of vincristine, doxorubicin (Adriamycin®, Bedford Laboratories), and dexamethasone (VAD) has been used in older adult, transplant-ineligible and transplant-eligible patients with myeloma for many years (Alexanian, Barlogie, & Tucker, 1990; Cavo et al., 2005; Rajkumar, 2005). VAD was one of the few effective chemotherapy regimens available in the past 20 years and became a standard regimen for transplant-eligible patients, as the three-drug therapy does not harm stem cell harvest. In recent years, this regimen has become scarcely used in older adult or transplant-ineligible patients because of the toxicity and relative ineffectiveness compared to newer agents with the potential for fewer side effects and better response rates (Rajkumar, 2005). Vincristine and doxorubicin are administered in this regimen by continuous infusion at the doses of 0.4 mg/day and 9 mg/m^2/day, respectively, on days 1–4 with standard doses of dexamethasone (40 mg PO/IV days 1–4, 9–12, and 17–20 of a 28-day cycle) and must be given via central venous catheter because doxorubicin is a vesicant (Cavo et al., 2005).

The efficacy of VAD in the era of novel agents has been questioned. One study suggests that dexamethasone was responsible for the efficacy of VAD and that doxorubicin and vincristine provided very little, if any, contribution toward efficacy (Alexanian et al., 1992). To determine whether newer agents such as thalidomide are as effective as upfront myeloma therapy, Cavo et al. (2005) compared the infusional VAD regimen to the oral TD regimen in 200 patients. Participants who received TD had a significantly higher response rate (76%) than those receiving IV VAD (52%). With the neurotoxicity seen with vincristine, the steroid side effect profile of high-dose dexamethasone, cost, inconvenience, and infection risk associated with implanted central venous catheter placement, most institutions do not use VAD in patients with newly diagnosed disease any longer, and it is not considered standard of care (Rajkumar, 2005).

As an alternative regimen designed to address the side effects of high-dose steroids given in the VAD regimen and the inconvenience of a four-day continuous infusion, pegylated liposomal doxorubicin replaced doxorubicin in the

VAD regimen in the 1990s. Pegylated liposomal doxorubicin is a nonvesicant anthracycline given on day 1 of a 28-day cycle as a 1.5-hour infusion in combination with reduced-dose dexamethasone; 40 mg PO is given on only days 1–4 of a 28-day cycle. The same dose of vincristine 2 mg IV push is given on day 1 of therapy. The reduced intensity and dose of steroids attempts to address concerns of steroid-related side effects, which may negatively affect quality of life. In addition, patients receiving the regimen with pegylated liposomal doxorubicin have experienced less cumulative cardiac toxicity, which is seen with doxorubicin, and achieved similar response rates as those receiving the VAD regimen (Hussein et al., 2006).

Nurses should be aware that although VAD has been used for many years, it is no longer the best front-line option for transplant-eligible or transplant-ineligible patients, given the plethora of newer, more effective therapies. Major side effects of VAD include myelosuppression and constipation, which may be attributed to doxorubicin, and neurotoxicity secondary to vincristine, which may provide little if any contribution to the regimen. Nausea and vomiting may occur but generally is mild and can be prevented with the administration of antiemetic agents. Oral mucositis can develop, and good oral hygiene is encouraged. Cardiotoxicity may occur; nurses should be aware of the cumulative dose of doxorubicin prior to each infusion, as patients should not receive a cumulative dose of greater than 550 mg/m^2. Baseline left ventricular ejection fraction should be obtained to assess for stable cardiac function. As discussed in previous sections, transplant-ineligible patients are often older, and high doses of dexamethasone used in the VAD regimen may lead to increased toxicity (Facon et al., 2006; Ludwig et al., 2007). As with any treatment decision that is to be made, the risks, benefits, and alternatives should be weighed carefully before proceeding with VAD therapy.

MAINTENANCE THERAPY

The role of maintenance therapy in patients with multiple myeloma who have not received high-dose therapy remains controversial, and no clear consensus exists. Clinical trials are ongoing to answer this question, which primarily focuses on individual patients' response to therapy. Maintenance has been incorporated into cancer treatment for years in an effort to prevent the reemergence of a malignant clone and maintain control of the disease. Interferon, corticosteroids, immunomodulatory agents, and proteasome inhibitors have all been studied to varying degrees, but of the novel agents, thalidomide has been the most widely studied maintenance agent in randomized, controlled trials following autologous high-dose chemotherapy. Despite this, debate is ongoing as to whether maintenance is actually a form of treatment and whether it should be used after induction chemotherapy in the nontransplant setting with the intention to control residual disease. In general, patients have few options following conventional therapy and transplantation, primarily based on their response to the treatment (Santos, Goodman, Byrnes, & Fernandez, 2004).

Thalidomide

Thalidomide is an active antimyeloma therapy and is safe for use in patients who are not candidates for a transplant. Several trials have examined the use of thalidomide as maintenance therapy. Short-term side effects, such as increased risk for thrombosis, constipation, sedation, and dizziness, and long-term side effects, such as neurotoxicity, provide a questionable risk-benefit ratio that should be balanced before maintenance with thalidomide is initiated.

In a prospective, randomized, controlled trial, 597 patients with myeloma were randomly assigned to one of three treatment arms following tandem high-dose chemotherapy. Patients were randomized to receive no maintenance (arm A), pamidronate 90 mg IV every four weeks (arm B), or pamidronate plus thalidomide at a mean dose of 200 mg/day PO (arm C). Maintenance began two months after receiving the second transplant. In this study, 67% of patients achieved a very good partial remission of greater than 90% reduction in serum monoclonal protein in arm C versus 55% in arm A. Despite the aggressive use of bisphosphonates, skeletal-related events in this trial were not statistically significant in any of the arms. In regard to cytogenetic risk, a subgroup analysis suggested that patients with the deletion of chromosome 13 or those who achieved very good partial remission after high-dose chemotherapy did not clearly benefit from thalidomide maintenance (Attal et al., 2006).

A second study evaluating the use of thalidomide as maintenance therapy was a trial that included 668 patients with newly diagnosed disease (Barlogie, Tricot, et al., 2006). Each was assigned to receive thalidomide throughout the entire treatment period (excluding during the transplantation and stem cell harvest) or not at all. Despite the improved complete response rates of the thalidomide group versus the control group (62% versus 43%, respectively), the OS of the patients was unchanged. These data suggest that for patients who undergo an intensive regimen of melphalan-based chemotherapy and tandem high-dose chemotherapy, the addition of thalidomide improved patient response rates but did not improve OS in this trial. In addition, the adverse effects associated with long-term high doses of thalidomide may be considerable for some and, thus, not acceptable. This is true especially when other treatment options, or in some instances observation, may be reasonable (Barlogie, Tricot, et al., 2006).

A third trial of 195 patients, all younger than 60 years old, investigated the use of thalidomide. Patients were randomized to treatment with ASCT followed by thalidomide maintenance or tandem ASCT without thalidomide. Patients assigned to the thalidomide maintenance arm received a second ASCT at disease progression rather than up front. Patients receiving thalidomide maintenance showed significantly higher three-year progression-free survival rates (85% versus 57%) and OS (85% versus 65%) after a median follow-up of 33 months (Abdelkefi et al., 2008).

A smaller retrospective analysis of 112 patients who received ASCT at a single institution were evaluated according to the type of preparative regimen they received and whether maintenance thalidomide had improved OS. Regardless of the type of induction regimen each patient received (busulfan, cyclophosphamide, VP-16, or melphalan), the median survival was superior in the group receiving thalidomide compared to in the group without thalidomide maintenance (79.6 months versus 39.6 months) (Brinker et al., 2006). Although this single-institution trial may suggest that there is a benefit to patients receiving thalidomide after transplant, further prospective trials are necessary to confirm this hypothesis.

The National Comprehensive Cancer Network (NCCN) guidelines for thalidomide maintenance in multiple myeloma consider the use of thalidomide as a single agent following ASCT as a category 1 recommendation, meaning there is a high level of evidence from randomized, controlled trials and uniform NCCN consensus. The combination of thalidomide and prednisone is a category 2A recommendation, meaning that although there is a lower level of evidence, uniform consensus recommends this type of maintenance. Each practitioner is strongly encouraged to consider current data to make an informed recommendation based on each patient's individual situation. When possible, participation in a clinical trial to evaluate the role of maintenance therapy is recommended (NCCN, 2008).

Bortezomib

Bortezomib has demonstrated efficacy when used to treat patients with newly diagnosed and relapsed disease. Although the use of bortezomib as a maintenance drug has been incorporated into several published clinical trials in relapsed myeloma and upfront use in the transplant-ineligible population (Richardson et al., 2007; San Miguel et al., 2008), its use after transplantation is still very much under investigation at the time of this publication. An ongoing phase II study evaluating the use of bortezomib as an induction and post-transplant maintenance regimen has shown promising preliminary results, but these are limited. At this time, the maintenance dosing and schedule of bortezomib is not clear, and it is not recommended outside of a clinical trial (Goyal, Uy, DiPersio, & Vij, 2007).

Lenalidomide

Lenalidomide, when used as a single agent, has shown effectiveness in relapsed disease (Richardson, Jagannath, et al., 2009). Based on prior clinical trial designs, patients who have received lenalidomide and dexamethasone have remained on the combination regimen until disease progression. Ongoing trials, including one large Cancer and Leukemia Group B trial and an Italian myeloma group study, are assessing its effectiveness as a maintenance regimen following transplantation.

Glucosteroids

For patients who have received standard combination therapy as the induction regimen for the treatment of multiple myeloma, steroids may play a role in maintaining an initial response. In a Southwest Oncology Group trial, patients received VAD chemotherapy and were randomized to different alternate-day schedules of oral prednisone. Two different dose levels of prednisone were used, either 10 mg PO every other day or 50 mg PO every other day for remission maintenance. Patients who received prednisone 50 mg PO every other day had improved progression-free survival (14 months versus 5 months) and improved OS (37 months versus 26 months) compared to patients who received 10 mg PO every other day. This suggests that using oral prednisone 50 mg every other day following induction chemotherapy may prolong progression-free survival intervals (Berenson et al., 2002) and is independent of whether the patient underwent transplantation.

Interferon

Interferon has been studied in patients with multiple myeloma, but this drug is seldom used in the maintenance phase because of its poor tolerability, conflicting efficacy data, high cost, and relatively low benefit associated with therapy (Sirohi, Treleaven, & Powles, 2002). Interferon is a less attractive option than other available novel agents, but a few studies are still evaluating its role and use in patients with myeloma.

CONCLUSION

Patients have undoubtedly benefited from the advances in myeloma clinical research in the past decades. Those who are ineligible for transplant or who decide not to pursue transplant have many different options that were not available in the past. An enormous amount of dedication is needed on behalf of investigators, patients, nurses, study coordinators, and support staff to complete a clinical trial. Each trial, no matter how big or small, provides valuable information for the next group of patients and researchers. Numerous clinical trials are ongoing, and each strives to find a more effective and better tolerated antimyeloma therapy with the hope of ultimately achieving a cure. Nurses will continue to play a critical role as they guide patients through the maze of treatment, improving outcomes and quality of life with their knowledge, education, and expertise.

REFERENCES

Abdelkefi, A., Ladeb, S., Torjman, L., Othman, T.B., Lakhal, A., Romdhane, N.B., … Abdela-dhim, A.B. (2008). Single autologous stem-cell transplantation followed by maintenance therapy with thalidomide is superior to double autologous transplantation in multiple myeloma: Results of a multicenter randomized clinical trial. *Blood, 111,* 1805–1810. doi:10.1182/blood-2007-07-101212

Alexanian, R., Barlogie, B., & Tucker, S. (1990). VAD-based regimens as primary treatment for multiple myeloma. *American Journal of Hematology, 33,* 86–89. doi:10.1002/ajh.2830330203

Alexanian, R., Dimopoulos, M.A., Delasalle, K., & Barlogie, B. (1992). Primary dexamethasone treatment of multiple myeloma. *Blood, 80,* 887–890.

Alexanian, R., Haut, A., Khan, A.U., Lane, M., McKelvey, E.M., Migliore, P.J., … Wilson, H.E. (1969). Treatment for multiple myeloma: Combination chemotherapy with different melphalan dose regimens. *JAMA, 208,* 1680–1685. doi:10.1001/jama.208.9.1680

Arlt, W., & Allolio, B. (2003). Adrenal insufficiency. *Lancet, 361,* 1881–1893. doi:10.1016/S0140-6736(03)13492-7

Attal, M., Harousseau, J.-L., Facon, T., Guilhot, F., Doyen, C., Fuzibet, J.G., … Bataille, R. (2003). Single versus double autologous stem-cell transplantation for multiple myeloma. *New England Journal of Medicine, 349,* 2495–2502. doi:10.1056/NEJMoa032290

Attal, M., Harousseau, J.-L., Leyvraz, S., Doyen, C., Hulin, C., Benboubkher, L., … Facon, T. (2006). Maintenance therapy with thalidomide improves survival in patients with multiple myeloma. *Blood, 108,* 3289–3294. doi:10.1182/blood-2006-05-022962

Attal, M., Harousseau, J.-L., Stoppa, A.M., Sotto, J.J., Fuzibet, J.G., Rossi, J.F., … Bataille, R. (1996). A prospective, randomized trial of autologous bone marrow transplantation and chemotherapy in multiple myeloma: Intergroupe Francais du Myelome. *New England Journal of Medicine, 335,* 91–97. doi:10.1056/NEJM199607113350204

Badros, A., Barlogie, B., Siegel, E., Morris, C., Desikan, R., Zangari, M., … Tricot, G. (2001). Autologous stem cell transplantation in elderly multiple myeloma patients over the age of 70 years. *British Journal of Haematology, 114,* 600–607. doi:10.1046/j.1365-2141.2001.02976.x

Barlogie, B., Kyle, R.A., Anderson, K.C., Greipp, P.R., Lazarus, H.M., Hurd, D.D., … Crowley, J.C. (2006). Standard chemotherapy compared with high-dose chemoradiotherapy for multiple myeloma: Final results of phase III US Intergroup Trial S9321. *Journal of Clinical Oncology, 24,* 929–936. doi:10.1200/JCO.2005.04.5807

Barlogie, B., Tricot, G., Anaissie, E., Shaughnessy, J., Rasmussen, E., van Rhee, F., … Crowley, J. (2006). Thalidomide and hematopoietic-cell transplantation for multiple myeloma. *New England Journal of Medicine, 354,* 1021–1030. doi:10.1056/NEJMoa053583

Berenson, J.R., Crowley, J.J., Grogan, T.M., Zangmeister, J., Briggs, A.D., Mills, G.M., … Salmon, S.E. (2002). Maintenance therapy with alternate-day prednisone improves survival in multiple myeloma patients. *Blood, 99,* 3163–3168. doi:10.1182/blood.V99.9.3163

Bergsagel, D.E., Sprague, C.C., Austin, C., & Griffith, K.M. (1962). Evaluation of new chemotherapeutic agents in the treatment of multiple myeloma. IV. L-Phenylalanine mustard (NSC-8806). *Cancer Chemotherapy Reports, 21,* 87–99.

Bergsagel, D.E., & Stewart, A.K. (2004). Conventional-dose chemotherapy of myeloma. In J.S. Malpas, D.E. Bergsagel, R. Kyle, & K. Anderson (Eds.), *Myeloma: Biology and management* (3rd ed., pp. 203–217). Philadelphia, PA: Saunders.

Brinker, B.T., Waller, E.K., Leong, T., Heffner, L.T., Jr., Redei, I., Langston, A.A., & Lonial, S. (2006). Maintenance therapy with thalidomide improves overall survival after autologous hematopoietic progenitor cell transplant with multiple myeloma. *Cancer, 106,* 2171–2180. doi:10.1002/cncr.21852

Cavo, M., Zamagni, E., Tosi, P., Tacchetti, P., & Cellini, C., Cangini, D., … Baccarani, M. (2005). Superiority of thalidomide and dexamethasone over vincristine-doxorubicin dexamethasone (VAD) as primary therapy in preparation for autologous transplantation for multiple myeloma. *Blood, 106,* 35–39. doi:10.1182/blood-2005-02-0522

Celgene Corp. (2006a). Revlimid (lenalidomide) [Package insert]. Summit, NJ: Author.

Celgene Corp. (2006b). Thalomid (thalidomide) [Package insert]. Summit, NJ: Author.

Centers for Disease Control and Prevention. (2008). *ACIP provisional recommendations for use of pneumococcal vaccines.* Retrieved from http://www.cdc.gov/vaccines/recs/provisional/downloads/pneumo-oct-2008-508.pdf

Chanan-Khan, A.A., Sonneveld, P., Schuster, M., Irwin, D., Stadtmauer, E.A., Facon, T., ... Richardson, P.G. (2006). Analysis of varicella zoster virus reactivation among bortezomib-treated patients in the APEX study [Abstract No. 3535]. *Blood, 108*(11). Retrieved from http://abstracts.hematologylibrary.org/cgi/content/abstract/108/11/3535

Child, J.A., Morgan, G.J., Davies, F.E., Owen, R.G., Bell, S.E., Hawkins, K., ... Selby, P.J. (2003). High-dose chemotherapy with hematopoietic stem-cell rescue for multiple myeloma. *New England Journal of Medicine, 348,* 1875–1883. doi:10.1056/NEJMoa022340

Colson, K., Doss, D.S., Swift, R., Tariman, J., & Thomas, T.E. (2004). Bortezomib, a newly approved proteasome inhibitor for the treatment of multiple myeloma: Nursing implications. *Clinical Journal of Oncology Nursing, 8,* 473–480. doi:10.1188/04.CJON.473-480

Cook, R.J., Vogl, D., Mangan, P.A., Cunningham, K., Luger, S., Porter, D.L., ... Stadtmauer, E.A. (2008). Lenalidomide and stem cell collection in patients with multiple myeloma [Abstract No. 8547]. *Journal of Clinical Oncology, 26*(Suppl. 15). Retrieved from http://meeting.ascopubs.org/cgi/content/abstract/26/15_suppl/8547

Cornwell, G.G., 3rd, Pajak, T.F., McIntyre, O.R., Kochwa, S., & Dosik, H. (1982). Influence of renal failure on myelosuppressive effects of melphalan: Cancer and Leukemia Group B experience. *Cancer Treatment Reports, 66,* 475–481.

Doss, D.S. (2006). Advances in oral therapy in the treatment of multiple myeloma. *Clinical Journal of Oncology Nursing, 10,* 514–520. doi:10.1188/06.CJON.514-520

Facon, T., Mary, J.-Y., Pegourie, B., Attal, M., Renaud, M., Sadoun, A., ... Bataille, R. (2006). Dexamethasone-based regimens versus melphalan-prednisone for elderly multiple myeloma patients ineligible for high-dose therapy. *Blood, 107,* 1292–1298. doi:10.1182/blood-2005-04-1588

Faiman, B. (2007). Clinical updates and nursing considerations for patients with multiple myeloma. *Clinical Journal of Oncology Nursing, 11,* 831–840. doi:10.1188/07.CJON.831-840

Faiman, B., Bilotti, E., Mangan, P.A., & Rogers, K. (2008). Steroid-associated side effects in patients with multiple myeloma: Consensus statement of the IMF Nurse Leadership Board. *Clinical Journal of Oncology Nursing, 12*(Suppl. 3), 53–63. doi:10.1188/08.CJON.S1.53-62

Gay, F., Hayman, S., Lacy, M.Q., Buadi, F., Gertz, M.A., Kumar, S., ... Rajkumar, S.V. (2009, December). *Superiority of lenalidomide-dexamethasone versus thalidomide-dexamethasone as initial therapy for newly diagnosed multiple myeloma* [Abstract No. 3884]. Poster presented at the 51st ASH Annual Meeting and Exposition, New Orleans, LA. Retrieved from http://ash.confex.com/ash/2009/webprogram/Paper20613.html

Goyal, S.D., Uy, G., DiPersio, J.R., & Vij, R. (2007). Bortezomib (BTZ) prior to and as maintenance therapy after autologous stem cell transplant (ASCT) in multiple myeloma (MM): Long-term follow-up of a phase II study [Abstract No. 8044]. *Journal of Clinical Oncology, 25*(Suppl. 18). Retrieved from http://meeting.ascopubs.org/cgi/content/abstract/25/18_suppl/8044

Harousseau, J.-L., Attal, M., Leleu, X., Troncy, J., Pegourie, B., Stoppa, A.M., ... Avet-Loiseau, H. (2006). Bortezomib plus dexamethasone as induction treatment prior to autologous stem cell transplantation in patients with newly diagnosed multiple myeloma: Results of an IFM phase II study. *Haematologica, 91,* 1498–1505.

Harousseau, J.-L., Mathiot, C., Attal, M., Marit, G., Caillot, D., Hullin, C., ... Moreau, P. (2008). Bortezomib/dexamethasone versus VAD as induction prior to autologous stem cell transplantation (ASCT) in previously untreated multiple myeloma (MM): Updated data from IFM 2005/01 trial [Abstract No. 8505]. *Journal of Clinical Oncology, 26*(Suppl.

15). Retrieved from http://www.asco.org/ASCOv2/Meetings/Abstracts?&vmview=abst_detail_view&confID=55&abstractID=35165

Hernandez, J.M., Garcia-Sanz, R., Golvano, E., Blade, J., Fernandez-Calvo, J., Trujillo, J., … San Miguel, J.F. (2004). Randomized comparison of dexamethasone combined with melphalan versus melphalan with prednisone in the treatment of elderly patients with multiple myeloma. *British Journal of Haematology, 127,* 159–164. doi:10.1111/j.1365-2141.2004.05186.x

Horner, M.J, Ries, L.A, Krapcho, M., Neyman, N., Aminou, R., Howlader, N., … Edwards, B.K. (Eds.). (2009). *SEER cancer statistics review, 1975–2006.* Bethesda, MD: National Cancer Institute. Retrieved from http://seer.cancer.gov/csr/1975_2006/

Hulin, C., Facon, T., Rodon, P., Pegourie, B., Benboubker, L., Doyen, C., … Moreau, P. (2009). Efficacy of melphalan and prednisone plus thalidomide in patients older than 75 years with newly diagnosed multiple myeloma: IFM 01/01 trial. *Journal of Clinical Oncology, 27,* 3664–3670. doi:10.1200/JCO.2008.21.0948

Hussein, M.A., Baz, R., Srkalovic, G., Agrawal, N., Suppiah, R., Hsi E., … Walker, E. (2006). Phase 2 study of pegylated liposomal doxorubicin, vincristine, decreased-frequency dexamethasone and thalidomide in newly diagnosed and relapsed-refractory multiple myeloma. *Mayo Clinic Proceedings, 81,* 889–895. doi:10.4065/81.7.889

Jagannath, S., Barlogie, B., Berenson, J.R., Singhal, S., Alexanian, R., Srkalovic, G., … Anderson, K.C. (2005). Bortezomib in recurrent and/or refractory multiple myeloma: Initial clinical experience in patients with impaired renal function. *Cancer, 103,* 1195–1200. doi:10.1002/cncr.20888

Jagannath, S., Durie, B.G.M., Wolf, J.L., Camacho, E.S., Irwin, D., Lutzky, J., … Vescio, R. (2006). Long-term follow-up of patients treated with bortezomib alone and in combination with dexamethasone as frontline therapy for multiple myeloma [Abstract No. 796]. *Blood, 108.* Retrieved from http://abstracts.hematologylibrary.org/cgi/content/abstract/108/11/796

Kim, S.J., Kim, K., Kim, B.S., Lee, H.J., Kim, H., Lee, N.R., … Shin, H.J. (2008). Bortezomib and the increased incidence of herpes zoster in patients with multiple myeloma. *Clinical Lymphoma and Myeloma, 8,* 237–240. doi:10.3816/CLM.2008.n.031

Kumar, S., & Rajkumar, S.V. (2006). Thalidomide and lenalidomide in the treatment of multiple myeloma. *European Journal of Cancer, 42,* 1612–1622. doi:10.1016/j.ejca.2006.04.004

Kumar, S.K., Rajkumar, S.V., Dispenzieri, A., Lacy, M.Q., Hayman, S.R., Buadi, F.K., … Gertz, M.A. (2008). Improved survival in multiple myeloma and the impact of novel therapies. *Blood, 111,* 2516–2520. doi:10.1182/blood-2007-10-116129

Kyle, R.A., & Rajkumar, S.V. (2004). Multiple myeloma. *New England Journal of Medicine, 351,* 1860–1873. doi:10.1056/NEJMra041875

Kyle, R.A., & Rajkumar, S.V. (2008). Multiple myeloma. *Blood, 111,* 2962–2972. doi:10.1182/blood-2007-10-078022

Ludwig, H., Tothova, E., Hajek, R., Drach, J., Adam, Z., Labar, B., … Hinke, A. (2007). Thalidomide-dexamethasone vs. melphalan-prednisone as first line treatment and thalidomide-interferon vs. interferon maintenance therapy in elderly patients with multiple myeloma [Abstract No. 529]. *Blood, 110.* Retrieved from http://abstracts.hematologylibrary.org/cgi/content/abstract/110/11/529

Merck & Co., Inc. (2007). *Zostavax prescribing information.* Retrieved from http://www.merck.com/product/usa/pi_circulars/z/zostavax/zostavax_pi.pdf

Miceli, T., Colson, K., Gavino, M., & Lilleby, K. (2008). Myelosuppression associated with novel therapies in patients with multiple myeloma: Consensus statement of the IMF Nurse Leadership Board. *Clinical Journal of Oncology Nursing, 12*(Suppl. 3), 13–19. doi:10.1188/08.CJON.S1.13-19

Mileshkin, L. Stark, R., Day, B., Seymour, J.F., Zeldis, J.B., & Prince, H.M. (2006). Development of neuropathy in patients with myeloma treated with thalidomide: Patterns of occurrence and the role of electrophysiologic monitoring. *Journal of Clinical Oncology, 24,* 4507–4514. doi:10.1200/JCO.2006.05.6689

Millennium Pharmaceuticals, Inc. (2007). Velcade (bortezomib) [Package insert]. Cambridge, MA: Author.

Mulkerin, D., Remick, S., Ramanathan, R., Hamilton, A., Takimoto, C., Davies, A., ... Wright, J. (2006). A dose-escalating and pharmacologic study of bortezomib in adult cancer patients with impaired renal function [Abstract No. 2032]. *Journal of Clinical Oncology, 24*(Suppl. 18). Retrieved from http://meeting.ascopubs.org/cgi/content/abstract/24/18_suppl/2032

Myeloma Trialists' Collaborative Group. (1998). Combination chemotherapy versus melphalan plus prednisone as treatment for multiple myeloma: An overview of 6,633 patients from 27 randomized trials. *Journal of Clinical Oncology, 16*, 3832–3842.

National Comprehensive Cancer Network. (2008). NCCN 2008 multiple myeloma clinical practice guidelines in oncology. In *The complete library of NCCN clinical practice guidelines in oncology* [CD-ROM]. Jenkintown, PA: Author.

Niesvizky, R., Jayabalan, D., Zafar, F., Christos, P., Pearse, R., Jalbrzikowski, J.B., ... Coleman, M. (2007). BiRD (Biaxin®/Revlimid®/dexamethasone) in myeloma (MM) [Abstract No. PO-714]. *Haematologica, 92*(Suppl. 2), 178.

Orlowski R.Z., Eswara, J.R., Lafond-Walker, A., Grever, M.R., Orlowski, M., & Dang, C.V. (1998). Tumor growth inhibition induced in a murine model of human Burkitt's lymphoma by a proteasome inhibitor. *Cancer Research, 58*, 4342–4348.

Palumbo, A., Bringhen. S., Caravita, T., Merla, E., Capparella, V., Callea, V., ... Galli, M. (2006). Oral melphalan and prednisone chemotherapy plus thalidomide compared with melphalan and prednisone alone in elderly patients with multiple myeloma: Randomised controlled trial. *Lancet, 367*, 825–831. doi:10.1016/S0140-6736(06)68338-4

Palumbo, A., Bringhen, S., Petrucci, M.T., Musto, P., Rossini, F., Nunzi, M., ... Boccadoro, M. (2004). Intermediate-dose melphalan improves survival of myeloma patients aged 50 to 70: Results of a randomized controlled trial. *Blood, 104*, 3052–3057. doi:10.1182/blood-2004-02-0408

Palumbo, A., Falco, P., Corradini, P., Falcone, A., Di Raimondo, F., Giuliani, N., ... Petrucci, M.T. (2007). Melphalan, prednisone, and lenalidomide treatment for newly diagnosed myeloma: A report from the GIMEMA—Italian Multiple Myeloma Network. *Journal of Clinical Oncology, 25*, 4459–4465. doi:10.1200/JCO.2007.12.3463

Palumbo, A., Rajkumar, S.V., Dimopoulos, M.A., Richardson, P.G., San Miguel, J., Barlogie, B., ... Hussein, M.A. (2008). Prevention of thalidomide- and lenalidomide-associated thrombosis in myeloma. *Leukemia, 22*, 414–423. doi:10.1038/sj.leu.2405062

Palumbo, A., Triolo, T., Argentino, C., Bringhen, S., Dominietto, A., Rus, C., ... Boccadoro, M. (1999). Dose-intensive melphalan with stem cell support (MEL100) is superior to standard treatment in elderly myeloma patients. *Blood, 94*, 1248–1253.

Pogach, L.M., Brietzke, S.A., Cowan, C.L., Conlin, P., Walder, D.J., & Sawin, C.T. (2004). Development of evidence-based clinical practice guidelines for diabetes: The Department of Veterans Affairs/Department of Defense guidelines initiative. *Diabetes Care, 27*(Suppl. 2), B82–B89. doi:10.2337/diacare.27.suppl_2.B82

Rajkumar, S.V. (2005). Multiple myeloma: The death of VAD as initial therapy. *Blood, 106*, 2–3. doi:10.1182/blood-2005-04-1451

Rajkumar, S.V., Blood, E., Vesole, D., Fonseca, R., & Greipp, P.R. (2006). Phase III clinical trial of thalidomide plus dexamethasone compared with dexamethasone alone in newly diagnosed multiple myeloma: A clinical trial coordinated by the Eastern Cooperative Oncology Group. *Journal of Clinical Oncology, 24*, 431–436. doi:10.1200/JCO.2005.03.0221

Rajkumar, S.V., Hussein, M., Catalano, J., Jedrzejcak, W., Sirkovich, S., Olesnyckyj, M., ... Blade, J. (2006). A randomized, double-blind, placebo-controlled trial of thalidomide plus dexamethasone versus dexamethasone alone as primary therapy for newly diagnosed multiple myeloma [Abstract No. 795]. *Blood, 108*. Retrieved from http://abstracts.hematologylibrary.org/cgi/content/abstract/108/11/795

Rajkumar, S.V., Jacobus, S., Callander, N., Fonseca, R., Vesole, M., Williams, M., ... Greipp, P.R. (2008). Randomized trial of lenalidomide plus high-dose dexamethasone versus lenalidomide plus low-dose dexamethasone in newly diagnosed myeloma (E4A03), a trial coordinated by the Eastern Cooperative Oncology Group: Analysis of response, survival, and outcome with primary therapy and with stem cell transplant [Abstract No. 8504]. *Journal of Clinical Oncology, 26*(Suppl.). Retrieved from http://www.asco.org/ASCOv2/Meetings/Abstracts?&vmview=abst_detail_view&confID=55&abstractID=36097

Richardson, P., Jagannath, S., Hussein, M., Berenson, J., Singhal, S., Irwin, D., ... Anderson, K.C. (2009). Safety and efficacy of single-agent lenalidomide in patients with relapsed and refractory multiple myeloma. *Blood, 114,* 772–778. doi:10.1182/blood-2008-12-196238

Richardson, P.G., Sonneveld, P., Schuster, M.W., Irwin, D., Stadtmauer, E.A., Facon, T., ... Anderson, K.C. (2007). Safety and efficacy of bortezomib in high-risk and elderly patients with relapsed multiple myeloma. *British Journal of Haematology, 137,* 429–435. doi:10.1111/j.1365-2141.2007.06585.x

Richardson, P.G., Sonneveld, P., Schuster, M.W., Stadtmauer, E.A., Facon, T., Harousseau, J.-L., ... San Miguel, J. (2009). Reversibility of symptomatic peripheral neuropathy with bortezomib in the phase III APEX trial in relapsed multiple myeloma: Impact of dose-modification guidelines. *British Journal of Haematology, 144,* 895–903. doi:10.1111/j.1365-2141.2008.07573.x

Rome, S., Doss, D.S., Miller, K.C., & Westphal, J. (2008). Thromboembolic events associated with novel therapies in patients with multiple myeloma: Consensus statement of the IMF Nurse Leadership Board. *Clinical Journal of Oncology Nursing, 12*(Suppl. 3), 21–28. doi:10.1188/08.CJON.S1.21-27

San Miguel, J.F., Schlag, R., Khuageva, N.K., Dimopoulos, M.A., Shpilberg, O., Kropff, M., ... Richardson, P.G. (2008). Bortezomib plus melphalan and prednisone for initial treatment of multiple myeloma. *New England Journal of Medicine, 359,* 906–917. doi:10.1056/NEJMoa0801479

Santos, E.S., Goodman, M., Byrnes, J.J., & Fernandez, H.F. (2004). Thalidomide effects in the post-transplantation setting in patients with multiple myeloma. *Hematology, 9,* 35–39. doi:10.1080/10245330310001652428

Singhal, S., Mehta, J., Desikan, R., Ayers, D., Roberson, P., Eddlemon, P., ... Crowley, J. (1999). Antitumor activity of thalidomide in refractory multiple myeloma. *New England Journal of Medicine, 341,* 1565–1571. doi:10.1056/NEJM199911183412102

Sirohi, B., Treleaven, J., & Powles, R. (2002). Role of interferon. In J. Mehta & S. Singhal (Eds.), *Myeloma* (pp. 383–396). London, England: Martin Dunitz.

Smith, L.C., Bertolotti, P., Curran, K., & Jenkins, B. (2008). Gastrointestinal side effects associated with novel therapies in patients with multiple myeloma: Consensus statement of the IMF Nurse Leadership Board. *Clinical Journal of Oncology Nursing, 12*(Suppl. 3), 37–52. doi:10.1188/08.CJON.S1.37-51

Tariman, J., Love, G., McCullagh, E., & Sandifer, S. (2008). Peripheral neuropathy associated with novel therapies in patients with multiple myeloma: Consensus statement of the IMF Nurse Leadership Board. *Clinical Journal of Oncology Nursing, 12*(Suppl. 3), 29–36. doi:10.1188/08.CJON.S1.29-35

Wiley, K.E. (2007). Multiple myeloma and treatment-related thromboembolism: Oncology nurses' role in prevention, assessment, and diagnosis. *Clinical Journal of Oncology Nursing, 11,* 847–851. doi:10.1188/07.CJON.847-851

Wilson, T.A., & Speiser, P. (2009). *Adrenal insufficiency.* Retrieved from http://emedicine.medscape.com/article/919077-overview

Zeldis, J.B., Williams, B.A., Thomas, S.D., & Elsayed, M.E. (1999). S.T.E.P.S.: A comprehensive program for controlling and monitoring access to thalidomide. *Clinical Therapeutics, 21,* 319–330. doi:10.1016/S0149-2918(00)88289-2

CHAPTER 7

Treatment of Newly Diagnosed, Transplant-Eligible Patients

Anna Liza Rodriguez, RN, MSN, MHA, OCN®

INTRODUCTION

After almost 30 years of clinical trial research, multiple myeloma remains incurable with a complete response (CR) rate of less than 10% (Kulkarni et al., 1999) and a median survival of only 30–36 months with conventional standard treatment of melphalan and prednisolone (Barlogie et al., 1997). Several studies in the early 1990s suggested that dose intensification followed by hematopoietic stem cell rescue results in higher CR rates and extended event-free survival (EFS). The superiority of high-dose chemotherapy with stem cell transplantation (SCT) over standard treatment established the role of high-dose chemotherapy with SCT as a safe and effective therapy for patients with multiple myeloma (Singhal, 2002). Various SCT strategies as treatment for patients with multiple myeloma continued to evolve over the years (see Figure 7-1). The refinement of SCT conditioning regimens, use of novel agents before and after transplant, combination of immunotherapy with SCT, and engineering of a better graft-versus-myeloma effect all hold promise for better responses to treatments and clinical outcomes. Table 7-1 describes the European Group for Blood and Marrow Transplantation (EBMT) response criteria for evaluating success of treatment.

SCT evolved over the years as a unique treatment modality using blood and bone marrow hematopoietic stem cells for diseases. Blood-derived stem cells result in faster hematologic recovery than marrow stem cells. Additionally, EFS and overall survival (OS) appear to be identical in patients with multiple myeloma who received blood or marrow-derived stem cells (Singhal, 2002). SCT is classified based on the relationship of the donor to

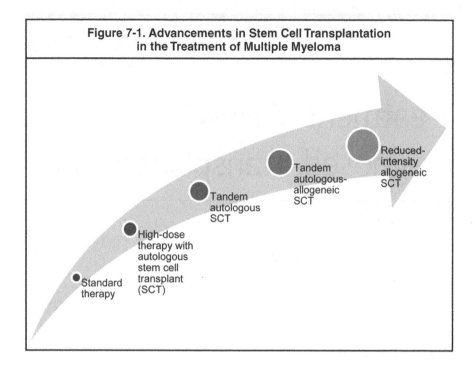

Figure 7-1. Advancements in Stem Cell Transplantation in the Treatment of Multiple Myeloma

the patient. An autologous SCT (ASCT) uses cells derived from the patient; allogeneic SCT (alloSCT) uses cells derived from a human-leukocyte antigen (HLA)-matched sibling or unrelated donors; and syngeneic SCT uses cells from an identical twin. Transplant-eligible patients with multiple myeloma can undergo either a single ASCT, tandem ASCT, myeloablative alloSCT, or nonmyeloablative (mini) alloSCT. Figure 7-2 illustrates the process of stem cell transplantation.

SINGLE OR TANDEM AUTOLOGOUS STEM CELL TRANSPLANTATION

Beginning in the 1990s, several nonrandomized and randomized clinical trials studied high-dose chemotherapy followed by ASCT as a treatment modality for patients with multiple myeloma (Attal et al., 1996; Blade et al., 2000; Child et al., 2003; Palumbo et al., 2004), comparing conventional chemotherapy to high-dose therapy (HDT) followed by ASCT. These studies demonstrated the superiority of HDT with ASCT in terms of response rates and EFS, but not all studies demonstrated OS advantage. A study by Fermand et al. (2005) with a median follow-up time of approximately 10 years did not provide evidence for the superiority of HDT over conventional chemotherapy in OS of patients ages 55–65 with symptomatic newly diagnosed multiple myeloma.

Table 7-1. European Group for Blood and Marrow Transplant Therapy Response Criteria

Response Criteria[a]	Monoclonal Protein[b]	Immunofixation Test	Bone Marrow Biopsy[b]	Lytic Bone Lesions[c]	Plasmacytomas
Complete response[a]	Absent in serum and urine	Negative	Less than 5% plasma cells in bone marrow aspirate	No increase in size or number of lytic bone lesions	Disappearance of soft tissue plasmacytomas
Near complete response	Absent in serum and urine	Positive	Less than 5% plasma cells in bone marrow aspirate	No increase in size or number of lytic bone lesions	Disappearance of soft tissue plasmacytomas
Partial response[a]	50% reduction in serum and greater than or equal to 90% reduction in urine. Reduction in 24-hour urine light-chain excretion by greater than or equal to 90% or to 200 mg	Positive	Greater than or equal to 50% reduction in plasma cells in bone marrow aspirate	No increase in size or number of lytic bone lesions	Greater than or equal to 50% reduction in size of soft tissue plasmacytomas
Minimal response[a]	24%–29% reduction in serum; 50%–89% reduction in 24-hour urine light chain or still exceeding 200 mg/24 hr	Positive	25%–49% reduction in plasma cells in bone marrow aspirate	No increase in size or number of lytic bone lesions	25%–49% reduction in size of soft tissue plasmacytomas
No change	Not meeting criteria of either minimal response or progressive disease				
Plateau	Stable values within 25% above or below value at the time response is assessed, maintained for at least three months				

[a] All response criteria components must be met unless otherwise indicated.
[b] Response must be maintained for a minimum of six weeks.
[c] Development of a compression fracture does not exclude response.

Note. Based on information from Blade et al., 1998.

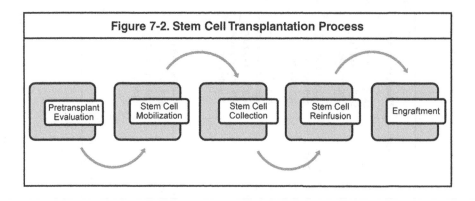

Figure 7-2. Stem Cell Transplantation Process

However, the study confirmed the benefits of HDT in terms of EFS and time without symptoms, treatments, and treatment toxicities. Similarly, long-term results of the prospective randomized clinical trial from the Spanish group PETHEMA showed significant increase in CR rate but no significant impact on progression-free survival (PFS) or OS (Blade et al., 2005). Moreover, a systematic review and meta-analysis of randomized clinical trials confirmed PFS benefit but not OS benefit for HDT with ASCT early in patients with multiple myeloma (Koreth et al., 2007). Despite HDT providing no significant benefit to OS, its ability to overcome tumor resistance demonstrated by superior response in CR rates ranging from 25%–50% and EFS advantage established HDT followed by ASCT as the standard management after induction therapy for patients with newly diagnosed symptomatic multiple myeloma (Blade et al., 2005; Fermand et al., 2005; National Comprehensive Cancer Network, 2009; Patriarca et al., 2009). Table 7-2 summarizes results of various randomized clinical trials of HDT versus conventional chemotherapy for multiple myeloma. Table 7-3 lists common conventional chemotherapy regimens for patients with multiple myeloma. Induction therapy including thalidomide preceding SCT and novel agents bortezomib and lenalidomide combined with corticosteroids, alkylators, and anthracyclines demonstrated very high response rates and complete response rates before and after ASCT with a positive impact on PFS (Bensinger, 2009; Palumbo & Rajkumar, 2009). The various combination regimens used for induction include thalidomide/dexamethasone and novel agents bortezomib/dexamethasone or lenalidomide/dexamethasone (Palumbo & Rajkumar, 2009) (see Table 7-4). Commonly used conditioning regimens include busulfan, cyclophosphamide, and etoposide or high-dose melphalan. High-dose melphalan at 200 mg/m^2 is the well-established transplant conditioning regimen for patients younger than age 65 years (Singhal, 2002).

Barlogie et al. (1997) investigated a more intensive therapy using tandem ASCT to improve outcomes. The "Total Therapy" (TT) was initiated in 1990 combining all therapeutic avenues available at that time to achieve maximum tumor cytoreduction in patients with newly diagnosed multiple myeloma.

Table 7-2. Relevant Randomized Controlled Trials of Upfront High-Dose Therapy Versus Standard-Dose Therapy for Myeloma[a]

Study ID, First Author, Year, and Sample Size	HDT Regimen (Conditioning Regimen)	Stem Cell Source	SDT Regimen	Conclusion
IFM90 Attal 1990 N = 200	VMCP/BVAP→(Mel140/TBI-8)	BM	VMCP/BVAP	OS: benefit EFS: benefit
MAG90 Fermand 1990 N = 185	VAMP→(Cc/Cy/VP/Mel140/TBI-12)	PBSC	VMCP	OS: no benefit EFS: benefit
MAG91 Fermand 1991 N = 190	VAMP→(Bu/Mel140 or Mel200)	PBSC	VMCP	OS: no benefit EFS: benefit
CIAM Facon 1992 N = 115	VAD/Mel140→(Mel140/TBI-12)	BM	VAD/Mel140	OS: no benefit PFS: NR
MRC7 Child 1993 N = 401	VAMPC→(Mel200 or Mel140/TBI [unspecified])	PBSC	ABCM	OS: benefit PFS: benefit
S9321 Barlogie 1993 N = 516	VAD→(Mel140/TBI-12)	PBSC	VAD→VBMCP	OS: no benefit PFS: no benefit
PETHEMA Blade 1994 N = 164	VBMCP/VBAD→(Mel200 or Mel140/TBI-12)	PBSC	VBMC/VBAD	OS: no benefit PFS: no benefit
HOVON Segeren 1995 N = 261	VAD→Mel70x2→(Cy60x4/TBI-9)	PBSC	VAD→Mel70x2	OS: no benefit EFS: no benefit
M97G Palumbo 1997 N = 194	VAD→(Mel100x2)	PBSC	MP	OS: benefit EFS: benefit

(Continued on next page)

Table 7-2. Relevant Randomized Controlled Trials of Upfront High-Dose Therapy Versus Standard-Dose Therapy for Myeloma[a] (Continued)

Study ID, First Author, Year, and Sample Size	HDT Regimen (Conditioning Regimen)	Stem Cell Source	SDT Regimen	Conclusion
IFM9906 Facon 2000 N = 248	VAD (Mel100x2)	PBSC	MPT	OS: no benefit EFS: no benefit

ABCM—doxorubicin, carmustine, cyclophosphamide, melphalan; BM—bone marrow; Bu/Mel—busulfan, melphalan; BVAP—carmustine, vincristine, doxorubicin, prednisone; Cc/Cy/VP/Mel140—lomustine, cyclophosphamide, etoposide, melphalan, XRT; Cy60—cyclophosphamide at 60 mg/kg; EFS—event-free survival; HDT—high-dose therapy and single autologous stem cell transplantation; Mel70/100/140/200—melphalan at 70/100/140/200 mg/m²; MP—melphalan, prednisone; MPT—melphalan, prednisone, thalidomide; NR—not reported; OS—overall survival; PBSC—peripheral blood stem cell; PFS—progression-free survival; SDT—nonmyeloablative standard-dose therapy; TBI-8/9/12—total body irradiation (XRT) at 8/9/12 Gy; VAD—vincristine, carmustine, doxorubicin, dexamethasone; VAMP—vincristine, doxorubicin, methylprednisolone; VAMPC—vincristine, doxorubicin, methylprednisolone, cyclophosphamide; VBAD—vincristine, carmustine, doxorubicin, dexamethasone; VBMCP—vincristine, carmustine, melphalan, cyclophosphamide, prednisone; VMCP—vincristine, melphalan, cyclophosphamide, prednisone

[a] The study ID, first author, year of initial patient enrollment, study size (n, number of patients randomized), median patient age (years) at enrollment, median β2M, percentage of patients with DS III disease, and median duration of follow-up are listed. Information on HDT regimen, source of stem cells, SDT regimen, and conclusions regarding OS and PFS benefit are also shown for each study.

Note. From "High-Dose Therapy With Single Autologous Transplantation Versus Chemotherapy for Newly Diagnosed Multiple Myeloma: A Systematic Review and Meta-Analysis of Randomized Controlled Trials," by J. Koreth, C. Cutler, B. Djulbegovic, R. Behl, R.L. Schlossmann, R.L., Munshi, N., ... Alyea, E.P., 2007, *Biology of Blood and Marrow Transplantation, 13,* p. 186. Copyright 2007 by American Society for Blood and Marrow Transplantation. Adapted with permission.

TT1 was a historical control, pair-mate study (subjects selected from both TT and among 1,123 patients are matched for the following major prognostic features: age, β2 microglobulin levels, and serum creatinine concentrations) comparing two sequential rounds of HDT with ASCT to Southwest Oncology Group patients treated with standard therapy. TT1 compared to standard therapy alone induced higher partial response rates (85% versus 52%, p < 0.0001), extended EFS (49 months versus 22 months, p < 0.0001), and longer OS (62+ months versus 48 months, p = 0.01). With TT1's promising outcomes, the researchers continued to lead innovations in tandem ASCT incorporating novel agents thalidomide (TT2 protocol) and bortezomib (TT3 protocol) (Barlogie et al., 2007) up front into a tandem transplant regimen. TT2 was superior to TT1 in CR duration, EFS, and OS after adjusting for prognostic variables in multivariate and pair-mate analyses (Zangari et al., 2008). TT3 affected two-year CR estimates greater than 90%, and with similar baseline prognostic factors, EFS (p = 0.0002) and CR duration (p = 0.003) were superior with TT3 versus TT2 with a strong trend noted for improved OS (p = 0.16) (Pineda-Roman et al., 2008).

Despite the promising results of tandem ASCT prior to the addition of novel agents before transplantation, a recent systematic review and meta-analysis of six randomized clinical trials with 1,803 patients investigated the efficacy of tandem versus single ASCT (Kumar, Kharfan-Dabala, Glasmacher, & Djulbegovic, 2009). Results showed that patients treated with tandem ASCT did not have better OS (hazard ratio [HR] = 0.94; 95% confidence interval [CI] = 0.77 to 1.14) or EFS (HR = 0.86; 95% CI = 0.70 to 1.05). Additionally, although there was a statistically significant response rate with tandem ASCT (risk ratio = 0.79, 95% CI = 0.67 to 0.93), the investigators highlighted a significant increase in treatment-related mortality (TRM).

Table 7-3. Conventional Chemotherapy Regimens

Regimen	Dose	Cycle
EDAP	Etoposide 100 mg/m^2/day CI days 1–4 Dexamethasone 40 mg/m^2/day PO days 1–5 Cytosine arabinoside 1 g/m^2 day 5 Cisplatin 20–25 mg/m^2/day CI days 1–4	Every 35–42 days
MP	Melphalan 8 mg/m^2/day PO days 1–4 Prednisone 40 mg/m^2/day PO days 1–7	Every 4–6 weeks
VMCP	Vincristine 1.4 mg/m^2 PO day 1 Melphalan 6 mg/m^2 IV days 1–4 Cyclophosphamide 600 mg/m^2 IV day 1 Prednisone 80 mg/m^2 PO days 1–4	Monthly dosing until stable plateau phase
VAMP	Vincristine 0.4 mg/day CI over 24 hours Doxorubicin 9 mg/m^2/day IV Methylprednisolone 0.4 g/day IV	Days 1–4, three to four cycles
VAD	Vincristine 1.2 mg/m^2 CI days 1–4 Doxorubicin 10 mg/m^2 CI days 1–4 Dexamethasone 40 mg PO daily days 1–4, 9–12, and 17–20	Repeat every 35 days
VBMPC	Vincristine 1.2 mg/m^2 IV day 1 Carmustine 20 mg/m^2 IV day 1 Melphalan 8 mg/m^2 days 1–4 Cyclophosphamide 400 mg/m^2 IV day 1 Prednisone 40 mg/m^2/day PO days 1–7	Repeat every 35–42 days

CI—continuous infusion; IV—intravenous; PO—by mouth

Note. Based on information from Fermand et al., 2005; Sirohi et al., 2004; Zomas & Dimopoulos, 2002.

Table 7-4. Induction Regimens for Multiple Myeloma

Regimen	Dose	Cycle
Thalidomide/dexamethasone	Thalidomide 100–200 mg PO days 1–28 Dexamethasone 40 mg PO days 1–4, 9–12, and 17–20 every 28 days or 35 days	Repeat every four weeks for four cycles
Bortezomib/dexamethasone	Bortezomib 1.3 mg/m^2 IV days 1, 4, 8, and 11 Dexamethasone 40 mg PO days 1–4 and 9–12. Reduce to days 1–4 only after first two cycles.	Repeat every three weeks for two to four cycles
Bortezomib/pegylated liposomal doxorubicin/dexamethasone	Bortezomib 1.3 mg/m^2 on days 1, 4, 8, and 11 Pegylated liposomal doxorubicin 30 mg/m^2 on day 4 Dexamethasone 40 mg PO days 1–4 and 15–18 for cycle 1 and days 1–4 for cycles 2–4	21-day cycle for four cycles
Bortezomib/thalidomide/dexamethasone	Bortezomib 1.3 mg/m^2 IV days 1, 4, 8, and 11 Thalidomide 200 mg PO on days 1–21 Dexamethasone 20 mg the day of and day after bortezomib	Repeat every three weeks for three cycles
Lenalidomide/dexamethasone	Lenalidomide 25 mg PO days 1–21 every 28 days Dexamethasone 40 mg PO days 1, 8, 15, and 22 every 28 days	Repeat every four weeks for two cycles

IV—intravenous; PO—by mouth

Note. Based on information from Palumbo & Rajkumar, 2009.

ALLOGENEIC STEM CELL TRANSPLANTATION

Myeloablative Allogeneic Transplantation

Although the treatment outcomes of patients with multiple myeloma following ASCT was encouraging, patients continued to relapse within five years and were unlikely to be cured. The role of alloSCT in patients with multiple myeloma has been studied to reduce relapse rate and improve survival because of an immunologically mediated graft-versus-myeloma effect similar to the graft-versus-leukemia effect (Mehta & Singhal, 1998). A single-center study compared responses of a large cohort of patients with multiple myeloma treated with myeloablative alloSCT with patients who received ASCT (Kuruvilla et al., 2007). Seventy-two patients underwent myeloablative alloSCT (58 related, 14 unrelated), and 86 patients underwent ASCT. Most patients received single-agent high-dose dexamethasone or vincristine, doxorubicin (Adriamycin®, Bedford Laboratories), and dexamethasone (VAD) therapy before SCT. Conditioning regimens were melphalan-based for all ASCT recipients, and the alloSCT recipients received a melphalan-based, total body irradiation–based, or other chemotherapeutic conditioning regimen. The results were not significant with the OS of the alloSCT cohort, reaching only 48.1% at 5 years and 39.9% at 10 years compared to 46.2% at 5 years and 30.8% at 10 years for the ASCT cohort (p = 0.94). The EFS of the alloSCT cohort was 33.3% at 5 years and 31.4% at 10 years compared to 32.9% and 15.2% for the ASCT cohort (p = 0.64). The reported TRM at one year was 22% in the alloSCT cohort and 14% in the ASCT cohort (p = 0.21). TRM appeared to be higher in the myeloablative alloSCT arm. A reduction in relapse occurred in patients who developed acute graft-versus-host disease (GVHD) but not chronic GVHD; however, neither acute nor chronic GVHD had a beneficial effect on EFS and OS. Other similar studies concluded that conventional myeloablative alloSCT is associated with TRM as high as 53% and a low survival rate (Barlogie, Tricot, et al., 2006). A case-matched retrospective review by Bjorkstrand et al. (1996) revealed TRM of 41% for alloSCT versus only 13% for ASCT (p = 0.0001). Mortality was mostly related to infections and GVHD-related complications (Harousseau, 2007). The high TRM with alloSCT is currently the major limitation to wider use of this potentially curative modality (Bensinger, 2007).

NONMYELOABLATIVE OR REDUCED-INTENSITY ALLOGENEIC STEM CELL TRANSPLANTATION

Because of the high toxicity associated with myeloablative alloSCT, researchers have investigated nonmyeloablative or reduced-intensity conditioning alloSCT. The rationale was to exploit the sensitivity of the multiple myeloma cell to irradiation and alkylating agents and the ability of the newly transplanted immunocompetent cells to mount a graft-versus-myeloma effect (Hunter et al., 2005). The goal was to utilize the antitumor effect of the graft-versus-myeloma reaction while reducing the treatment-related complications of high-dose conditioning by inducing maximum cytoreduction. Common regimens include high-dose chemotherapy (usually melphalan) with ASCT support followed by consolidation with reduced-intensity conditioning alloSCT (Bjorkstrand, 2005). Figure 7-3 lists various reduced-intensity conditioning regimens.

Bruno et al. (2007) studied the outcomes of tandem transplant protocols requiring an initial ASCT followed by a second ASCT or an allograft from an HLA-identical sibling. A total of 58 patients completed the autograft-allograft treatment, and 46 patients completed the double-autologous transplant regi-

---

Figure 7-3. Conditioning Regimens

- Melphalan
- Melphalan/total body irradiation (TBI)
- Melphalan/methylprednisolone
- Busulfan/cyclophosphamide
- Busulfan/cyclophosphamide/TBI
- Busulfan/cyclophosphamide/thiotepa
- Busulfan/melphalan/thiotepa
- Carmustine/etoposide/melphalan/TBI
- Fludarabine/melphalan
- Fludarabine/TBI
- Fludarabine/TBI/cyclophosphamide
- Fludarabine/alemtuzumab/TBI
- Busulfan/fludarabine/antithymocyte globulin

Note. Based on information from Fermand et al., 2005; Harousseau, 2007; Singhal, 2002.

---

men from September 1998 through July 2004. Patients with HLA-identical siblings received nonmyeloablative total body irradiation and sibling stem cells; patients without an HLA-identical sibling received two consecutive doses of myeloablative melphalan followed by ASCT. After a median follow-up of 45 months (range = 21–90), patients with HLA-matched siblings demonstrated a median OS of 80 months and EFS of 54 months compared to a median OS of 54 months and EFS of 29 months in the double-ASCT group. Interestingly, TRM did not differ significantly between the two groups. The disease-related mortality was significantly higher in the double-ASCT group (43% versus 7%, $p < 0.001$). The auto-allograft tandem transplant recipients appeared to have superior OS and EFS (Bruno et al., 2007; Carella et al., 2004). The superiority of reduced-intensity alloSCT was similarly highlighted in a study by the PETHEMA/GEM group (Rosinol et al., 2008) and a more recent study by the Gruppo Italiano Trapianti di Midollo group (Bruno et al., 2009). The tandem transplant approach with nonmyeloablative allografting allows prolonged survival and long-term disease control in patients. The reduced-intensity conditioning regimen for alloSCT reduced TRM to 10%–20% with approximately 40%–50% CR rates (Blade & Rosinol, 2009).

Although alloSCT using matched related donors has demonstrated reduced relapse rates and improved survival, only 25%–30% of patients have a matched sibling donor (Ballen et al., 2005). Another option is SCT using matched unrelated donors. The results of a study using myeloablative SCT with matched unrelated donors demonstrated poor survival with a five-year OS of only 9% and a high TRM at 42% because of infection, GVHD, and other toxicities (Ballen et al.).

However, when nonmyeloablative unrelated donor transplantation was utilized following cytoreductive ASCT, responses were significantly better. A study by Georges et al. (2007) to determine long-term outcome of unrelated donor nonmyeloablative hematopoietic cell transplantation in patients with poor-risk multiple myeloma concluded that unrelated hematopoietic cell transplantation is an effective treatment approach, with low non-relapse mortality, high CR rates, and prolonged disease-free survival. A total of 24 patients were enrolled, 17 (71%) of whom had chemotherapy-refractory disease and 14 (58%) of whom had experienced disease relapse or progression after previous ASCT. Thirteen patients underwent planned ASCT followed with unrelated transplantation, and 11 patients proceeded directly to unrelated transplantation. All 24 patients were treated with fludarabine (90 mg/m^2) and 2 gray (Gy) of total body irradiation before HLA-matched unrelated SCT. At three years, OS and PFS rates were 61% and 33%, respectively. Patients who received tandem autologous unrelated transplantation had superior OS at 77% and PFS at 51% compared to only 44% OS and 11% EFS in patients who proceeded directly to unrelated donor transplantation (for PFS, p = 0.03).

MAINTENANCE THERAPY FOLLOWING STEM CELL TRANSPLANTATION

Although treatment with HDT followed by SCT improves CR, EFS, and OS, a plateau in the survival curves is not achieved, and a majority of the patients relapse and die. Maintenance therapies following SCT are important in achieving prolonged survival.

Interferon

Interferon alfa-2 was investigated as maintenance therapy following transplantation in patients with multiple myeloma but yielded no significant benefits (Harousseau, 2008a).

Thalidomide

Thalidomide has been extensively investigated as a viable maintenance therapy following ASCT. In a phase II study, Sahebi et al. (2006) enrolled 29 patients to receive maintenance thalidomide following a single ASCT. Patients were started on 50 mg/day for six to eight weeks following SCT with gradual dose escalation to a targeted 400 mg/day, continued until disease progression or six months after achieving CR for a maximum total duration of 18 months. Results showed an estimated two-year OS at 83% and PFS at 49%. The median tolerated dose was 200 mg/day.

Spencer et al. (2009) evaluated the benefits of 12-month low-dose thalidomide therapy following a single ASCT. Results revealed that the three-year PFS rate was 42%, and the OS was 86%. However, thalidomide did not benefit patients with chromosome 13 deletion (Harousseau, 2008b). In a recent trial (IFM 99-02), patients younger than 65 years of age were randomized to receive, after SCT, either no maintenance, pamidronate, or pamidronate plus thalidomide (Attal et al., 2006). The study showed that 55% of patients in the no maintenance arm achieved a complete or very good partial response, versus 57% and 67% in the pamidronate and pamidronate plus thalidomide arms, respectively. Additionally, the three-year postrandomization probability of EFS was 36%, 37%, and 52%, and the four-year postdiagnosis probability of survival was 77%, 74%, and 87% in the no maintenance, pamidronate, and pamidronate plus thalidomide arms, respectively. This study clearly indicates a superior post-transplant outcome with maintenance therapy of pamidronate plus thalidomide.

Bortezomib

Bortezomib appears to be active in patients with and without chromosome 13 deletion and is being evaluated in ongoing maintenance therapy trials. A study investigating bortezomib administered before ASCT and as a weekly maintenance therapy after transplantation in 40 patients demonstrated an overall response rate of 83% and CR plus a very good partial response rate of 50% without adverse effects on mobilization or engraftment (Uy et al., 2009). The most frequently reported adverse events associated with bortezomib are fatigue, weakness, malaise, nausea, diarrhea, constipation, vomiting, peripheral neuropathy, pyrexia, thrombocytopenia, neutropenia, psychiatric disorders, and anorexia or decreased appetite (Curran & McKeage, 2009).

Lenalidomide

Lenalidomide, a thalidomide derivative that stimulates host antimyeloma natural killer cell immunity, induces very little neurologic toxicity and currently is being tested as maintenance therapy after ASCT (Kumar, Hayman, & Kyle, 2007; Palumbo et al., 2008) or tandem ASCT (Barlogie et al., 2008).

CONCLUSION

The treatment of multiple myeloma is changing, driven by the advances in ASCT, reduced-intensity alloSCT, the advent of novel therapies, and newer combination regimens. Clinical outcomes have improved along with these advances. It is essential for oncology nurses to maintain a comprehensive knowledge base about the changing paradigms in the treatment of multiple myeloma in order to provide thorough assessments, individualized care planning, and extensive patient education. Oncology nurses play a significant role in maximizing the therapeutic benefits of available treatment options for patients with multiple myeloma.

REFERENCES

Attal, M., Harousseau, J.-L., Leyvraz, S., Doyen, C. Hulin, C., Benboubkher, L., ... Facon, T. (2006). Maintenance therapy with thalidomide improves survival in patients with multiple myeloma. *Blood, 108,* 3289–3294. doi:10.1182/blood-2006-05-022962

Attal, M., Harousseau, J.L., Stoppa, A.M., Sotto, J.J., Fuzibet, J.G., Rossi, J.F., ... Bataille, R. (1996). A prospective randomized trial of autologous bone marrow transplantation and chemotherapy in multiple myeloma. Intergroupe Francais du Myelome. *New England Journal of Medicine, 335,* 91–97. doi:10.1056/NEJM199607113350204

Ballen, K.K., King, R., Carston, M., Kollman, C., Nelson, G., Lim, S., ... Vesole, D.H. (2005). Outcome of unrelated transplants in patients with multiple myeloma. *Bone Marrow Transplantation, 35,* 675–681. doi:10.1038/sj.bmt.1704868

Barlogie, B., Anaissie, E., van Rhee, F., Haessler, J., Hollmig, K., Pineda-Roman, M., ... Shaughnessy, J.D., Jr. (2007). Incorporating bortezomib into upfront treatment for multiple myeloma: Early results of total therapy 3. *British Journal of Haematology, 138,* 176–185. doi:10.1111/j.1365-2141.2007.06639.x

Barlogie, B., Anaissie, E.J., Shaughnessy, J.D., Jr., van Rhee, F., Pineda-Roman, M., Haessler, J., ... Crowley, J. (2008). Ninety percent sustained complete response (CR) rate projected 4 years after onset of CR in gene expression profiling (GEP)-defined low-risk multiple myeloma (MM) treated with total therapy 3 (TT3): Basis for GEP-risk-adapted TT4 and TT5 [Abstract No. 162]. *Blood, 112.* Retrieved from http://abstracts.hematologylibrary.org/cgi/content/abstract/112/11/162?maxtoshow=&HITS=10&hits=10&RESULTFOR MAT=&fulltext=lenalidomide+and+maintenance&searchid=1&FIRSTINDEX=20&sorts pec=relevance&resourcetype=HWCIT

Barlogie, B., Jagannath, S., Vesole, D.H., Naucke, S., Cheson, B., Mattox, S., ... Tricot, G. (1997). Superiority of tandem autologous transplantation over standard therapy for previously untreated multiple myeloma. *Blood, 89,* 789–793.

Barlogie, B., Tricot, G., Anaissie, E., Shaughnessy, J., Rasmussen, E., van Rhee, F., ... Crowley, J. (2006). Thalidomide and hematopoietic-cell transplantation for multiple myeloma. *New England Journal of Medicine, 354,* 1021–1030. doi:10.1056/NEJMoa053583

Bensinger, W.I. (2007). Is there still a role for allogeneic stem-cell transplantation in multiple myeloma? *Best Practice and Research: Clinical Haematology, 20,* 783–795. doi:10.1016/j.beha.2007.09.007

Bensinger, W.I. (2009). Role of autologous and allogeneic stem cell transplantation in myeloma. *Leukemia, 23,* 442–448. doi:10.1038/leu.2008.396

Bjorkstrand, B. (2005). Stem cell transplantation in multiple myeloma. *Hematology, 10*(Suppl. 1), 26–28. doi:10.1080/10245330512331389809

Bjorkstrand, B.B., Ljungman, P., Svensson, H., Hermans, J., Alegre, A., Apperley, J., ... Gahrton, G. (1996). Allogeneic bone marrow transplantation versus autologous stem cell transplantation in multiple myeloma: A retrospective case-matched study from the European Group for Blood and Marrow Transplantation. *Blood, 88,* 4711–4718.

Blade, J., Esteve, J., Rives, S., Martinez, C., Rovira, M., Urbano-Ispizua, A., ... Montserrat, E. (2000). High-dose therapy autotransplantation/intensification vs continued standard chemotherapy in multiple myeloma in first remission. Results of a non-randomized study from a single institution. *Bone Marrow Transplantation, 26,* 845–849. doi:10.1038/sj.bmt.1702622

Blade, J., & Rosinol, L. (2009). Changing paradigms in the treatment of multiple myeloma. *Haematologica, 94,* 163–166. doi:10.3324/haematol.2008.002766

Blade, J., Rosinol, L., Sureda, A., Ribera, J.M., Diaz-Mediavilla, J., Garcia-Larana, J., ... San Miguel, J. (2005). High-dose therapy intensification compared with continued standard chemotherapy in multiple myeloma patients responding to the initial chemotherapy: Long-term results from a prospective randomized trial from the Spanish cooperative group PETHEMA. *Blood, 106,* 3755–3759. doi:10.1182/blood-2005-03-1301

Blade, J., Samson, D., Reece, D., Apperley, J., Bjorkstrand, B., Gahrton, G., ... Vesole, D. (1998). Criteria for evaluation disease response and progression in patients with multiple myeloma treated by high-dose therapy and haemopoietic stem cell transplantation. Myeloma subcommittee of the EBMT. European Group for Blood and Marrow Transplant. *British Journal of Haematology, 102,* 1115–1123. doi:10.1046/j.1365-2141.1998.00930.x

Bruno, B., Rotta, M., Patriarca, F., Mattei, D., Allione, B., Carnevale-Schianca, F., ... Boccadoro, M. (2009). Nonmyeloablative allografting for newly diagnosed multiple myeloma: The experience of the Gruppo Italiano Trapianti di Midollo. *Blood, 113,* 3375–3382. doi:10.1182/blood-2008-07-167379

Bruno, B., Rotta, M., Patriarca, F., Mordini, N., Allione, B., Carnevale-Schianca, F., ... Boccadoro, M. (2007). A comparison of allografting with autografting for newly diagnosed myeloma. *New England Journal of Medicine, 356,* 1110–1120. doi:10.1056/NEJMoa065464

Carella, A.M., Beltrami, G., Corsetti, M.T., Scalzulli, P., Carella, A.M., & Musto, P. (2004). A reduced intensity conditioning regimen for allografting following autografting is feasible and has strong anti-myeloma activity. *Haematologica, 89,* 1534–1536.

Child, J.A., Morgan, G.J., Davies, F.E., Owen, R.G., Bell, S.E., Hawkins, K., ... Selby, P.J. (2003). High-dose chemotherapy with hematopoietic stem-cell rescue for multiple myeloma. *New England Journal of Medicine, 348,* 1875–1883. doi:10.1056/NEJMoa022340

Curran, M.P., & McKeage, K. (2009). Bortezomib: A review of its use in patients with multiple myeloma. *Drugs, 69,* 859–888. doi:10.2165/00003495-200969070-00006

Fermand, J.P., Katsahian, S., Divine, M., Leblond, V., Dreyfus, F., Macro, M., ..., Ravaud, P. (2005). High-dose therapy and autologous blood stem-cell transplantation compared with conventional treatment in myeloma patients aged 55 to 65 years: Long-term results of a randomized control trial from the Group Myelome-Autogreffe. *Journal of Clinical Oncology, 23,* 9227–9233. doi:10.1200/JCO.2005.03.0551

Georges, G., Maris, M., Maloney, D.G., Sandmaier, B.M., Sorror, M.L., Shizuru, J.A., ... Storb, R. (2007). Nonmyeloablative unrelated donor hematopoietic cell transplantation for the treatment of patients with poor-risk, relapsed, or refractory multiple myeloma. *Biology of Blood and Marrow Transplantation, 13,* 423–432. doi:10.1016/j.bbmt.2006.11.011

Harousseau, J.-L. (2007). The allogeneic dilemma. *Bone Marrow Transplantation, 40,* 1123–1128. doi:10.1038/sj.bmt.1705810

Harousseau, J.-L. (2008a). Maintenance treatment in multiple myeloma. *Annals of Oncology, 19*(Suppl. 4), 54–55. doi:10.1093/annonc/mdn197

Harousseau, J.-L. (2008b). New treatments in multiple myeloma: Beyond optimal treatment. *Annals of Oncology, 19*(Suppl. 5), v68–v70. doi:10.1093/annonc/mdn314

Hunter, H.M., Peggs, K., Powles, R., Rahemtulla, A., Mahendra, P., Cavenagh, J., ... Russell, N.H. (2005). Analysis of outcome following allogeneic haemopoietic stem cell transplantation for myeloma using myeloablative conditioning—Evidence for a superior outcome using melphalan combined with total body irradiation. *British Journal of Haematology, 128,* 496–502. doi:10.1111/j.1365-2141.2004.05330.x

Koreth, J., Cutler, C., Djulbegovic, B., Behl, R., Schlossmann, R.L., Munshi, N., ... Alyea, E.P. (2007). High-dose therapy with single autologous transplantation versus chemotherapy for newly diagnosed multiple myeloma: A systematic review and meta-analysis of randomized controlled trials. *Biology of Blood and Marrow Transplantation, 13,* 183–196. doi:10.1016/j.bbmt.2006.09.010

Kulkarni, S., Powles, R.L., Treleaven, J.G., Singhal, S., Saso, R., Horton, C., ... Mehta, J. (1999). Impact of previous high-dose therapy on outcome after allografting for multiple myeloma. *Bone Marrow Transplantation, 23,* 675–680. doi:10.1038/sj.bmt.1701634

Kumar, A., Kharfan-Dabaja, M.A., Glasmacher, A., & Djulbegovic, B. (2009). Tandem versus single autologous hematopoietic cell transplantation for the treatment of multiple myeloma: A systemic review and meta-analysis. *Journal of the National Cancer Institute, 101,* 100–106. doi:10.1093/jnci/djn439

Kumar, S.K., Hayman, S.R., & Kyle, R.A. (2007). Autologous stem cell transplantation in the elderly including pre- and post-treatment options. *Bone Marrow Transplantation, 40,* 1115–1121. doi:10.1038/sj.bmt.1705800

Kuruvilla, J., Shepherd, J.D., Sutherland, H.J., Nevill, T.J., Nitta, J., Le, A., ... Song, K.W. (2007). Long-term outcome of myeloablative allogeneic stem cell transplantation for multiple myeloma. *Biology of Blood and Marrow Transplantation, 13,* 925–931. doi:10.1016/j.bbmt.2007.04.006

Mehta, J., & Singhal, S. (1998). Graft-versus-myeloma. *Bone Marrow Transplantation, 22,* 835–843. doi:10.1038/sj.bmt.1701459

National Comprehensive Cancer Network. (2009). NCCN 2009 multiple myeloma clinical practice guidelines in oncology. In *The complete library of NCCN clinical practice guidelines in oncology* [CD-ROM]. Jenkintown, PA: Author.

Palumbo, A., Bringhen, S., Petrucci, M.T., Musto, P., Rossini, F., Nunzi, M., ... Boccadoro, M. (2004). Intermediate-dose melphalan improves survival of myeloma patients aged 50 to 70: Results of a randomized controlled trial. *Blood, 104,* 3052–3057. doi:10.1182/blood-2004-02-0408

Palumbo, A., Falco, P., Gay, F., Montefusco, V., Crippa, C., Patriarca, F., ... Boccadoro, M. (2008). Bortezomib-doxorubicin-dexamethasone as induction prior to reduced intensity autologous transplantation followed by lenalidomide as consolidation/maintenance in elderly untreated myeloma patients [Abstract No. 159]. *Blood, 112.* Retrieved from http://abstracts.hematologylibrary.org/cgi/content/abstract/112/11/159?maxtoshow=&HITS=10&hits=10&RESULTFORMAT=&fulltext=lenlidomide%2C+maintenance%2C+transplant&searchid=1&FIRSTINDEX=0&volme=112&issue=11&resourcetype=HWCIT

Palumbo, A., & Rajkumar, S.V. (2009). Treatment of newly diagnosed myeloma. *Leukemia, 23,* 449–456. doi:10.1038/leu.2008.325

Patriarca, F., Petrucci, M.T., Bringhen, S., Baldini, L., Caravita, T., Corradini, P., ... Palumbo, A. (2009). Considerations in the treatment of multiple myeloma: A consensus statement from Italian experts. *European Journal of Haematology, 82,* 93–105. doi:10.1111/j.1600-0609.2008.01179.x

Pineda-Roman, M., Zangari, M., Haessler, J., Anaissie, E., Tricot, G., van Rhee, F., ... Barlogie, B. (2008). Sustained complete remissions in multiple myeloma linked to bortezomib in total therapy 3: Comparison with total therapy 2. *British Journal of Haematology, 140,* 625–634. doi:10.1111/j.1365-2141.2007.06921.x

Rosinol, L., Perez-Simon, J.A., Sureda, A., de la Rubia, J., de Arriba, F., Lahuerta, J.J., ... Blade, J. (2008). A prospective PETHEMA study of tandem autologous transplantation versus autograft followed by reduced-intensity conditioning allogeneic transplantation in newly diagnosed multiple myeloma. *Blood, 112,* 3591–3593. doi:10.1182/blood-2008-02-141598

Sahebi, F., Spielberger, R., Kogut, N.M., Fung, H., Falk, P.M., Parker, P., ... Somlo, G. (2006). Maintenance thalidomide following single cycle autologous peripheral blood stem cell transplant in patients with multiple myeloma. *Bone Marrow Transplantation, 37,* 825–829. doi:10.1038/sj.bmt.1705339

Singhal, S. (2002). High-dose therapy and autologous transplantation. In J. Mehta & S. Singhal (Eds.), *Myeloma* (pp. 327–347). London, England: Martin Dunitz.

Sirohi, B., Raje, N., & Powles, R. (2004). Autologous hematopoietic stem cell transplantation for multiple myeloma and AL amyloidosis. In K. Atkinson, R. Champlin, J. Ritz, W.E. Fibbe, P. Ljungman, & M.K. Brenner (Eds.), *Clinical bone marrow and blood stem cell transplantation* (3rd ed., pp. 620–651). New York, NY: Cambridge University Press.

Spencer, A., Prince, H.M., Roberts, A.W., Prosser, I.W., Bradstock, K.F., Coyle, L., ... Kennedy, N. (2009). Consolidation therapy with low-dose thalidomide and prednisolone prolongs the survival of multiple myeloma patients undergoing a single autologous stem-cell transplantation procedure. *Journal of Clinical Oncology, 27,* 1788–1793. doi:10.1200/JCO.2008.18.8573

Uy, G.L., Goyal, S.D., Fisher, N.M., Oza, A.Y., Tomasson, M.H., Stockerl-Goldstein, K., ... Vij, R. (2009). Bortezomib administered pre-auto-SCT and as maintenance therapy post transplant for multiple myeloma: A single institution phase II study [Abstract]. *Bone Marrow Transplantation, 43*, 793–800. doi:10.1038/bmt.2008.384

Zangari, M., van Rhee, F., Anaissie, E., Pineda-Roman, M., Haessler, J., Crowley, J., & Barlogie, B. (2008). Eight-year median survival in multiple myeloma after total therapy 2: roles of thalidomide and consolidation chemotherapy in the context of total therapy 1. *British Journal of Haematology, 141*, 433–444. doi:10.1111/j.1365-2141.2008.06982.x

Zomas, A., & Dimopoulos, M.A. (2002). Conventional treatment of myeloma. In J. Mehta & S. Singhal (Eds.), *Myeloma* (pp. 313–326). London, England: Martin Dunitz.

CHAPTER 8

Treatment of Relapsed or Refractory Multiple Myeloma

Beth Faiman, RN, MSN, APRN-BC, AOCN®

INTRODUCTION

Patients with multiple myeloma are living longer than ever because of, in part, better supportive care and myriad newer and emerging therapies (Kumar et al., 2008). The improved survival and advances made in the past decade are the result of the hard work on behalf of nurses, study coordinators, support staff, patients, and providers who have participated in the clinical trials that described the efficacy of these agents. Nurses are dedicated to battling myeloma and strive to conquer the side effects and the disease itself. Many successes in the past 10 years have led to the discovery of and U.S. Food and Drug Administration (FDA) approval of three key agents: thalidomide (Celgene Corp., 2009b), bortezomib (Millennium Pharmaceuticals, Inc., 2009), and lenalidomide (Celgene Corp., 2009a). Each of these agents has a slightly different mechanism of action and a unique side effect profile. For this reason, many clinical trials have combined at least one of these drugs with other existing regimens or novel agents for use in patients with relapsed multiple myeloma (see Table 8-1). This chemotherapy combination approach provides treatment teams with the opportunity to extend remissions and continue to suppress the malignant plasma cell clone through treatment of the disease.

The natural course of myeloma is one that is characterized by an indolent period of asymptomatic monoclonal gammopathy, which is then followed by a series of remissions and relapses until patients will unfortunately become refractory to therapy (Rajkumar & Dispenzieri, 2008). An abnormal overproduction of a malignant protein results in organ damage, which is an important aspect to consider when diagnosing a patient with myeloma. Criteria for diagnosis of myeloma can be remembered by the CRAB acronym, which stands for calcium elevation, renal insufficiency, anemia, and bone lesions (Greipp et al., 2005). Remission is an important goal of any cancer therapy, and often

Table 8-1. Summary of Available Agents and Time to Progression in the Treatment of Patients With Relapsed or Refractory Multiple Myeloma

Treatment Regimen	Dose Schedule	TTP, Response, or Survival	Major Side Effects and Nursing Monitoring	References
Bortezomib plus dexamethasone (APEX trial)	Bortezomib 1.3 mg/m² IV days 1, 4, 8, and 11 Dexamethasone 20/40 mg PO the day before and after bortezomib days 1, 2, 4, 5, 8, 9, 11, and 12 Give for eight three-week cycles, followed by bortezomib on days 1, 8, 15, and 22 for three five-week cycles.	• TTP 6.2 months with bortezomib • One-year survival 80% • Overall survival 29.8 months	• Myelosuppression, gastrointestinal toxicities, peripheral neuropathy, increased risk of HSV reactivation • Acyclovir or valacyclovir is recommended. • Obtain CBC with differential before each cycle. • Regimen is safe in patients with renal failure. • Watch for steroid side effects with high-dose dexamethasone. • Premedicate with 5-HT$_3$ receptor antagonist (ondansetron, granisetron) to prevent nausea.	Jagannath et al., 2006; Richardson et al., 2005

(Continued on next page)

Table 8-1. Summary of Available Agents and Time to Progression in the Treatment of Patients With Relapsed or Refractory Multiple Myeloma (Continued)

Treatment Regimen	Dose Schedule	TTP, Response, or Survival	Major Side Effects and Nursing Monitoring	References
Bortezomib plus PLD	Bortezomib 1.3 mg/m² IV days 1, 4, 8, and 11 and doxorubicin 30 mg/m² day 4 IV Repeat every 21 days.	• 9.3 months TTP with PLD and bortezomib	Grade 3 or higher adverse events: myelosuppression and GI toxicities, no further details reported • Obtain CBC with differential prior to each dose of bortezomib. • No dose reductions are necessary if renal insufficiency is present. • Risk of HSV reactivation is increased (acyclovir or valacyclovir recommended). • Educate patient to prevent PPE. • Educate patient about oral hygiene to prevent mucositis with PLD. • Premedicate patient with 5-HT₃ receptor antagonist (ondansetron, granisetron) to prevent nausea.	Orlowski et al., 2007
Lenalidomide plus dexamethasone	Lenalidomide 25 mg PO daily for 21 days and dexamethasone 40 mg PO days 1–4, 9–12, and 17–20 Repeat every 21 days.	• TTP 11.1 months • Median overall survival 29.6 months • Overall survival of 42 months when taken earlier in the disease	Neutropenia, thrombocytopenia, anemia, pneumonia, VTE • Obtain CBC with differential every 2 weeks for the first 12 weeks of treatment, then monthly. • Modify doses for grade 3 toxicities (myelosuppression, GI toxicities). • Assess for rash/itchy scalp at the start of therapy. • Risk stratify patient for VTE.	Stadtmauer et al., 2009; Weber et al., 2007

(Continued on next page)

Table 8-1. Summary of Available Agents and Time to Progression in the Treatment of Patients With Relapsed or Refractory Multiple Myeloma (Continued)

Treatment Regimen	Dose Schedule	TTP, Response, or Survival	Major Side Effects and Nursing Monitoring	References
Lenalidomide plus bortezomib and dexamethasone	Bortezomib 1.0 mg/m² IV days 1, 4, 8, and 11, lenalidomide 15 mg PO days 1–14, and dexamethasone 40 mg PO/IV (cycles 1–4) followed by 20 mg (cycles 5–8) on day of/day after bortezomib dosing. Give up to eight 21-day cycles.	• ORR: 84%; median duration of response: 24 weeks	Myelosuppression, fatigue, mild GI toxicities (no nausea, vomiting), risk for VTE • Obtain CBC with differential prior to each dose of bortezomib. • Adjust lenalidomide dose appropriately if renal insufficiency is present. • Risk-stratify patient for VTE. • Watch for nausea; vomiting was rare in clinical trials.	Anderson et al., 2009
DCEP	Cyclophosphamide 400 mg/m² daily for four days, cisplatin 15 mg/m² daily for four days; and etoposide 40 mg/m² daily for four days given as a 24-hour infusion IV dexamethasone 40 mg daily days 1–4 Administer G-CSF daily, beginning 24 hours after therapy until WBC recovery. Repeat every 28 days.	• ORR 18%	Neutropenia, thrombocytopenia, anemia, pneumonia, GI toxicities • Obtain CBC with differential weekly. • Must use central line for doxorubicin infusion. • Premedicate patient with 5-HT₃ receptor antagonist (ondansetron, granisetron) to prevent nausea. • Assess patient for rash/itchy scalp at the start of therapy. • Risk stratify patient for VTE.	Dadacaridou et al., 2007

(Continued on next page)

Table 8-1. Summary of Available Agents and Time to Progression in the Treatment of Patients With Relapsed or Refractory Multiple Myeloma (Continued)

Treatment Regimen	Dose Schedule	TTP, Response, or Survival	Major Side Effects and Nursing Monitoring	References
DT-PACE	Dexamethasone 40 mg PO daily for four days Thalidomide 400 mg PO daily at night Four-day continuous infusion of Cisplatin 10 mg/m²/day Doxorubicin 10 mg/m²/day Cyclophosphamide 400 mg/m²/day Etoposide 40 mg/m²/day Mix cisplatin, cyclophosphamide, and etoposide in 1 L 0.9% NS and infuse doxorubicin separately in 50 ml D5W via central line. Repeat every 4–6 weeks if ANC > 1,000/mcl and platelet count > 100,000/mcl.	• PR after two cycles of DT-PACE was 32%; 49% in patients able to tolerate 100% of the dose.	Neutropenia, thrombocytopenia, anemia, pneumonia, GI toxicities, VTE • Obtain CBC with differential weekly. • Use central line for doxorubicin infusion. • Premedicate patient with 5-HT₃ receptor antagonist (ondansetron, granisetron) to prevent nausea. • Assess patient for rash/itchy scalp at the start of therapy. • Risk stratify patient for VTE (increased risk with thalidomide and doxorubicin).	Lee et al., 2003

ANC—absolute neutrophil count; CBC—complete blood count; D5W—dextrose 5% in water; 5-HT₃—5-hydroxytryptamine-3; G-CSF—granulocyte–colony-stimulating factor; GI—gastrointestinal; HSV—herpes simplex virus; IV—intravenously; mcl—microliter; NS—normal saline; ORR—overall response rate; PLD—pegylated liposomal doxorubicin; PO—by mouth; PPE—palmar-plantar erythrodysesthesia; PR—partial response; TTP—time to progression; VTE—venous thromboembolism; WBC—white blood cell

Note. Thalidomide dose is currently limited to 200 mg/day due to neurotoxicity.

patients will achieve remission from most types of antimyeloma therapy, but relapse is always a concern.

Many experts currently disagree as to the degree of remission required for overall survival and the goals of therapy associated with treating the disease (Lonial, 2007). Myeloma is a chronic illness and one for which cure is not possible for most, so some patients feel that control of the disease while balancing toxicity and quality-of-life issues is most important (Rajkumar, 2008). Others strive to eliminate the malignant clone by undergoing aggressive combinations of chemotherapy, novel agents, and transplantation. The benefit of this aggressive approach is an impressive 10% cure rate at 10 years as seen in the University of Arkansas Total Therapy trials, but the price to pay is greater toxicities than with other agents (Barlogie et al., 2008).

Although no consensus exists as to the degree of response from therapy that a patient should achieve, or how aggressive an initial regimen may be, a complete remission (CR) allows for disappearance of the monoclonal protein. In many studies, patients who have achieved CR have the longest remission, so many clinical trials focus on this end point (Lonial, 2007). The International Myeloma Working Group established response criteria in order to standardize and uniformly analyze outcomes in multiple myeloma treatment, which is important to be aware of when discussing relapse in patients with multiple myeloma. Three main categories most often noted in clinical practice roughly include CR, which is defined as disappearance of the abnormal protein with negative immunofixation of the serum and/or urine; very good partial remission, where patients achieve a 90% or greater reduction from baseline abnormal protein values in the serum plus a urine protein level of less than 100 mg/24 hours; and partial remission, which is defined as a 50%–90% reduction in the abnormal protein in serum or urine (Durie et al., 2006).

SYMPTOMATIC AND ASYMPTOMATIC RELAPSE

There is a difference between *symptomatic* and *asymptomatic* relapse of multiple myeloma in individuals who have been previously treated (Durie et al., 2003). Patients are considered to have relapsed myeloma if there is a steady increase in the amount of protein in the serum or urine from the lowest detectable point once a remission has been achieved, as obtained on two different laboratory evaluations at four-week intervals. If no signs and no end-organ damage are present, then often the treatment may be continued until symptoms develop that reflect the CRAB criteria. In the absence of new end-organ damage, the patient is characterized as having progressive disease, or asymptomatic relapse. Asymptomatic relapse also may occur with the reappearance of monoclonal protein in the blood or urine in patients who had achieved a CR or disappearance of the abnormal protein.

Myeloma is incurable, but many approaches are available to patients with relapsed disease. One approach in asymptomatic patients or those with progressive disease would be to watch and wait for signs of CRAB-related organ damage to develop. Patients may remain on therapy until an increasing paraprotein is detected on two different blood or urine samples. There are nuances to myeloma therapy at relapse, but therapy usually is not changed until patients develop signs of symptomatic disease relapse. However, this is at the physician's or practitioner's discretion (Durie et al., 2003). Nurses should be familiar with criteria for relapse before starting a new therapy and nursing interventions (see Table 8-2). Nearly all patients will ultimately relapse from their primary induction therapy.

IMAGING IN PATIENTS WITH RELAPSED MULTIPLE MYELOMA

As the 19th century was drawing to a close, the German physicist Wilhelm Conrad Roentgen made the discovery of x-rays. It was not long after Roentgen's

Table 8-2. Definition of Relapse, Criteria, and Nursing Considerations			
Relapse Category	Laboratory and Imaging	Criteria for Relapse	Nursing Considerations
Progressive disease (PD) (asymptomatic relapse)	PD requires two consecutive serum or urine tests four weeks apart. Additional tests: • CBC and differential • CMP • SPEP • UPEP • 24-hour urine for protein • Bone marrow biopsy (optional) • Skeletal survey to rule out lesions	Increase of greater than 25% from baseline in • Serum M component (the absolute increase must be greater than 0.5 g/dl) • Urine M component (the absolute increase must be greater than 200 mg/24 hours) • Bone marrow plasma cell percentage: absolute percentage must be greater than 10% • New bone lesions or hypercalcemia with serum calcium greater than 11.5 mg/dl	Patients who are experiencing PD may not have symptoms of relapse and can be at risk for psychological impairment (fear of impending new treatment, depression, anxiety) and physiologic impairment from sequelae of relapse. • Acknowledge what they are feeling. • Reinforce that laboratory parameters will be monitored closely on a monthly basis to assess for disease stabilization or confirm relapse. • Discuss next steps with the healthcare team if relapse is confirmed. Reinforce plan to the patient. If hypercalcemia, see next page.

(Continued on next page)

Table 8-2. Definition of Relapse, Criteria, and Nursing Considerations (Continued)

Relapse Category	Laboratory and Imaging	Criteria for Relapse	Nursing Considerations
Clinical relapse (symptomatic relapse)	Requires two consecutive serum or urine tests four weeks apart with serum M component increase of greater than 1 g/dl (if starting M component is greater than 5 g/day) • CBC and differential • CMP • SPEP • UPEP • 24-hour urine for protein • Bone marrow biopsy (optional) • Skeletal survey to rule out lesions	CRAB criteria: • Calcium elevation: hypercalcemia (greater than 11.5 mg/dl) • Renal: rise in serum creatinine by 2 mg/dl or more related to M protein (especially in light-chain disease) • Anemia: decrease in hemoglobin of greater than 2 g/dl • Bone: development of new soft tissue plasmacytomas or bone lesions, or increase in the size of existing plasmacytomas or bone lesions	HCM • Determine the degree of severity. Mild can be managed as an outpatient. • Consider other causes such as medications (diuretics, supplements) or hyperparathyroidism. • Encourage aggressive oral or IV fluids. • Avoid calcium supplements. • Administer pamidronate disodium, zoledronic acid IV, or calcitonin (renal failure). • Severe HCM requires hospital admission to correct. Steroids such as dexamethasone should be initiated to treat multiple myeloma. Renal: Monitor creatinine, encourage aggressive hydration, if severe, obtain kidney ultrasound to rule out hydronephrosis Anemia: Administer ESAs or blood transfusion (if symptomatic). Bone: Consider stability of bone, palliation of bone pain with pain medications, and radiation therapy.

CBC—complete blood count; CMP—complete metabolic panel; ESAs—erythropoiesis-stimulating agents; M—monoclonal; HCM—hypercalcemia of malignancy; IV—intravenous; SPEP—serum protein electrophoresis with M component; UPEP—urine protein electrophoresis with M component

Note. Based on information from Durie et al., 2006; Major et al., 2001; Miceli et al., 2008; Yeh & Berenson, 2006.

discovery that scientists demonstrated the disappearance of moles and tumors, but a better understanding of the physics of radiation was needed. Dr. Vera Peters' work focused on Hodgkin disease, and in 1950, she became the first physician to develop a cure. Because of Peters' earlier findings, hematologic malignancies and their application to patients with multiple myeloma were better understood (Ng & Mauch, 2005).

Assessment of bone disease is a critical first step to identify the need for radiation treatment in patients with multiple myeloma (Berenson, 2004). The development of bone lesions or plasmacytomas may occur in previously treated patients and may be the first indicator of relapsed disease. Up to 90% of patients will have destruction occur at any time in their disease. Bone lytic lesions most often affect the spine (49%), skull (35%), pelvis (34%), ribs (33%), and humerus (Roodman, 2008).

Plain film radiography, or x-rays, can be used to identify single painful areas of bone destruction. Lesions or thinned areas of the bone may be found on x-ray and further staging. Multiple myeloma is a widespread disease, and it is important to identify areas of bone loss that may not be painful in addition to identifying symptomatic, painful areas. Skeletal survey is an imaging technique that includes x-rays of the skull, pelvis, long bones, and extremities and will demonstrate myeloma-related bone damage. Lytic lesions or plasmacytomas may be detected on x-ray if bone loss has occurred in one area of the body. Although patients may sometimes be asymptomatic and not have pain from a destructive lesion, the majority will experience pain at the site of bone damage (Roodman, 2008).

Magnetic resonance imaging is useful in the evaluation of suspicious lesions noted on x-ray, in the evaluation of spinal metastases, or in the assessment of vertebral compression fractures (VCFs). A VCF is defined as a break in the vertebral body that causes it to collapse. This loss of height of a vertebral body causes the spinal column above it to bend forward. A VCF in patients with multiple myeloma will occur as a result of a plasmacytoma that is causing bone destruction or because of increased osteoclastic activity from the disease (Dudeney, Lieberman, Reinhardt, & Hussein, 2002).

Radiation to the site of a VCF is indicated if a tumor is suspected and if a lesion or plasmacytoma is found on imaging. Radiation is effective in palliating pain or decreasing the tumor size, but other procedures may be used to correct the vertebral body deformity. Percutaneous balloon kyphoplasty or vertebroplasty may be an option for patients with metastatic or advanced disease, even in the presence of a poorer performance status, as an adjunct to radiation. Vertebral augmentation with polymethyl methacrylate, or bone cement, may help to stabilize the deformity and prevent future fractures from occurring (Hussein et al., 2008). These two approaches have few complications and provide patients with immediate pain relief in most instances. It is important to note that although a VCF may occur in a patient with multiple myeloma and often is related to the tumor, it also may be the result of osteoporosis and unrelated to the cancer.

In this instance, balloon kyphoplasty or vertebroplasty may be warranted, but radiation would be of no benefit.

USE OF RADIATION THERAPY IN RELAPSED MULTIPLE MYELOMA

Plasma cells are sensitive to the effects of radiation (Rowell & Tobias, 1991; Weber, 2005) and radiation has long been considered an effective treatment modality for patients with myeloma-related bone disease (Munshi, Tricot, & Barlogie, 2001), providing local control in 80% of patients. Radiation may be curative in a small percentage of patients who present with a solitary plasmacytoma of the bone (SPB), but this is rare and only occurs in approximately 5% of patients (Weber, 2005). The primary presenting symptom of patients with SPB is pain, and a plasma cell tumor often is affixed to bone. The difference between multiple myeloma and SPB is that patients with SPB are without widespread evidence of plasma cell dyscrasia and lack monoclonal protein in the serum or urine or have increased bone marrow plasma cells. Patients without additional evidence of plasma cell dyscrasias have a relatively low risk of recurrence or progression to overt multiple myeloma, as approximately 70% will remain without recurrence of the tumor (Hu & Yahalom, 2000).

Radiation for patients with myeloma is most often administered with palliative intent to provide relief from a painful lesion or tumor. Radiation may be administered in patients who may not be candidates for systemic treatment or as an adjunct to systemic therapy. In patients with refractory myeloma, other indications for radiation may be to prevent an impending fracture, to provide pain relief of actual pathologic fractures, or to reduce a tumor on the spine that may be causing a spinal cord compression with neurologic compromise. Multiple myeloma is a hematologic malignancy, and the goal of treatment of active multiple myeloma with systemic therapy is to prevent further lesions or tumors from forming (Berenson, 2004).

Many types of radiation exist, but external beam radiation therapy is very commonly used in patients with relapsed myeloma. The dose delivered and the number of fractions depends on the location of the tumor, but in general, the usual dose is 4,000–5,000 centigray (cGy). Although some consider these to be standard radiation doses, Ozsahin et al. (2006) suggested that little benefit is derived from doses greater than 3,000 cGy. Patients with painful lesions may receive the radiation dose over days to weeks depending on the location and intention of therapy and the overall intention of radiation, which in the relapsed group is palliation.

While local field external beam radiation therapy is one well-recognized and effective palliative treatment option, stereotactic or CyberKnife® (Accuray Inc.) radiosurgery is an emerging concept that may be used in patients with myeloma and symptomatic lesions or tumors. Stereotactic radiosurgery delivers a carefully calculated, high dose of radiation to individual tumor sites in a single fraction. In contrast to external beam radiation, stereotactic and CyberKnife radiosurgery is less likely to expose surrounding tissue structures to damaging radiation. In one study, 26 patients without spinal canal compromise who were diagnosed with a VCF experienced pain relief from a procedure that combined balloon kyphoplasty and spinal radiosurgery (Gerszten et al., 2005). Another group evaluated the safety of radiosurgery in patients with a neurologic deficit and radiation-sensitive tumors such as multiple myeloma. In this study, 84% of patients were clinically stable or improved following radiosurgery (Lee et al., 2007). This study and others suggest that radiosurgery may be a viable treatment option for patients with or without spinal cord compromise and a new form of treatment in patients with multiple myeloma.

It is rare for patients with myeloma to receive total body irradiation or hemibody radiation, given the toxicities and little clinical benefit (Hu & Yahalom, 2000). Nursing care of patients receiving involved-field radiation includes alleviating side effects related to the radiated field. Patients with head and neck radiation may have trouble swallowing or eating and may be prone to mouth sores. Good oral hygiene is encouraged. Patients receiving mediastinal radiation may develop nausea or loss of appetite as radiation may irritate the esophagus. Fatigue is a common side effect of cumulative radiation therapy, and patients must educated about managing their activities. Pain medications may be warranted if patients are required to remain in an uncomfortable position during the radiation session and to enhance comfort afterward, but it also may be warranted if severe mouth sores or radiation burns develop.

THE ROLE OF BISPHOSPHONATES

One last consideration in patients with relapsed disease who are receiving radiation to the bone is related to supportive care and the use of bisphosphonates. As mentioned, most patients with multiple myeloma will have destructive bone lesions or diffuse osteopenia at diagnosis or at relapse. Bone disease may lead to hypercalcemia of malignancy or an increase in skeletal-related events or fractures. Bone disease results from the stimulation of osteoclast activating growth factors that cause bone destruction, cytokine release that further leads to bone destruction, and the lack of osteoblastic response that is necessary to rebuild bone. Nurses should be aware that treatment with IV bisphosphonates such as pamidronate and zoledronic acid on a monthly basis is recommended for a duration of up to two years in patients with documented bone disease, which includes osteopenia or widespread lytic lesions. Because patients may temporarily discontinue bisphosphonates after two years of stable disease, bisphosphonates may be resumed at the time of relapse (Kyle et al., 2007).

Renal impairment is common in patients with relapsed multiple myeloma, and a reduced dosage or longer infusion of bisphosphonates is indicated in the setting of preexisting mild to moderate renal impairment (estimated creatinine clearance of 30–60 ml/min). The usual dose of zoledronic acid is 4 mg IV over 15–45 minutes in patients with normal renal function, but dosage adjustments are recommended for patients with even mild renal impairment (Novartis Pharmaceuticals Corp., 2008b). Pamidronate 90 mg IV is administered over four to six hours and is recommended for patients with extensive bone disease and existing severe renal impairment (serum creatinine level of 3 mg/dl (265 μmol/L) or an estimated creatinine clearance of 30 ml/min (Novartis Pharmaceuticals Corp., 2008a). Increasing or prolongation of the interval between bisphosphonate infusions and slowing the infusion rate can further reduce the risk of chronic renal toxicity.

Nursing management of patients receiving bisphosphonates includes side effect education and assessment for complications. Maintenance of good hydration is important in patients receiving IV bisphosphonates as well as monitoring of the serum creatinine before each dose to assess for renal dysfunction (Kyle et al., 2007). Flu-like symptoms after bisphosphonate infusion are rare but usually are responsive to acetaminophen 650–1,000 mg PO every four to six hours after the infusion. Monitoring and surveillance for osteonecrosis of the jaw (ONJ) is encouraged. ONJ is a rare but serious condition of avascular necrosis of the maxilla or mandible that may occur with prolonged infusions of bisphosphonates. Signs of ONJ include jaw or tooth pain, and exposed bone may be identified on physical examination in severe cases. If ONJ symptoms occur, initial treatment should consist of antibiotic therapy and avoidance of extractions (Cafro et al., 2008).

Prevention of ONJ is preferred, and clinicians should follow some key recommendations. Baseline and routine dental examinations every six months should be discussed and implemented before initiating bisphosphonates. Montefusco et al. (2008) studied the effects of various types and schedules of antibiotic prophylaxis for dental procedures in patients receiving bisphosphonates versus standard care. One group was randomized to receive amoxicillin-clavulanate 2 g/day PO or levofloxacin 500 mg/day PO from one day before to three days after any dental procedure. In patients receiving antibiotic prophylaxis, incidence of infection was decreased with dental procedures such as cleaning, implants, and extractions. Although more studies are needed to evaluate antibiotic prophylaxis, the low cost and potential benefit may warrant implementing this intervention in patients who are receiving IV bisphosphonates and undergoing dental procedures (Montefusco et al., 2008).

Radiation in patients with relapsed or refractory multiple myeloma often is necessary to provide comfort and local control of the disease. Adjunct procedures such as percutaneous balloon kyphoplasty or vertebroplasty may provide additional symptomatic pain relief. Bisphosphonates may effectively treat hypercalcemia of malignancy and are indicated in relapsed multiple myeloma to help strengthen bones and prevent future fractures or skeletal-related events. Prompt identification of new sites of disease is warranted to deliver appropriate intervention using systemic therapy or a supportive therapy such as bisphosphonates or localized radiation. Few therapeutic options were available to patients with relapsed multiple myeloma and bone disease in the past, but several options for systemic treatment are now widely available.

TREATMENT MODALITIES FOR RELAPSED MULTIPLE MYELOMA

It is generally recommended that if patients had achieved a response to their initial therapy and the response lasted longer than six months after therapy had stopped, the initial treatment can be repeated. If this is not an option, patients will be offered many of the novel therapies earlier on in the disease, be recommended for autologous stem cell transplantation if they did not pursue transplantation up front and are candidates, or be encouraged to participate in a clinical trial (Rajkumar & Dispenzieri, 2008). Once the up-front therapies have been exhausted, a few treatments are available that have been studied in relapsed disease that can provide various degrees of remission and response.

Bortezomib

Bortezomib emerged as a first-in-class proteasome inhibitor with a novel mechanism of action. As compared to traditional chemotherapeutic agents, bortezomib has many different actions, including inhibition of NF-κB, which is a protein complex that acts as a transcription factor (Harousseau, 2008). Its efficacy in newly diagnosed multiple myeloma has been established (Jagannath et al., 2006; San Miguel et al., 2008), and bortezomib has been successfully used in patients with relapsed disease as well. Richardson et al. (2003) first reported its efficacy in patients with relapsed multiple myeloma, and the same year, the FDA approved bortezomib for treatment of those patients.

Pursuant to efficacy data from the initial trials, Richardson et al. (2005) initiated a multicenter study, called the APEX (Assessment of Proteasome Inhibition for Extending Remissions) trial, using bortezomib alone or in combination with dexamethasone in patients with relapsed multiple myeloma. Patients were randomized to receive bortezomib plus dexamethasone (BD) or dexamethasone alone in this phase III trial. The dose of bortezomib was 1.3 mg/m^2 IV on days 1, 4, 8, and 11 of therapy. If there was suboptimal response after four cycles of bortezomib, then patients were given dexamethasone 20 mg PO the day of and day after bortezomib. The one-year survival rate was 80% in patients receiving bortezomib and 66% in those receiving dexamethasone. As a result, the study was terminated early, and all patients who were initially randomized to dexamethasone were offered bortezomib regardless of disease status. An updated efficacy analysis after a median follow-up of 22 months showed a median survival of 30 months versus 24 months with dexamethasone alone (Richardson et al., 2007).

Side effects of bortezomib are manageable, and nurses are charged with providing education and monitoring of treatment-related side effects. Appropriate laboratory monitoring, especially for hematologic parameter, for patients receiving bortezomib is important. A complete blood count should be obtained prior to each dose of bortezomib to assess for leukopenia, anemia, or thrombocytopenia. An increased risk of herpes zoster virus (HZV) reactivation was noted in clinical trials up to 13%. Patients who are receiving bortezomib should also receive prophylactic doses of acyclovir or valacyclovir (Kim et al., 2008). Dosage reductions according to the package insert should be considered for moderate to severe leukopenia, anemia, or thrombocytopenia or any other significant side effects that may be related to bortezomib and affect function or quality of life (Millennium Pharmaceuticals, Inc., 2009). Bortezomib is safe for use in patients with renal insufficiency and/or concurrent renal failure, and dose modifications are unnecessary (San Miguel et al., 2008).

In a multicenter retrospective analysis of patients with renal failure who had a median serum creatinine level of 6.8 mg/dl, patients received bortezomib alone or in combination with other agents such as dexamethasone, liposomal doxorubicin, or thalidomide. Of the 20 patients with renal failure, three out of four had improved renal function following bortezomib-based therapy, which was thought to be caused by the addition of bortezomib to the regimen (Chanan-Khan et al., 2007). In addition, these patients were able to stop dialysis because of the improved kidney function. Bortezomib is well tolerated and should be considered in patients with relapsed myeloma alone or in combination with dexamethasone as a viable treatment option, especially in the setting of renal disease or renal failure.

Gastrointestinal effects of bortezomib also are common but preventable. Although the emetogenic potential of bortezomib is low compared to other forms of chemotherapy, nausea and vomiting can be prevented with prophylactic antiemetics and dietary modifications (Colson, Doss, Swift, Tariman, & Thomas, 2004). Increased dietary fiber or psyllium dietary fiber supplement may help decrease the number of diarrhea stools. Intermittent stool samples and laboratory evaluation for *Clostridium* or other serious gastrointestinal infections should be performed. It is important to assess stools for *Clostridium difficile* and culture in patients with recurrent diarrhea, especially if the diarrhea is accompanied by nausea, fever, or abdominal cramping (Smith, Bertolotti, Curran, & Jenkins, 2008).

Clinically significant peripheral neuropathy as a result of bortezomib can be a dose-limiting toxicity and is a common reason for discontinuation (Tariman, Love, McCullagh, & Sandifer, 2008). Clinically apparent neuropathy may be present at baseline as a result of the disease or after prior treatment (Richardson et al., 2005, 2007). Severe (grade 3 or 4) peripheral neuropathy has been reported in greater than 10% of patients receiving bortezomib therapy. The mechanism of bortezomib-induced peripheral neuropathy is not widely understood, but one group recently noted that a possible mechanism contributing to peripheral neuropathy and cellular toxicity following proteasome inhibition was an increase in tubulin polymerization and microtubule stabilization in tissue culture cells (Poruchynsky et al., 2008).

Nurses may be familiar with chemotherapy-induced peripheral neuropathy, as this form of neuropathy is noted in approximately 40%–60% of patients receiving different classes of chemotherapy drugs. Bortezomib now joins the taxanes, platinum compounds, vinca alkaloids, and thalidomide, as each have been implicated in causing neuropathy (Wolf, Barton, Kottschade, Grothey, & Loprinzi, 2008). Neuropathy can cause symptoms of numbness, tingling, burning, and pain and in severe cases, weakness in a stocking-and-glove pattern (Colson et al., 2004; Tariman et al., 2008). Patients with relapsed or refractory multiple myeloma may experience baseline neuropathy as a result of the disease itself or prior treatments, but regardless of the etiology, nurses should assess for painful or decreased sensation in the peripheral extremities before each dose of bortezomib. Appropriate dose modifications for neuropathy symptoms have not been shown to decrease efficacy. Rather, reducing the dose of bortezomib in patients with severe neuropathy allowed patients to remain on therapy (Richardson et al., 2005).

Bortezomib and Liposomal Doxorubicin

Bortezomib has been combined with pegylated liposomal doxorubicin (PLD), and the FDA approved the combination for use in patients with relapsed myeloma based on its efficacy. In a phase II study to evaluate this steroid-free regimen, patients were assigned to one of either two groups. Both groups received bortezomib on days 1, 4, 8, and 11 of a 21-day cycle, but the other group received PLD at a dose of 30 mg/m² on day 4 of therapy in addition to bortezomib. Results showed that bortezomib plus PLD significantly increased time to progression to 9.3 months compared to a time to progression of 6.5 months with bortezomib alone. Patients with relapsed disease generally tolerate this regimen well (Orlowski et al., 2007), and the most common side effects of therapy are myelosuppression (thrombocytopenia and neutropenia), nausea, diarrhea, constipation, and fatigue.

Other manageable side effects unique to the bortezomib plus PLD combination include stomatitis and hand-foot syndrome (also referred to as palmar-plantar erythrodysesthesia [PPE]). These side effects occurred in less than 15% of patients receiving the combination therapy, and only 5% had serious stomatitis or hand-foot syndrome. Although a low percentage of patients experienced these toxicities, ongoing nursing assessment, patient education, and adjustments to the dose or dose schedule can reduce the severity and frequency of these occurrences.

The first step to management of stomatitis includes good oral hygiene. Rinses with a baking soda solution may prevent the development of mouth sores. Once mouth sores develop, a swish-and-swallow mix of topical viscous lidocaine–based preparations with or without nystatin and/or tetracycline can relieve pain. Patients should avoid rinses that contain alcohol. Acyclovir may be initiated if viral infection, such as with herpes zoster virus, is suspected, or the dose may be increased if patients were already on prophylactic doses of acyclovir. If patients continue to experience persistent stomatitis symptoms, the dose and schedule of PLD should be considered, as these symptoms may impair quality of life (Yee, 1998).

PPE is a side effect of PLD therapy that may lead to burn-like rash on the hands and feet. PPE often results in a painful sloughing of skin that can vary from a slight peel to a severe burn. The mechanism responsible for PPE is not clear, but one theory is that localized extravasation of liposomes through capillaries in the skin will cause a vesicant-type burn that leads to PPE (Alberts & Garcia, 1997). Patients should be discouraged from immersing hands in water for long periods of time within 24–48 hours of PLD administration and should avoid repetitive activities and exercise. Minimizing sun exposure and applying direct heat to any one area, such as in wearing heavy socks and restrictive clothing, is cautioned against (Richards, 2008; von Moos et al., 2008).

Nurses can recommend cold compresses and cushioning to the affected area, and over-the-counter analgesics such as acetaminophen may help decrease pain. It is important to note that patients with multiple myeloma who are experiencing painful PPE should avoid nonsteroidal anti-inflammatory drugs (NSAIDs). NSAIDs such as naproxen, ibuprofen, and celecoxib have been implicated in contributing to acute renal failure in patients with multiple myeloma (Blade et al., 1998; Goldschmidt, Lannert, Bommer, & Ho, 1998; Shpilberg, Douer, Ehrenfeld, Engelberg, & Ramot, 1990). The mechanism of renal failure is likely multifactorial. Variables such as a decline in baseline renal function, presence of light chains in the urine, or dehydration may contribute to acute renal failure, but two theories have been proposed. First, NSAIDs inhibit vasodilatory prostaglandin synthesis, which is necessary to maintain appropriate glomerular filtration rate. Impaired prostaglandin synthesis in patients with multiple myeloma may further compromise renal functionality. Second, inhibition of these substances could lead to toxic cast precipitation within the kidney tubules that leads to impaired renal function. Regardless of the mechanism, the use of NSAIDs in patients with multiple myeloma should be avoided (Ronco, Aucouturier, & Mougenot, 2007).

If acetaminophen does not relieve pain, prescription narcotic or non-narcotic analgesics should be considered. Analgesia in acute pain syndromes such as PPE is critical to improve mental and social functioning, increase mobility when the feet are affected, decrease the risk of infections such as pneumonia from inactivity, and prevent other inactivity-related complications such as venous thromboembolism (VTE). When recommending analgesia, it is important to recognize the needs of each patient and perform a comprehensive pain and psychosocial assessment. Acetaminophen and a mild opioid combination regimen is recommended for short-term use, but if significant skin damage has occurred, long-acting opioids may be needed for relief of severe pain (National Comprehensive Cancer Network, 2009).

The use of pyridoxine has been anecdotally reported in patients with multiple myeloma. The pain associated with PPE generally is transient; pyridoxine may provide relief of mild PPE symptoms, although the rationale for this remains unclear. Several case reports described the efficacy of pyridoxine in patients receiving a continuous infusion of 5-fluorouracil and intermittent infusions of PLD without treatment delay or dosage reduction (Fabian et al., 1990; Vukelja, Lombardo, James, & Weiss, 1989). A suggested starting dosage of pyridoxine is 50 mg/day, and no adverse effects were reported with a higher dosage of 150 mg/day (Hussein et al., 1998; Patel, 1999).

Lenalidomide and Dexamethasone

The combination of lenalidomide and dexamethasone (LD) has been studied since 2002. In June 2006, the FDA approved the use of lenalidomide in combination with dexamethasone in patients with relapsed or refractory multiple myeloma (Chen et al., 2009). This was based on the results of a large, international, phase III randomized trial that took place in North America (Weber et al., 2007). In the North American trial, patients in the United States and Canada were eligible to participate if they had received at least one previous therapy and had experienced disease progression. Each participant was randomly assigned to receive oral doses of lenalidomide 25 mg or placebo on days 1–21 of a 28-day cycle. Both groups also received dexamethasone 40 mg PO on days 1–4, 9–12, and 17–20 for the first four cycles, which were then followed by dexamethasone on days 1–4 of a 28-day cycle for maintenance. The median time to progression was 11.1 months in patients who received LD compared to 4.7 months in patients who received dexamethasone alone. Furthermore, a median OS of 29.6 months was seen in patients receiving LD versus 20.2 months in those receiving dexamethasone alone (Weber et al., 2007).

Prior to FDA approval of lenalidomide in April 2005, patient advocacy groups had petitioned the FDA to allow the manufacturers of lenalidomide to develop an expanded access program. This allowed patients with relapsed and refractory multiple myeloma who were unable to participate in a clinical trial the opportunity to receive lenalidomide. Many patients were enrolled in the expanded access program, and 1,438 patients who received lenalidomide followed the same dose and schedule of the previously referenced international trial (Weber et al., 2007). In this group, hematologic, gastrointestinal, and thrombotic effects were similar to those seen in the larger trials. The median time for patients to remain on treatment was 15.4 weeks, and the median dose was 25 mg of lenalidomide. The safety data collected in the expanded access program echoed the data reported in the larger trial and suggested that the combination of LD is superior to dexamethasone alone and is safe for use in patients with relapsed multiple myeloma (Chen et al., 2009).

Two other studies have commented on the use of lenalidomide as a single agent without dexamethasone or for use earlier in the disease course (Richardson et al., 2009; Stadtmauer et al., 2009). In one study, 222 patients received lenalidomide 30 mg/day once daily (days 1–21, every 28 days) until disease progression or intolerance to the side effects. More than 67% of patients had received three or more prior treatment regimens. At least 44% of these heavily pretreated patients experienced a minimal response or better with lenalidomide alone. The incidence of myelosuppression was similar to prior studies and, surprisingly, the incidence of VTE, when lenalidomide was used as a single agent, was less than in combination in other trials. These data support the use of lenalidomide without dexamethasone in the treatment of patients with relapsed multiple myeloma (Richardson et al., 2009).

In a study to assess the difference between the use of lenalidomide early or later in the disease course, researchers evaluated the use of lenalidomide after patients received one prior therapy. When lenalidomide was used earlier in the disease course after one prior therapy, patients showed prolonged median TTP of 17.1 versus 10.6 months (p = 0.026) and improved progression-free survival of 14.1 versus 9.5 months (p = 0.047) compared with those who received two or more therapies. OS was significantly prolonged for patients treated with lenalidomide plus dexamethasone with one prior therapy, compared with patients treated later in the disease course with a median OS of 42 months versus 35.8 months (p = 0.041). This analysis showed no differences in toxicity, dose reductions, or discontinuations, despite longer treatment. Therefore, LD is both effective and tolerable for second-line multiple myeloma therapy, and the greatest benefit of OS occurred with earlier use (Stadtmauer et al., 2009).

Common side effects of this combination of LD include myelosuppression, gastrointestinal toxicities such as constipation alternating with diarrhea, and an increased risk of VTE. All of these side effects in most relapsed multiple myeloma trials were more common in the lenalidomide group than in the placebo group. An important nursing consideration when caring for patients who have multiple myeloma and are receiving lenalidomide is to counsel against pregnancy. Lenalidomide is a potential teratogen with a chemical structure that closely resembles thalidomide, which warrants caution, although no data show that lenalidomide causes birth defects in humans at the present time (Kumar & Rajkumar, 2006).

To address the concern of birth defects and safeguard against the risk of fetal exposure in women of childbearing potential, the Celgene Corp. administers the RevAssist® program. RevAssist is a restricted access program developed to address the need for safety and education when prescribing lenalidomide. Patients must be counseled before the start of lenalidomide therapy and on an ongoing basis in regard to black box warnings, such as being aware of the increased risk of VTE, avoiding becoming pregnant if they are female and of childbearing potential, and for males, preventing a female from becoming pregnant. Two forms of birth control are required at all times, and patients cannot donate blood or sperm while taking lenalidomide. Counseling against fetal exposure to lenalidomide should be ongoing and occur prior to monthly prescription refills at the minimum (Celgene Corp., 2009a).

Myelosuppression is a common side effect of LD, but appropriate dosing schedules may lessen the likelihood of blood counts becoming critically low. Inappropriate dosing of lenalidomide in patients with renal insufficiency or renal failure may lead to myelosuppression (Niesvizky et al., 2007). Niesvizky et al. (2007) observed that patients who received the oral combination of clarithromycin, lenalidomide, and dexamethasone and had concurrent renal dysfunction with a creatinine clearance of less than 40 ml/min experienced more significant myelosuppression than those with normal renal function. Further evaluation of data in several clinical trials has led to updated dosing guidelines in the lenalidomide package insert (Celgene Corp., 2009a).

Lenalidomide is safe in renal dysfunction and when given to a patient on dialysis, but it is important to initiate the appropriate dose and implement routine monitoring of serum creatinine clearance. Nurses should monitor serum creatinine levels in patients with compromised renal function and assess worsening renal failure that may warrant additional dose reduction. Dosage reductions based on decreased renal function should be considered in all patients with multiple myeloma (see Table 8-3). A complete blood count and differential should be obtained at least every two weeks at the beginning of therapy; serum creatinine should be monitored at the time of each blood draw (Celgene Corp., 2009a).

Gastrointestinal side effects of lenalidomide were reportedly mild and mainly included constipation and diarrhea, which were present in 39% and 29% of patients, respectively. Nausea and vomiting are extremely rare, and only mild nausea and vomiting were transient and reported in 22% of patients in the initial phase III registration trial. Physical effects related to oral therapies can lead to decreased adherence to treatment regimens and may produce negative psychological effects, which may include anxiety and depression;

Table 8-3. Dose Modifications for Lenalidomide in Multiple Myeloma	
Renal Function	**Dose of Lenalidomide[a]**
Creatinine clearance (CrCl) = 30–60 ml/min	10 mg every 24 hours
CrCl < 30 ml/min (not requiring dialysis)	15 mg PO every 48 hours
CrCl < 30 ml/min (requiring dialysis)	5 mg once daily on dialysis days The dose should be administered following dialysis.

For the first 12 weeks of therapy, nurses should obtain
• CBC and differential every two weeks
• Basic chemistry panel to assess for renal dysfunction.

These laboratory values should be obtained monthly before refilling each dose of lenalidomide.

Note. Based on information from Celgene Corp., 2009a; Miceli et al., 2008.

nurses must be aware of the severity complaints that may affect patients' well-being (Richards, 2009; Smith et al., 2008).

Most adverse gastrointestinal effects of lenalidomide are manageable with dietary education and over-the-counter preparations that target the complaint. Before any intervention can be recommended, a thorough patient history is critical and must be documented. This will establish a time course for when the constipation or diarrhea began and allows the nurse to evaluate medications that may lead to increased constipation, such as analgesics, certain cardiac medications, and diuretics, which may lead to dehydration. Examination of the abdomen for the presence and character of bowel sounds, accompanied by palpation of the abdomen to evaluate the presence of abdominal pain, may be indicated for prolonged periods of constipation (Smith et al., 2008).

Once a history and examination are performed, dietary modifications, over-the-counter preparations, and herbal remedies may be discussed. Patients who note constipation as the greatest concern may increase their dietary fiber and add senna-containing laxatives. More potent over-the-counter medications for constipation may be indicated but often are not needed in patients receiving lenalidomide. Diarrhea may occur in patients receiving lenalidomide but in clinical trials was often noted to be mild and transient. Bulking agents such as a psyllium dietary fiber supplement (Metamucil®, Procter & Gamble) or mild antidiarrheal agents can be used to manage diarrhea (Richards, 2009).

It is important for nurses to educate patients that appropriate dietary modifications may affect diarrhea or constipation. By keeping a food diary, patients may notice a correlation with certain foods that trigger an episode of diarrhea or lead to constipation. It is important with either diarrhea or constipation that patients are instructed to increase fluid intake and avoid becoming dehydrated. Avoidance of consumption of excessive alcohol and caffeinated beverages also is encouraged for mild to moderate gastrointestinal symptoms.

Another nursing consideration for patients who are receiving lenalidomide and dexamethasone is to educate them on the increased risk of VTE. Patients with relapsed multiple myeloma in a large, randomized trial had an increased risk of VTE. Early in the trial, thrombosis rates were 12%, but once aspirin was added, the rates of DVT significantly ($p < 0.001$) decreased (Weber et al., 2007). Intervention and management of these side effects are the same as with patients receiving thalidomide and should be discussed with patients routinely. Guidelines exist for the prevention, diagnosis, and management of VTE associated with lenalidomide and thalidomide (Palumbo et al., 2008; Rome, Doss, Miller, & Westphal, 2008).

Bortezomib, Lenalidomide, and Dexamethasone

Bortezomib and lenalidomide are two of the most effective therapies for multiple myeloma currently available, and an ongoing phase I/II trial evaluated this combination in previously treated patients (Anderson et al., 2009). After the maximum tolerated doses of each of these drugs were determined in a phase I trial, Anderson et al. (2009) reported the efficacy and safety of this regimen based on the maximum tolerated doses. In the study, each of the patients received up to eight 21-day cycles of lenalidomide 15 mg PO (days 1–14), bortezomib 1 mg/m^2 IV (days 1, 4, 8, and 11), and dexamethasone 40/20 mg PO (cycles 1–4/5–8, the day of and day after bortezomib dosing). A maintenance phase of treatment was initiated for patients who were still responding and exhibited unacceptable toxicities. This included lenalidomide days 1–14, bortezomib days 1 and 8, and dexamethasone 10 mg days 1, 2, 8, and 9. Maintenance continued until disease progression or toxicity. A total of 64 patients were recruited, and of these, 33 continued on maintenance and 22 discontinued therapy (11 because of progressive disease). The overall response rate was an impressive 84% in this heavily pretreated population, and the median duration of response was 24 weeks.

Side effects of the bortezomib, lenalidomide, and dexamethasone combination consisted mostly of mild myelosuppression, gastrointestinal effects (e.g., nausea, diarrhea, constipation), and peripheral neuropathy, as would be expected with this regimen. One person developed pneumonia and another developed DVT while on aspirin therapy. The combination of bortezomib, lenalidomide, and dexamethasone has shown effectiveness in patients with newly diagnosed multiple myeloma, and although studies are ongoing, it appears to be effective in heavily pretreated patients. Based on its efficacy, the combination should be considered in relapsed multiple myeloma even in patients who have been treated previously with either bortezomib, lenalidomide, or dexamethasone (Anderson et al., 2009).

Cyclophosphamide, Dexamethasone, Etoposide, and Cisplatin

The combination of cyclophosphamide, dexamethasone, etoposide, and cisplatin (CDEP) was evaluated in the mid-1990s for use in patients as a salvage regimen following transplantation (Munshi et al., 1996). In a study of 57 patients with multiple myeloma who relapsed after undergoing transplantation, CDEP reduced the tumor mass by 75% in 40% of the patients and induced CR in 13% of patients. The effectiveness of thalidomide was emerging (Singhal et al., 1999), and researchers at the University of Arkansas added this novel agent to the CDEP regimen. After a median follow-up of 17 months, patients had a response rate of 18% after three cycles of CDEP, and the response rate doubled to 36% with the addition of thalidomide (Barlogie et al., 2001). Although CDEP had induced remission in a small number of patients, response rates were relatively low compared to CDEP plus thalidomide.

More recently, this regimen was evaluated in patients with refractory multiple myeloma (Dadacaridou et al., 2007). CDEP was administered to 11 patients and included cyclophosphamide 400 mg/m^2 daily for four days, cisplatin 15 mg/m^2 daily for four days, and etoposide 40 mg/m^2 daily for four days given as a 24-hour infusion. Patients received dexamethasone 40 mg IV bolus daily on days 1–4. Granulocyte–colony-stimulating factor was administered daily beginning 24 hours after therapy until white blood cell recovery. The course was repeated every 28 days. The overall response rate of this regimen was 58.3% with a median response duration of nine months. Despite a relatively low response rate in the era of novel agents, CDEP represents an opportunity for another therapeutic option in patients who have been previously treated.

Italian researchers studied reduced doses of CDEP prior to stem cell mobilization (Lazzarino et al., 2001) and proposed a reduced dosing schedule before stem cell mobilization. Corso et al. (2005) studied 152 patients with newly diagnosed multiple myeloma and treated each patient with two cycles of CDEP from 2000 to 2004. Although this was a pretransplant regimen, lower doses of CDEP had not previously been studied in patients with relapsed multiple myeloma. Based on these results, a less intensive dosing schedule may be given to patients with relapsed multiple myeloma, which may allow for similar efficacy, outpatient administration, and fewer toxicities (Corso et al., 2005).

The most common toxicity of the CDEP regimen is moderate to severe myelosuppression, which improves by the end of the treatment cycle. Nurses can anticipate that patients should have a complete blood count and differential at least weekly if not more regularly following the CDEP regimen, depending on the baseline blood cell counts. Filgrastim or pegfilgrastim should be implemented to facilitate white blood cell count recovery, and nurses can anticipate the white blood cells to nadir between days 10 and 14 of each cycle. Because patients are at risk for neutropenia and fever, they must be educated about this risk, prevention of infection, and when to call the nurse or go to the emergency department. Practicing strict hand-washing techniques and avoiding people with colds or signs of overt illness are important. Nurses also must reinforce prompt reporting of a febrile episode. Neutropenia and fever can pose a potentially life-threatening event and must be taken seriously (Miceli, Colson, Gavino, & Lilleby, 2008).

Severe anemia and thrombocytopenia can be managed by red blood cell or platelet transfusions if bone marrow recovery is not imminent and patients are symptomatic. Nurses should educate patients regarding the increased risk of bleeding and must closely monitor blood counts. Fatigue associated with anemia is common, and nurses can discuss with patients the importance of managing activities during the week after chemotherapy. Severe anemia may lead to dizziness, hypotension, and cardiac dysfunction especially in patients with a history of renal insufficiency or cardiac conduction abnormalities (Silverberg, Blum, Peer, & Iaina, 1998).

Erythropoiesis-stimulating agents (ESAs) can be used in the management of anemia to maintain the blood hemoglobin level higher than 10 g/dl. According to the National Comprehensive Cancer Network (NCCN) guidelines for the treatment of anemia, darbepoetin can be initiated at a dose of 2.25 mcg/kg subcutaneous (SC) weekly or 500 mcg SC every three weeks as a fixed dose (NCCN, 2009). In addition, epoetin alfa can be given at a dose of 150 units three times weekly and up to 40,000 units SC weekly. It is important to note that while patients are receiving long-term erythropoietin therapy, functional iron deficiency may develop. As such, serum iron, ferritin, and serum total iron-binding capacity tests are recommended prior to initiating oral iron therapy. In addition, ESAs have been implicated in increasing the risk of thrombosis in patients with multiple myeloma. Therefore, clinicians should assess the severity of anemia and balance the risks of ESA therapy versus blood transfusion or observation with the benefits of therapy (Zonder, 2006).

Dexamethasone, Thalidomide, Cisplatin, Doxorubicin, Cyclophosphamide, and Etoposide

Relapse will ultimately occur in the vast majority of patients with multiple my-eloma regardless of which therapy is selected. One combination chemotherapy regimen that produces remission in patients with previously treated multiple myeloma is that of dexamethasone, thalidomide, cisplatin, doxorubicin, cyclo-phosphamide, and etoposide, known as DT-PACE (Lee et al., 2003). In this regi-men, investigators at the University of Arkansas who studied the CDEP regimen noted that when thalidomide was added to CDEP, the response rate doubled. Lee et al. (2003) added thalidomide and doxorubicin to the aforementioned CDEP program to improve drug synergy and patient response. In this study, 236 patients with relapsed multiple myeloma each received a regimen that consisted of high-dose dexamethasone 40 mg PO daily for four days; thalidomide 400 mg PO at night days 1–28; a four-day continuous infusion of cisplatin 10 mg/m^2/day (total dose per cycle 40 mg/m^2), doxorubicin 10 mg/m^2/day (total dose per cycle 40 mg/m^2), cyclophosphamide 400 mg/m^2/day (total dose per cycle 1,600 mg/m^2), and etoposide 40 mg/m^2/day (total dose 160 mg/m^2). The daily dose of cisplatin, cyclophosphamide, and etoposide was combined in 1,000 ml of 0.9% normal saline, and doxorubicin was infused separately in more than 50 ml of 5% dextrose in water each day. Infusions were administered via a central venous access device in the outpatient setting by using a portable infusion pump. Each cycle of DT-PACE was repeated every four to six weeks, provided the patient's absolute neutrophil count had recovered to more than 1,000/microliter (mcl) and platelet count was more than 100,000/mcl. The results showed that the partial remission rate after two cycles of DT-PACE was 32%, but patients who were able to tolerate 100% of the dose for at least two cycles had a partial remission rate of 49% or better. This suggests that better response rates occurred in patients with previously treated multiple myeloma who were able to take full doses of DT-PACE (Lee et al., 2003).

As expected, patients who received this combination chemotherapy regi-men experienced mild to moderate nonhematologic and hematologic side effects. Nonhematologic toxicities in this trial included nausea and vomiting, mucositis, and hypophosphatemia, but none of these were severe and were rarely noted. Thromboprophylaxis was initiated after a high incidence of DVT (15%) was noted with this regimen. One of the most common neurologic complaints was paresthesias and numbness in hands and feet, which improved with dose reduction of thalidomide (Zangari et al., 2002).

CONCLUSION

The introduction of novel agents in the previous decade has provided patients with myeloma the ability to not only live a longer life but also to have a better quality of life. Kumar et al. (2008) reviewed 2,981 patients with newly diagnosed multiple myeloma from the Mayo Clinic and examined survival trends over time. The patients diagnosed in the past decade had a 50% survival advantage, with an overall survival of 44.8 months if diagnosed in the past decade, versus 29.9 months for patients who were diagnosed in the prior decade. This illustrates that patients are living longer, and, because of improved supportive care agents, better patient identification and management, and ongoing research, the number of therapeutic combinations will continue to grow. Researchers are forever in search of a cure for multiple myeloma. Even when that time arrives, nurses will remain integral to the healthcare team and improvement of patient outcomes.

REFERENCES

Alberts, D.S., & Garcia, D.J. (1997). Safety aspects of pegylated liposomal doxorubicin in patients with cancer. *Drugs, 54*(Suppl. 4), 30–35.

Anderson, K.C., Jagannath, S., Jakubowiak, A., Lonial, S., Raje, N., Alsina, M., ... Richardson, P. (2009). Lenalidomide, bortezomib, and dexamethasone in relapsed/refractory multiple myeloma (MM): Encouraging outcomes and tolerability in a phase II study [Abstract No. 8536]. *Journal of Clinical Oncology, 27*(Suppl. 15). Retrieved from http://www.asco.org/ASCOv2/Meetings/Abstracts&confID=65&abstractID=32787

Barlogie, B., Anaissie, E.J., van Rhee, F., Shaughnessy, J.D., Jr., Haessler, J., Pineda-Roman, M., ... Crowley, J.J. (2008). Total therapy (TT) for myeloma (MM)—10% cure rate with TT1 suggested by >10 yr continuous complete remission (CCR): Bortezomib in TT3 overcomes poor-risk associated with T(4;14) and DelTP53 in TT2 [Abstract No. 8516]. *Journal of Clinical Oncology, 26*(Suppl.). Retrieved from http://www.asco.org/ASCOv2/Meetings/Abstracts?&vmview=abst_detail_view&confID=55&abstractID=35972

Barlogie, B., Zangari, M., Spencer, T., Fassas, A., Anaissie, E., Badros, A., ... Tricot, G. (2001). Thalidomide in the management of multiple myeloma. *Seminars in Hematology, 38*, 250–259.

Berenson, J.R. (2004). Management of skeletal complications. In J.S. Malpas, D.E. Bergsagel, R. Kyle, & K. Anderson (Eds.), *Myeloma biology and management* (3rd ed., pp. 239–249). Philadelphia, PA: Saunders.

Blade, J., Fernandes-Llama, P., Bosch, F., Montoliu, J., Lens, X.M., Montoto, S., ... Montserrat, E. (1998). Renal failure in multiple myeloma: Presenting features and predictors of outcome in 94 patients from a single institution. *Archives of Internal Medicine, 158*, 1889–1893.

Cafro, A.M., Barbarano, L., Nosari, A.M., D'Avanzo, G., Nichelatti, M., Bibas, M., ... Andriani, A. (2008). Osteonecrosis of the jaw in patients with multiple myeloma treated with bisphosphonates: Definition and management of the risk related to zoledronic acid. *Clinical Lymphoma and Myeloma, 8*, 111–116.

Celgene Corp. (2009a). Revlimid (lenalidomide) [Package insert]. Summit, NJ: Author.

Celgene Corp. (2009b). Thalomid (thalidomide) [Package insert]. Summit, NJ: Author.

Chanan-Khan, A.A., Kaufman, J.L., Mehta, J., Richardson, P.G., Miller, K.C., Lonial, S., ... Singhal, S. (2007). Activity and safety of bortezomib in multiple myeloma patients with advanced renal failure: A multicenter retrospective study. *Blood, 109*, 2604–2606. doi:10.1182/blood-2006-09-046409

Chen, C., Reece, D.E., Siegel, D., Niesvizky, R., Boccia, R.V., Stadtmauer, E.A., ... Rajkumar, V. (2009). Expanded safety experience with lenalidomide plus dexamethasone in relapsed or refractory myeloma. *British Journal of Hematology, 146*, 164–170. doi:10.1111/j.1365-2141.2009.07728.x

Colson, K., Doss, D.S., Swift, R., Tariman, J., & Thomas, T.E. (2004). Bortezomib, a newly approved proteasome inhibitor for the treatment of multiple myeloma: Nursing implications. *Clinical Journal of Oncology Nursing, 8*, 473–480. doi:10.1188/04.CJON .473-480

Corso, A., Mangiacavalli, S., Nosari, A., Castagnola, A., Zappasodi, P., Cafro, A.M., ... Lazzarino, M. (2005). Efficacy, toxicity and feasibility of a shorter schedule of DCEP regimen for stem cell mobilization in multiple myeloma. *Bone Marrow Transplantation, 36*, 951–954. doi:10.1038/sj.bmt.1705166

Dadacaridou, M., Papanicolaou, X., Maltesas, D., Megalakaki, C., Patos, P., Panteli, K., ... Mitsouli-Mentzikof, C. (2007). Dexamethasone, cyclophosphamide, etoposide and cisplatin (DCEP) for relapsed or refractory multiple myeloma patients. *Journal of the Balkan Union of Oncology, 12*, 41–44.

Dudeney, S., Lieberman, I.H., Reinhardt, M.K., & Hussein, M. (2002). Kyphoplasty in the treatment of osteolytic vertebral compression fractures as a result of multiple myeloma. *Journal of Clinical Oncology, 20*, 2382–2387. doi:10.1200/JCO.2002.09.097

Durie, B.G., Kyle, R.A., Belch, A., Bensinger, W., Blade, J., Boccadoro, M., ... Van Ness, B. (2003). Myeloma management guidelines: A consensus report from the Scientific Advisors of the International Myeloma Foundation. *Hematology Journal, 4*, 379–398. doi:10.1038/sj.thj.6200312

Durie, B.G., Harousseau, J.-L., Miguel, J.S., Blade, J., Barlogie, B., Anderson, K., ... Rajkumar, S.V. (2006). International uniform response criteria for multiple myeloma. *Leukemia, 20*, 1467–1473. doi:10.1038/sj.leu.2404284

Fabian, C.J., Molina, R., Slavik, M., Dahlberg, S., Giri, S., & Stephens, R. (1990). Pyridoxine therapy for palmar-plantar erythrodysesthesia associated with continuous 5-fluorouracil infusion. *Investigational New Drugs, 8*, 57–63. doi:10.1007/BF00216925

Gerszten, P.C., Germanwala, A., Burton, S.A., Welch, W.C., Ozhasoglu, C., & Vogel, W.J. (2005). Combination kyphoplasty and spinal radio surgery: A new treatment paradigm for pathological fractures. *Journal of Neurosurgery: Spine, 3*, 296–301. doi:10.3171/ spi.2005.3.4.0296

Goldschmidt, H., Lannert, H., Bommer, J., & Ho, A.D. (2000). Multiple myeloma and renal failure. *Nephrology, Dialysis, Transplantation, 15*, 301–304. doi:10.1093/ndt/15.3.301

Greipp, P.R., San Miguel, J., Durie, B.G., Crowley, J.J., Barlogie, B., Blade, J., ... Westin, J. (2005). International staging system for multiple myeloma. *Journal of Clinical Oncology, 23*, 3412–3420. doi:10.1200/JCO.2005.04.242

Harousseau, J.-L. (2008). Induction therapy in multiple myeloma. *Hematology: American Society of Hematology Education Program Book, 2008*, 306–312. doi:10.1182/asheducation-2008.1.306

Hu, K., & Yahalom, J. (2000). Radiotherapy in the management of plasma cell tumors. *Oncology, 14*, 101–108, 111.

Hussein, M.A., Wood, L., Saluan, M.A., Lee, E.J., Fletcher, R., & Schiffer, C.A. (1998). Efficacy of pyridoxine to ameliorate percutaneous toxicity associated with Doxil [Abstract No. 4143]. *Proceedings of the American Society of Hematology, 92*, 265b.

Hussein, M.A., Vrionis, F.D., Allison, R., Berenson, J., Berven, S., Erdem, E., ... Durie, B.G.M. (2008). The role of vertebral augmentation in multiple myeloma: International

Myeloma Working Group Consensus Statement. *Leukemia, 22,* 1479–1484. doi:10.1038/leu.2008.127

Jagannath, S., Durie, B.G.M., Wolf, J.L., Camacho, E.S., Irwin, D., Lutzky, J., ... Vescio, R. (2006). Long-term follow-up of patients treated with bortezomib alone and in combination with dexamethasone as frontline therapy for multiple myeloma [Abstract No. 796]. *Blood, 108.* Retrieved from http://abstracts.hematologylibrary.org/cgi/content/abstract/108/11/796

Kim, S.J., Kim, K., Kim, B.S., Lee, H.J., Kim, H., Lee, N.R., ... Shin, H.J. (2008). Bortezomib and the increased incidence of herpes zoster in patients with multiple myeloma. *Clinical Lymphoma, Myeloma and Leukemia, 8,* 237–240. doi:10.3816/CLM.2008.n.031

Kumar, S., & Rajkumar, S.V. (2006). Thalidomide and lenalidomide in the treatment of multiple myeloma. *European Journal of Cancer, 42,* 1612–1622. doi:10.1016/j.ejca.2006.04.004

Kumar, S.K., Rajkumar, S.V., Dispenzieri, A., Lacy, M.Q., Hayman, S.R., Buadi, F.K., ... Gertz, M.A. (2008). Improved survival in multiple myeloma and the impact of novel therapies. *Blood, 111,* 2516–2520. doi:10.1182/blood-2007-10-116129

Kyle, R.A., Yee, G.C., Somerfield, M.R., Flynn, P.J., Halabi, S., Jagannath, S., ... Anderson, K. (2007). American Society of Clinical Oncology 2007 clinical practice guideline update on the role of bisphosphonates in multiple myeloma. *Journal of Clinical Oncology, 25,* 2464–2472. doi:10.1200/JCO.2007.12.1269

Lazzarino, M., Corso, A., Barbarano, L., Alessandrino, E.P., Cairoli, R., Pinotti, G., ... Morra, E. (2001). DCEP (dexamethasone, cyclophosphamide, etoposide, and cisplatin) is an effective regimen for peripheral blood stem cell collection in multiple myeloma. *Bone Marrow Transplantation, 28,* 835–839. doi:10.1038/sj.bmt.1703240

Lee, C.-K., Barlogie, B., Munshi, N., Zangari, M., Fassas, A., Jacobson, J., ... Tricot, G. (2003). DTPACE: An effective, novel combination chemotherapy with thalidomide for previously treated patients with myeloma. *Journal of Clinical Oncology, 21,* 2732–2739. doi:10.1200/JCO.2003.01.055

Lee, I., Ryu, S., Gates, M., Jain, R., James, K., Nerenz, D., & Rock, J. (2007). *Spinal canal compromise: Is radiosurgery a reasonable treatment alternative?* [Abstract No. 40830]. Retrieved from http://www.aans.org/library/article.aspx?ShowMenu=false&ShowPrint=false&ArticleId=40830

Lonial, S. (2007). Designing risk-adapted therapy for multiple myeloma: The Mayo perspective. *Mayo Clinic Proceedings, 82,* 279–281. doi:10.4065/82.3.279

Major, P., Lortholary, A., Hon, J., Abdi, E., Mills, G., Menssen, H.D., ... Seaman, J. (2001). Zoledronic acid is superior to pamidronate in the treatment of hypercalcemia of malignancy: A pooled analysis of two randomized, controlled clinical trials. *Journal of Clinical Oncology, 19,* 558–567.

Miceli, T., Colson, K., Gavino, M., & Lilleby, K. (2008). Myelosuppression associated with novel therapies in patients with multiple myeloma: Consensus statement of the IMF Nurse Leadership Board. *Clinical Journal of Oncology Nursing, 12*(Suppl. 3), 13–20. doi:10.1188/08.CJON.S1.13-19

Millennium Pharmaceuticals, Inc. (2009). Velcade (bortezomib) [Package insert]. Retrieved from http://www.velcade.com/full_prescrib_velcade.pdf

Montefusco, V., Gay, F., Spina, F., Miceli, R., Maniezzo, M., Teresa Ambrosini, M., ... Corradini, P. (2008). Antibiotic prophylaxis before dental procedures may reduce the incidence of osteonecrosis of the jaw in patients with multiple myeloma treated with bisphosphonates. *Leukemia and Lymphoma, 49,* 2156–2162. doi:10.1080/10428190802483778

Munshi, N.C., Desikan, K.R., Jagannath, S., Siegel, D., Bracy, D., Tricot, G., & Barlogie, B. (1996). Dexamethasone, cyclophosphamide, etoposide and cis-platinum (DCEP), an effective regimen for relapse after high-dose chemotherapy and autologous transplantation (AT) [Abstract 2231]. *Blood, 88*(Suppl. 1), 586a.

Munshi, N.C., Tricot, G., & Barlogie, B. (2001). Plasma cell neoplasms. In V.T. De Vita Jr., S. Hellman, & S.A. Rosenberg (Eds.), *Cancer: Principles and practice of oncology* (6th ed., pp. 2465–2493). Philadelphia, PA: Lippincott Williams & Wilkins.

National Comprehensive Cancer Network. (2009). *NCCN Clinical Practice Guidelines in Oncology™: Cancer- and chemotherapy-induced anemia* [v.2.2010]. Retrieved from http://www.nccn.org/professionals/physician_gls/PDF/anemia.pdf

Niesvizky, R., Jayabalan, D., Zafar, F., Christos, P., Pearse, R., Jalbrzikowski, J.B., ... Coleman, M. (2007). BiRD (Biaxin®/Revlimid®/dexamethasone) in myeloma (MM) [Abstract No. PO-714]. *Haematologica, 92*(Suppl. 2), 178.

Ng, A.K., & Mauch, P.M. (2005). Radiation therapy in the treatment of hematologic malignancies. In R. Hoffman, E.J. Benz, S.J. Shattil, B. Furie, J.H. Cohen, L.E. Silberstein, & P. McGlave (Eds.), *Hematology: Basic principles and practice* (4th ed., pp. 899–906). Philadelphia, PA: Elsevier Churchill Livingstone.

Novartis Pharmaceuticals Corp. (2008a). Aredia (pamidronate disodium) [Package insert]. Retrieved from http://www.pharma.us.novartis.com/product/pi/pdf/aredia.pdf

Novartis Pharmaceuticals Corp. (2008b). Zometa (zoledronic acid) [Package insert]. Retrieved from http://www.us.zometa.com/info/prescribe.jsp

Orlowski, R.Z., Nagler, A., Sonneveld, P., Blade, J., Hajek, R., Spencer, A., ... Harousseau, J.-L. (2007). Randomized phase III study of pegylated liposomal doxorubicin plus bortezomib compared with bortezomib alone in relapsed or refractory multiple myeloma: Combination therapy improves time to progression. *Journal of Clinical Oncology, 25*, 3892–3901. doi:10.1200/JCO.2006.10.5460

Ozsahin, M., Tsang, R.W., Poortmans, P., Belkacemi, Y., Bolla, M., Dincbas, F.O., ... Zouhair, A. (2006). Outcomes and patterns of failure in solitary plasmacytoma: A multicenter Rare Cancer Network study of 258 patients. *International Journal of Radiation Oncology, Biology, Physics, 64*, 210–217. doi:10.1016/j.ijrobp.2005.06.039

Palumbo, A., Rajkumar, S.V., Dimopoulos, M.A., Richardson, P.G., San Miguel, J., Barlogie, B., ... Hussein, M.A. (2008). Prevention of thalidomide- and lenalidomide-associated thrombosis in myeloma. *Leukemia, 22*, 414–423. doi:10.1038/sj.leu.2405062

Patel, J.S. (1999). Pyridoxine for hand-foot syndrome. *Hospital Pharmacy, 34*, 605–609.

Poruchynsky, M.S., Sackett, D.L., Robey, R.W., Ward, Y., Annunziata, C., & Fojo, T. (2008). Proteasome inhibitors increase tubulin polymerization and stabilization in tissue culture cells: A possible mechanism contributing to peripheral neuropathy and cellular toxicity following proteasome inhibition. *Cell Cycle, 7*, 940–949.

Rajkumar, S.V. (2008). Treatment of myeloma: Cure vs control. *Mayo Clinic Proceedings, 83*, 1142–1145. doi:10.4065/83.10.1142

Rajkumar, S.V., & Dispenzieri, A. (2008). Multiple myeloma. In M.D. Abeloff, J.O. Armitage, J.E. Niederhuber, M.E. Kastan, & W.G. McKenna (Eds.), *Abeloff's clinical oncology* (4th ed., pp. 2323–2352). Philadelphia, PA: Saunders.

Richards, T. (2008). The nurse's role in improving compliance. *Oncology Nurse, 8*, 5–8.

Richards, T. (2009). Managing the side effects of lenalidomide and bortezomib. *Community Oncology, 6*, 55–58.

Richardson, P., Jagannath, S., Hussein, M., Berenson, J., Singhal, S., Irwin, D., ... Anderson, K.C. (2009). Safety and efficacy of single-agent lenalidomide in patients with relapsed and refractory multiple myeloma. *Blood, 114*, 772–778. doi:10.1182/blood-2008-12-196238

Richardson, P.G., Barlogie, B., Berenson, J., Singhal, S., Jagannath, S., Irwin, D., ... Anderson, K.C. (2003). A phase 2 study of bortezomib in relapsed, refractory myeloma. *New England Journal of Medicine, 348*, 2609–2617. doi:10.1056/NEJMoa030288

Richardson, P.G., Sonneveld, P., Schuster, M.W., Irwin, D., Stadtmauer, E.A., Facon, T., ... Anderson, K.C. (2005). Bortezomib or high-dose dexamethasone for relapsed multiple myeloma. *New England Journal of Medicine, 352*, 2487–2498. doi:10.1056/NEJMoa043445

Richardson, P.G., Sonneveld, P., Schuster, M.W., Irwin, D., Stadtmauer, E.A., Facon, T., ... Anderson, K.C. (2007). Safety and efficacy of bortezomib in high-risk and elderly patients with relapsed multiple myeloma. *British Journal of Haematology, 137*, 429–435. doi:10.1111/j.1365-2141.2007.06585.x

Rome, S., Doss, D., Miller, K., & Westphal, J. (2008). Thromboembolic events associated with novel therapies in patients with multiple myeloma: Consensus statement of the IMF Nurse Leadership Board. *Clinical Journal of Oncology Nursing, 12,* 21–28. doi:10.1188/08. CJON.S1.21-27

Ronco, P.M., Aucouturier, P., & Mougenot, B. (2007). Monoclonal gammopathies: Myeloma, amyloidosis and related disorders. In R.W. Schrier (Ed.), *Diseases of the kidney and urinary tract* (8th ed., Vol. III, pp. 1941–1985). Philadelphia, PA: Lippincott Williams & Wilkins.

Roodman, G.D. (2008). Skeletal imaging and management of bone disease. *Hematology: American Society of Hematology Education Program Book, 2008,* 313–319. doi:10.1182/ash-education-2008.1.313

Rowell, N.P., & Tobias, J.S. (1991). The role of radiotherapy in the management of multiple myeloma. *Blood Reviews, 5,* 84–89.

San Miguel, J.F., Schlag, R., Khuageva, N.K., Dimopoulos, M.A., Shpilberg, O., Kropff, M., ... Richardson, P.G. (2008). Bortezomib plus melphalan and prednisone for initial treatment of multiple myeloma. *New England Journal of Medicine, 359,* 906–917. doi:10.1056/ NEJMoa0801479

Shpilberg, O., Douer, D., Ehrenfeld, M., Engelberg, S., & Ramot, B. (1990). Naproxen-associated acute renal failure in myeloma. *Nephron, 55,* 448–449. doi:10.1159/000186023

Silverberg, D., Blum, M., Peer, G., & Iaina, A. (1998). Anemia during the predialysis period: A key to cardiac damage in renal failure. *Nephron, 80,* 1–5. doi:10.1159/000045118

Singhal, S., Mehta, J., Desikan, R., Ayers, D., Roberson, P., Eddlemon, P., ... Crowley, J. (1999). Antitumor activity of thalidomide in refractory multiple myeloma. *New England Journal of Medicine, 341,* 1565–1571. doi:10.1056/NEJM199911183412102

Smith, L.C., Bertolotti, P., Curran, K., & Jenkins, B. (2008). Gastrointestinal side effects associated with novel therapies in patients with multiple myeloma: Consensus statement of the IMF Nurse Leadership Board. *Clinical Journal of Oncology Nursing, 12*(Suppl. 3), 37–52. doi:10.1188/08.CJON.S1.37-51

Stadtmauer, E.A., Weber, D.M., Niesvizky, R., Belch, A., Prince, M.H., San Miguel, J.F., ... Dimopoulos, M.A. (2009). Lenalidomide in combination with dexamethasone at first relapse in comparison with its use as later salvage therapy in relapsed or refractory multiple myeloma. *European Journal of Haematology, 82,* 426–432. doi:10.1111/j.1600-0609.2009.01257.x

Tariman, J.D., Love, G., McCullagh, E., & Sandifer, S. (2008). Peripheral neuropathy associated with novel therapies in patients with multiple myeloma: Consensus statement of the IMF Nurse Leadership Board. *Clinical Journal of Oncology Nursing, 12*(Suppl. 3), 29–36. doi:10.1188/08.CJON.S1.29-35

von Moos, R., Thuerlimann, B.J.K., Aapro, M., Rayson, D., Harrold, K., Sehouli, J., ... Hauschild, A. (2008). Pegylated liposomal doxorubicin-associated hand-foot syndrome: Recommendations of an international panel of experts. *European Journal of Cancer, 44,* 781–790. doi:10.1016/j.ejca.2008.01.028

Vukelja, S.J., Lombardo, F.A., James, W.D., & Weiss, R.B. (1989). Pyridoxine for palmar-plantar erythrodysesthesia syndrome. *Annals of Internal Medicine, 111,* 688–689.

Weber, D.M. (2005). Solitary bone and extramedullary plasmacytoma. *Hematology: American Society of Hematology Education Program Book, 2005,* 373–376. doi:10.1182/asheducation-2005.1.373

Weber, D.M., Chen, C., Niesvizky, R., Wang, M., Belch, A., Stadtmauer, E.A., ... Knight, R.D. (2007). Lenalidomide plus dexamethasone for relapsed multiple myeloma in North America. *New England Journal of Medicine, 357,* 2133–2142. doi:10.1056/NEJMoa070596

Wolf, S., Barton, D., Kottschade, L., Grothey, A., & Loprinzi, C. (2008). Chemotherapy-induced peripheral neuropathy: Prevention and treatment strategies. *European Journal of Cancer, 44,* 1507–1515. doi:10.1016/j.ejca.2008.04.018

Yee, S. (1998). *Prevention and management of Doxil-related side effects: Basic strategies* [Abstract No. 281]. Retrieved from http://search.asco.org/ASCOv2/Meetings/ Abstracts?&vmview=abst_detail_view&confID=31&abstractID=5712

Yeh, H.S., & Berenson, J.R. (2006). Treatment for myeloma bone disease. *Clinical Cancer Research, 12,* 6279s–6284s. doi:10.1158/1078-0432.CCR-06-0681

Zangari, M., Siegel, E., Barlogie, B., Anaissie, E., Saghafifar, F., Fassas, A., … Tricot, G. (2002). Thrombogenic activity of doxorubicin in myeloma patients receiving thalidomide: Implications for therapy. *Blood, 100,* 1168–1171. doi:10.1182/blood-2002-01-0335

Zonder, J.A. (2006). Thrombotic complications of myeloma therapy. *Hematology: Education Program of the American Society of Hematology, 2006,* 348–355. doi:10.1182/asheducation -2006.1.348

Management and Evaluation of Patients Receiving High-Dose Chemotherapy With Stem Cell Transplantation

Anna Liza Rodriguez, RN, MSN, MHA, OCN®

INTRODUCTION

Several randomized trials have shown the superiority of stem cell transplantation (SCT) with high-dose chemotherapy over conventional chemotherapy. High-dose chemotherapy affords maximum cytoreduction in patients with multiple myeloma. Stem cell transplant rescue is imperative for bone marrow recovery following myeloablative chemotherapy. It is critical that oncology nurses develop the expertise to prevent and manage complications associated with high-dose chemotherapy with SCT.

Stem cells are progenitor hematopoietic cells with the capacity to repopulate marrow spaces, differentiating to various blood cell lineages. Peripheral blood has gradually replaced bone marrow as the preferred source of stem cells since the discovery of the peripheral blood progenitor cells in the hematopoietic reconstitution (Reddy, 2005). Table 9-1 explains how SCT is categorized based on the origin of the stem cells. The SCT process begins with a comprehensive evaluation of the patient to determine eligibility for SCT and type of SCT followed by stem cell mobilization, stem cell collection, stem cell processing and cryopreservation, and reinfusion or transplantation. Figure 9-1 lists common exclusion criteria for stem cell transplantation. See Figure 7-2 in Chapter 7 for an illustration of the stem cell transplant process. Figure 9-2 lists the various stem cell transplantation options in patients with multiple myeloma.

Table 9-1. Categories of Stem Cell Transplantation			
Category	Stem Cell Source	Advantages	Disadvantages
Autolo-gous	Patient	Readily available stem cells Decreased incidence and severity of side effects Earlier engraftment Absence of graft-versus-host disease (GVHD)	Potentially contaminated cells Earlier relapse because of lack of graft-versus-tumor (GVT) effect
Allogeneic	Related (sibling) or matched unrelated donor	Replacement of diseased or damaged marrow with healthy cells GVT effect	Organ toxicity GVHD
Syngeneic	Identical twin	Same as with autologous stem cell transplantation	Lack of GVT effect
Note. Based on information from Niess & Duffy, 2004.			

Figure 9-1. Exclusion Criteria* for Stem Cell Transplantation
• Serum creatinine greater than 0.25 mmol/L • Serum bilirubin greater than 40 mmol/L • Left ventricular ejection fraction less than 50% • Poor performance status
*This list is not exhaustive and may vary per program. Note. Based on information from Flowers & Sullivan, 2004.

PATIENT EVALUATION

Patients undergo a comprehensive evaluation prior to stem cell transplantation largely because of the life-threatening complications of the procedure. Figure 9-3 lists the goals of the pretransplant evaluation. Both the recipient and the donor complete a series of examinations (see Table 9-2). General considerations for transplant eligibility include chemotherapy-sensitive disease, adequate organ function, and no life-threatening viral exposures or comorbidities (Niess & Duffy, 2004). Special attention is given to the determination of organ dysfunctions that could exclude the patient from myeloablative conditioning or increase regimen-related toxicity (Flowers & Sullivan, 2004). Based on the patient's eligibility, the stem cell transplant strategy and plan of care are determined. Comprehensive patient education is performed during the initial stage of the transplantation process to ensure a detailed review of

Figure 9-2. Stem Cell Transplant Options in Patients With Multiple Myeloma

- Myeloablative single autologous SCT (ASCT)
- Tandem transplant
  - Double myeloablative ASCT
  - Myeloablative ASCT and myeloablative human leukocyte antigen (HLA)-matched allogeneic SCT (alloSCT)
  - Myeloablative ASCT and myeloablative HLA-matched matched unrelated donor SCT
  - Myeloablative ASCT and reduced-intensity conditioning HLA-matched alloSCT
  - Myeloablative ASCT and reduced-intensity conditioning matched unrelated donor alloSCT
- Myeloablative alloSCT
- Reduced-intensity conditioning alloSCT

Figure 9-3. Goals of Pretransplant Comprehensive Patient Evaluation

- Obtain informed consent.
- Confirm diagnosis and status of underlying disease.
- Assess patient and donor physical and psychological functioning.
- Assess patient and family psychosocial and support structure.
- Assess patient organ functioning.
- Confirm human leukocyte antigen typing.
- Establish the transplant type (autologous, allogeneic).
- Establish the transplant protocol/regimen (myeloablative, nonmyeloablative).
- Identify and treat coexisting comorbidities.
- Provide patient education.

Note. Based on information from Flowers & Sullivan, 2004; Niess & Duffy, 2004.

Table 9-2. Patient and Donor Evaluation

Evaluation	Patient	Donor
Review of records	X	X
History and physical assessment • History of illness • History of hematologic problems • Cancer history • Transfusion history • Adverse anesthesia reaction • Current medication • Allergies • Risk factors for HIV or viral hepatitis infection • Pregnancy history for females	X	X
Review of original diagnostic tests • Review of slides, pathology report, imaging tests	X	

(Continued on next page)

Table 9-2. Patient and Donor Evaluation *(Continued)*

Evaluation	Patient	Donor
Bone marrow aspirate and core biopsies • Aspirate for flow cytometry to determine clonality • Aspirate for cytogenetics or fluorescence in situ hybridization study • Plasma cell labeling index to determine proliferative rate of plasma cells	X	
Laboratory tests • Complete blood count with platelet and reticulocyte counts • Comprehensive chemistry panel including electrolytes, blood urea nitrogen, creatinine, alkaline phosphatase, alanine aminotransaminase, aspartate aminotransferase, bilirubin, lactic dehydrogenase, cholesterol, triglycerides, immunoglobulin levels • Coagulation tests: partial thromboplastin time, activated partial thromboplastin time • Serology for cytomegalovirus, HIV, hepatitis B virus, hepatitis C virus, human T-lymphocyte virus 1 and 2, herpes simplex virus, varicella zoster virus, Epstein-Barr virus	X X X X	X X X X
HLA and blood typing • Including DNA studies and leukocyte crossmatch	X	X
Imaging • Chest x-ray[a] • Magnetic resonance imaging • Computed tomography scan • Skeletal survey • Bone scan	X X X X X	X
Electrocardiogram[a]	X	X
Cardiac ejection studies	X	
Pulmonary function tests	X	
Special consults • Social worker • Nutritionist	X X	
Multiple myeloma–specific tests • Quantitative immunoglobulin • Serum and 24-hour urine protein electrophoresis • Serum and urine immunofixation • C-reactive protein and serum beta-2 microglobulin	X X X X	

[a] Donor evaluation only as appropriate

Note. Based on information from Flowers & Sullivan, 2004; National Comprehensive Cancer Network, 2009b; Niess & Duffy, 2004.

the natural history of the underlying disease, alternative therapies, results of all diagnostic tests and evaluations, the stem cell transplant process and associated risks, and post-transplant recovery. Figure 9-4 lists pretransplant support and prophylaxis as indicated.

HUMAN LEUKOCYTE ANTIGEN TYPING

The degree of match in human leukocyte antigen (HLA) typing between the patient (recipient) and the stem cell donor predicts the severity of complications and patient outcome after allogeneic SCT (alloSCT). The selection of both sibling and unrelated donors is based on tissue typing of the HLA, also called the major histocompatibility complex. Six major antigens exist in class I HLA (A, B, C) and class II HLA (DR, DQ, DP). Each parent accounts for one haplotype (a group of alleles of different genes on a single chromosome) to make up the combination of class I and class II antigens expressed by a person—an HLA phenotype consisting of two sets of the six major antigens. The donor search is focused on finding donors with a 10 out of 10 allele match. Other donor considerations include gender, weight, and overall health. Favorable donor characteristics include being male, being young, being at a healthy weight, and being in excellent overall health (DeMeyer, 2009).

STEM CELL MOBILIZATION

The peripheralization or mobilization of progenitor cells occurs as stem cells shift from the bone marrow to the circulatory system, rendering them easily accessible by apheresis (Korbling, 2004). Two techniques for increas-

---

Figure 9-4. Pretransplant Support and Prophylaxis

Pneumocystis prophylaxis
- Trimethoprim-sulfamethoxazole (TMP-SMX)
- Dapsone if TMP-SMX not tolerated
- Aerosolized pentamidine

Cytomegalovirus (CMV) prevention
- Transfuse CMV-seronegative and leukocyte-depleted blood products only.
- Ganciclovir if positive CMV antigenemia
- Foscarnet if CMV viremia occurs while on ganciclovir

Herpes simplex virus (HSV) prevention
- Acyclovir
- Valacyclovir

Antibacterial prophylaxis
- Started when absolute neutrophil count falls below 0.5×10^9/L
- Quinolone antibiotic, usually levofloxacin

Antifungal prophylaxis
- Fluconazole

ing the number of circulating stem cells in the peripheral bloodstream are chemotherapy priming and cytokine priming. Chemotherapy priming, as the term suggests, uses chemotherapy. Cytokine priming uses granulocyte–colony-stimulating factor (G-CSF) or granulocyte-macrophage–colony-stimulating factor (GM-CSF). Filgrastim and pegfilgrastim have been used for stem cell mobilization. Studies indicated approximately a 14-fold increase in circulating stem cells using chemotherapy mobilization alone (To et al., 1992), an 18-fold increase using GM-CSF, and approximately a 60-fold increase using a combination of GM-CSF and chemotherapy (Socinski et al., 1988). Combined cytokine and chemotherapy mobilization works synergistically, resulting in a higher stem cell yield.

In autologous SCT (ASCT), cytokine priming is indicated for patients who are unable to tolerate additional chemotherapy. A prospective randomized clinical trial comparing the efficacy of chemotherapy plus either G-CSF or GM-CSF for peripheral blood stem cell mobilization, followed by ASCT in patients with multiple myeloma, showed that mobilization with chemotherapy plus G-CSF versus GM-CSF resulted in similar CD34+ progenitor collections (Arora et al., 2004) (see Chapter 2 for more detailed information about CD34+ progenitor cells). The most common dose of GM-CSF is 125–250 mcg/m²/day, and the most common dose of G-CSF is 5–10 mcg/kg/day. Patients tolerate G-CSF better than GM-CSF. Additionally, the use of G-CSF-mobilized peripheral stem cells is documented to decrease the time to recovery of granulocytes and platelets after ASCT (Korbling, 2004). Recently, study data indicated feasibility and efficacy of stem cell mobilization using pegfilgrastim and filgrastim, with greater ease and cost-effectiveness associated with the former (Tricot et al., 2008). Chemotherapy mobilization combined with growth factor administration is the preferred mobilization strategy. Figure 9-5 lists common mobilization regimens for multiple myeloma. Allogeneic donors are mobilized with hematopoietic growth factors.

Management of patients undergoing stem cell mobilization includes symptom management of toxicities to the mobilization regimen. For high-dose cyclophosphamide regimens, hyperhydration of 4 liters of normal saline continuous infusion over 24 hours is started 12 hours before the cyclophosphamide infusion and continued 12 hours after to prevent hemorrhagic cystitis. Uroprotectants such as mesna are administered before and after the cyclophosphamide infusion. The total dose of mesna is equal to the total cyclophosphamide dose and is administered daily in three divided doses during cyclophosphamide infusion. Antiemetics are provided as ordered to manage chemotherapy-related nausea and vomiting. Patients' complete blood counts are monitored to determine hematologic toxicities. Neutropenic and thrombocytopenic precautions are instituted as needed. Blood products are transfused as indicated. The most common side effects associated with the use of growth factors usually are dose related and include bone pain, fever, and body malaise. Acetaminophen usually is administered. Other reported symptoms include chills, headache, nausea, vomiting, diarrhea, edema, rash,

Figure 9-5. Common Mobilization Regimens in Multiple Myeloma
Low-dose cyclophosphamide (CY) plus granulocyte–colony-stimulating factor (G-CSF) • CY 1–2 g/m^2 • G-CSF 10 mcg/kg Intermediate-dose CY plus G-CSF • CY 3–4 g/m^2 • G-CSF 5 mcg/kg High-dose CY plus G-CSF • CY 4–7 g/m^2 • G-CSF 5 mcg/kg VAD plus G-CSF • Doxorubicin 9 mg/m^2/day days 1–5 • Vincristine 0.4 mg/day days 1–5 • Dexamethasone 40 mg/day days 1–5 • G-CSF 10 mcg/kg days 10–15 CHOP with or without G-CSF • Doxorubicin 90 mg/m^2 day 1 • Cyclophosphamide 1,500 mg/m^2 day 1 • Vincristine 2 mg/day day 1 • Prednisone 80 mg/m^2 day 1–5 • G-CSF 5 mcg/kg/day D-CEP plus G-CSF • Dexamethasone 40 mg for four days • Cyclophosphamide 400 mg/m^2 days 1–4 • Etoposide 40 mg/m^2 days 1–4 • Cisplatin 10 mg/m^2 days 1–4 • G-CSF 5 mcg/kg/day 48 hours after end of D-CEP infusion
Note. Based on information from Corso et al., 2002; Lefrere et al., 2006; Lerro et al., 2003.

irritation at injection site, dyspnea, pleural or pericardial effusion, and nasal congestion, usually resolving upon discontinuation of the growth factor (Schmit-Pokorny, 2004).

STEM CELL COLLECTION

The general consensus among clinicians is that the minimum peripheral CD34+ cell count should be 2–5 × 10^6 CD34+/kg body weight. A predictor of CD34+ harvest yield is the hematopoietic progenitor cell count (Vogel, Kopp, Kantz, & Einsele, 2002). The number of CD34+ cells in the peripheral blood is also a guide to optimal timing to harvest (Basquiera et al., 2006). A blood CD34+ concentration of 15–40/microliter is believed to produce a sufficient CD34+ cell yield (Korbling, 2004). In most patients, the required minimal cell dose of 2.5–5 × 10^6/kg CD34+ cells can be collected in one or two apheresis collections (Reddy, 2005). A few ASCT recipients who mobilize stem cells poorly will require several attempts of apheresis procedures. Allogeneic donor stem cell collections usually are completed in one or two apheresis procedures. Cell separator machines such as the Cobe® Spectra (CaridianBCT, Inc.), Haemonetics V50® (Haemonetics) and the Fenwal CS-3000® (Fenwal, Inc.) are commonly used (Schmit-Pokorny, 2004).

Although antecubital peripheral IV lines may be used to collect stem cells, a thick-walled, large-bore catheter (14G), yielding the highest flow rate during apheresis, is preferred (Schmit-Pokorny, 2004). Venous access sites for apheresis include the jugular vein, the inferior vena cava, the femoral vein, and the subclavian vein. The subclavian vein usually is the preferred site. Immediately after catheter placement, the nurse should carefully assess the site for oozing or frank bleeding from the site, as additional sutures may be required to halt the bleeding. Swelling and discoloration or bruising from the site may indicate hematoma and necessitate removal of the catheter. Ongoing assessment throughout the duration of catheter placement is performed to monitor for signs and symptoms of infection, occlusion, and catheter-related venous thrombosis. Erythema, tenderness, swelling, and drainage at the insertion site along with fevers can indicate IV line infection. The nurse should obtain IV line site drainage and blood cultures peripherally and through all central line lumens. Antibiotics usually are prescribed when cultures are positive. Signs of occlusion include swelling and an inability to flush the line with patient repositioning. The nurse must administer alteplase (2 mg/2 ml) into the lumen of the occluded catheter, allow it to dwell for 30 minutes, and then aspirate the catheter (may repeat once). The IV line must be removed if occlusion is not resolved.

During the stem cell collection procedure, approximately 12–15 liters of blood are processed, taking two to four hours. Hematologic complications can arise during the procedure, including anemia and transient thrombocytopenia. Transfusion of blood components may be required as ordered. Other complications include transient hypotension (Goldberg et al., 1995) and symptomatic citrate toxicity as the sodium citrate used to prevent blood from clotting in the apheresis machine binds to ionized calcium (Schmit-Pokorny, 2004). The nurse should assess baseline calcium levels prior to stem cell collection. If calcium is low, the nurse must obtain an order for calcium replacement. It is important to assess the patient for hypotension, tachycardia, light-headedness, diaphoresis, and dysrhythmias. Additionally, the nurse must notify the physician with any abnormal finding and hold stem collection until symptoms resolve or until the patient is stable. Table 9-3 lists general considerations prior to stem cell collection.

STEM CELL PROCESSING AND CRYOPRESERVATION

After stem cell collection, cells are further tested for sterility and infectious diseases. The AABB (formerly known as American Association of Blood Banks) and other transplant-related organizations recommend the following tests (AABB et al., 2007).

Table 9-3. General Considerations Before Starting Stem Cell Collection	
Indicator	**Parameter**
Venous access	Patency established
Colony-stimulating growth factor	Administered two hours prior to collection
Hemoglobin prior to start of collection	9–11 g/dl or per institutional protocol
Platelets prior to start of collection	Greater than 40,000/microliter for autologous donors or per institutional protocol 120,000/microliter for normal donors or per institutional protocol
Note. Based on information from Korbling, 2004, Schmit-Pokorny, 2004.	

- HIV type 1 and 2
- Hepatitis B virus
- Hepatitis C virus
- Human T-cell lymphotropic virus type I and II
- Cytomegalovirus
- *Treponema pallidum* (syphilis)
- ABO blood group and Rh type
- HLA type
- Screening for hemoglobinopathies

The cells are then appropriately labeled and cryopreserved. Dimethyl sulfoxide (DMSO) is the most commonly used cryoprotectant in the cryopreservation of stem cells (Szer, 2004). DMSO stabilizes the cell membrane, preventing ice crystal formation and destruction during freezing and thawing. A 10% DMSO concentration plus 5% human serum albumin is a typical freezing mixture. However, recent studies investigating long-term cryopreservation of autologous stem cells concluded that 5% DMSO is the optimal concentration for cryopreservation (Bakken, 2006; Liseth et al., 2009). After the addition of the cryoprotectant, the stem cells are stored in a −80°F degree freezer for 24 hours and then placed in the vapor phase of liquid nitrogen for long-term storage.

STEM CELL TRANSPLANTATION

Before SCT, a preparative or conditioning regimen is administered. The most commonly used conditioning regimens for ASCT in patients with multiple myeloma are melphalan alone at 200 mg /m² or melphalan 140 mg/m² with or without total body irradiation (TBI) because of the high sensitivity of multiple myeloma cells to both melphalan and TBI. In alloSCT, immunosuppressive therapy to prevent graft-versus-host disease usually is started the day before transplantation (day −1). Corticosteroids, cyclosporine, tacrolimus, mycophenolate mofetil, and methotrexate are the most commonly used immunosuppressive agents during SCT.

Infusion of DMSO-cryopreserved stem cells can cause toxic reactions such as nausea, vomiting, flushing, fever, chills, dyspnea, anaphylaxis, cardiac dysfunction, acute renal failure, and hypertension (Bakken, 2006; Liseth et al., 2009; Szer, 2004). The severity of reactions is related to the concentration of DMSO used. Therefore, premedication with antipyretics, antihistamines, and corticosteroids commonly is administered. Aggressive hydration with fluids and sodium bicarbonate before and throughout the procedure may be administered to alkalinize urine and prevent renal damage from hemolyzed red cells. The stem cell reinfusion is performed at the patient's bedside as shown in Figure 9-6. Careful monitoring of the patient during and immediately after the reinfusion procedure is critical. Nurses need to monitor the patient's vital signs, including pulse oximetry at least every 15 minutes during the infusion and continuing until two hours after. The nurse should observe for any adverse DMSO toxicities, especially an anaphylactic reaction, and stop the infusion for any signs of anaphylaxis. It is critical that the nurse notifies the physician immediately and administers emergency medications

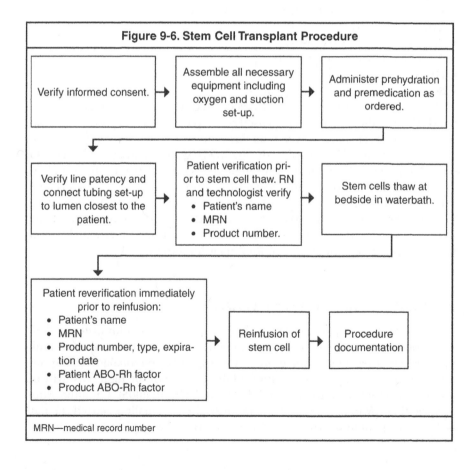

Figure 9-6. Stem Cell Transplant Procedure

Verify informed consent. → Assemble all necessary equipment including oxygen and suction set-up. → Administer prehydration and premedication as ordered.

Verify line patency and connect tubing set-up to lumen closest to the patient. → Patient verification prior to stem cell thaw. RN and technologist verify
• Patient's name
• MRN
• Product number. → Stem cells thaw at bedside in waterbath.

Patient reverification immediately prior to reinfusion:
• Patient's name
• MRN
• Product number, type, expiration date
• Patient ABO-Rh factor
• Product ABO-Rh factor → Reinfusion of stem cell → Procedure documentation

MRN—medical record number

(corticosteroids, antihistamines, diuretics, epinephrine, and vasopressors) and oxygen therapy as ordered (McAdams & Burgunder, 2004; Rodriguez, Tariman, Enecio, & Estrella, 2007). Lastly, institutional policies and procedures during respiratory or cardiac arrest must be strictly followed.

Fresh hematopoietic stem cells typically are used with alloSCT, especially in matched unrelated donor transplantation. The cells usually are taken directly from the donor, processed, and then delivered to the recipient transplant center for immediate reinfusion. Fresh stem cell reinfusion poses less risk for adverse reactions because of the absence of DMSO; however, potential reactions similar to a blood transfusion reaction may still occur, especially if ABO incompatibility between patient and donor exists (McAdams & Burgunder, 2004). The nurse should maintain vigilance in patient observation during the reinfusion process and provide appropriate symptom management.

Immediately after the reinfusion, the nurse must continue to observe the patient and provide education on garlic-like odor, which usually resolves within 24–48 hours, if the patient received cryopreserved products. The patient's urine may be red-tinged as a result of the breakdown of red cells in the stem cell product (McAdams & Burgunder, 2004).

ENGRAFTMENT OR RECOVERY PHASE

The engraftment phase is evidenced by a gradual but steady increase in blood counts. The duration of the patient's white blood cell count recovery is dependent on the rate of recipient or host cell disappearance and the rate of appearance of mature cells generated from the newly infused stem cells. Figure 9-7 describes the phases of engraftment following alloSCT.

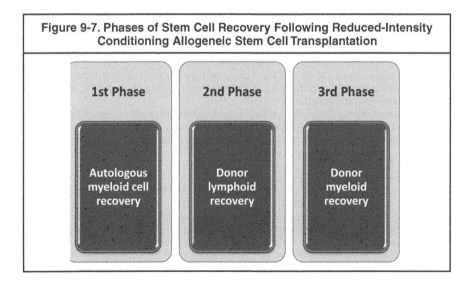

Figure 9-7. Phases of Stem Cell Recovery Following Reduced-Intensity Conditioning Allogeneic Stem Cell Transplantation

1st Phase	2nd Phase	3rd Phase
Autologous myeloid cell recovery	Donor lymphoid recovery	Donor myeloid recovery

CONCLUSION

The care of the patient with multiple myeloma following SCT is complex. Figure 9-8 summarizes the management of patients with multiple myeloma during the SCT procedure. Table 9-4 describes the management of long-term complications of SCT. Prevention, early assessment, and treatment of complications are essential in caring for the transplant recipient. Astute assessment ensures timely symptom management, thus ensuring patient safety and comfort.

Figure 9-8. Summary of Management of the Patient Undergoing High-Dose Chemotherapy and Stem Cell Transplantation

Pretransplant
- Obtain informed consent after full disclosure of the disease process, therapies, risks, and benefits.
- Provide detailed patient education regarding all phases of the treatment plan. Assess patient's comprehension. Reinforce teaching. Provide verbal, written, and electronic patient education resources.
- Ensure patient compliance with diagnostic testing appointments. Review results of examinations and tests with attending physician. All abnormal and critical findings must be reviewed with the transplant team.
- Assess patient's psychosocial and support systems to identify any psychosocial issues that may affect discharge planning and care at home following transplantation.
- Pretransplant supportive care includes
  - Care of the patient's venous access device ensuring patency
  - Transfusion support with blood products as needed depending on hemoglobin and platelet values
  - Appropriate infection prophylaxis. Explain to patient the importance of infection prophylaxis in reducing the number and severity of opportunistic infections.

Stem Cell Mobilization
- Monitor patient and donor for toxicities related to chemotherapy and growth factors.
- Monitor patient's complete blood counts for hematologic toxicities related to chemotherapy and institute appropriate precautions (e.g., neutropenic, thrombocytopenic). Provide blood product transfusion support as needed.
- For cyclophosphamide-based regimens, aggressive hydration is required to prevent hemorrhagic cystitis. Hydration is usually started 12 hours before cyclophosphamide infusion and continues 12 hours after. Administer uroprotectants. Strictly monitor urine output and check for blood. Instruct patient on frequent voiding. Occasionally, continuous bladder irrigation is required.
- Patients and healthy donors should be frequently assessed for side effects related to colony-stimulating factors. Monitor for flu-like symptoms: fever, chills, arthralgias, myalgias, chills, headache, and malaise. Administer acetaminophen.

Stem Cell Collection
- Perform venous access device care to prevent complications.
- Monitor patients for signs of hypocalcemia. Check ionized calcium level, and administer calcium supplement as indicated.
- Because the extracorporeal volume is greater during apheresis, patient or donor may experience symptoms of hypovolemia. Monitor blood pressure, and administer IV fluids as needed.

(Continued on next page)

Figure 9-8. Summary of Management of the Patient Undergoing High-Dose Chemotherapy and Stem Cell Transplantation *(Continued)*

- Apheresis generally is not started for autologous stem cell transplant recipients if the platelet level falls below 20,000/dl because of the transient thrombocytopenia associated with the procedure. Monitor patient for signs and symptoms of bleeding, and administer platelets as needed.

Stem Cell Reinfusion

- Administer hydration hours before reinfusion. Fluids usually contain sodium bicarbonate to alkalinize urine and prevent renal damage related to red cell lysis during the reinfusion.
- Administer premedication including an antipyretic, antihistamine, and corticosteroid to prevent adverse reactions during stem cell reinfusion.
- Monitor patient for signs and symptoms of toxicities related to the cryopreservative dimethyl sulfoxide, such as nausea, vomiting, flushing, fevers, chills, dyspnea, respiratory distress, cardiac arrhythmias, and hypertension. Slow the rate of infusion. For more severe reactions, including anaphylaxis, stop the infusion, notify the physician, and administer emergency medications as indicated. Activate institution-specific emergency teams in the event of respiratory or cardiac arrest.
- For fresh stem cell infusion, observe patient for signs and symptoms of blood transfusion or acute hemolytic reaction.

Note. Based on information from McAdams & Burgunder, 2004; Rodriguez et al., 2007; Schmit-Pokorny, 2004.

Table 9-4. Summary of Complications and Management Following Stem Cell Transplantation

Complication	Manifestation	Intervention/Management
Hematologic complications	Neutropenia	Institute neutropenic precautions. Administer prophylactic antibiotics/antifungal medications as ordered. Institute neutropenic protocol with initial temperature spike (pan culture, IV antibiotics within one hour of initial temperature spike) and thrombocytopenic precautions. Administer colony-stimulating factors as ordered.
	Thrombocytopenia	Monitor for signs of bleeding. Institute thrombocytopenic precautions. Administer platelets as ordered.

(Continued on next page)

Table 9-4. Summary of Complications and Management Following Stem Cell Transplantation *(Continued)*

Complication	Manifestation	Intervention/Management
	Anemia	Administer blood products as needed.
Hepatorenal complications	Veno-occlusive disease: • Elevated liver enzymes • Hepatomegaly • Pain • Fluid retention • Coagulopathies	Monitor liver enzymes. Provide supportive therapy: pain medication, low-dose heparin.
	Renal insufficiency and acute renal failure	Monitor intake and output. Monitor serum urea and creatinine. Provide supportive therapy.
Gastrointestinal complications	Mucositis	Provide meticulous oral hygiene after meals and at bedtime. Provide and instruct patient regarding use of mouth rinses. Administer pain medications as ordered.
	Nausea and vomiting	Administer antiemetics as ordered, preferably before meals. Modify diet: bland, cold or room temperature, low-fat foods; no foods with heavy odors.
	Diarrhea	Monitor strict intake and output. Monitor for signs and symptoms of fluid and electrolyte imbalance. Modify diet; bowel rest may be indicated for severe diarrhea.
Respiratory complications	Diffuse alveolar hemorrhage, idiopathic pneumonia syndrome, bronchiolitis obliterans, pulmonary fibrosis, transfusion-related acute lung injury (TRALI)	Monitor for signs and symptoms of respiratory distress.

(Continued on next page)

Table 9-4. Summary of Complications and Management Following Stem Cell Transplantation *(Continued)*

Complication	Manifestation	Intervention/Management
Infectious complications	Sepsis is a life-threatening consequence in the profoundly immunosuppressed transplant recipient. A patient with sepsis presents with two or more of the following: • Temperature higher than 100.4°F • Heart rate greater than 90 beats/minute • White blood cell count greater than 12,000 or less than 4,000. • Hypotension.	Monitor patient for clinical signs of infection. Administer prophylactic antibiotics, antifungal medications, and *Pneumocystis carinii* (now renamed *Pneumocystis jiroveci*) pneumonia prophylaxis. Obtain vital signs every four hours. Maintain vascular access devices per protocol, and monitor insertion site for any signs and symptoms of infection.
Engraftment syndrome	This is a potentially lethal syndrome associated with prompt hematologic recovery after autologous stem cell transplantation (SCT). It occurs less commonly in allogeneic SCT. The syndrome manifests as noninfectious fever with skin rash, capillary leak, and pulmonary infiltrates. Symptoms occur immediately after stem cell reinfusion in the early pre-engraftment phase (range days +4 to +22).	Initiate corticosteroid therapy as ordered.
Graft-versus-host disease (GVHD) (allogeneic SCT patients only)	Clinically divided into acute and chronic GVHD. Acute GVHD presents during the first 100 days after transplant and most commonly affects the liver, skin, gastrointestinal tract, and immune system. Common presentations include dermatitis and hepatitis. GVHD of the gut presents with abdominal pain, nausea, vomiting, diarrhea, and hyperbilirubinemia. Endoscopic findings indicate mucosal erythema and sloughing. Chronic GVHD presents 100 days after transplant and is more variable in manifestation but commonly involves the skin. Cutaneous manifestations include sclerodermatous or lichenoid skin changes with generalized erythema, plaques, and desquamation.	Administer systemic immunosuppressants; monitor for therapeutic level. Administer poly/monoclonal antibody-based therapies. Administer phototherapy. Provide local/topical therapy: oral, topical corticosteroids. Provide supportive management: pain medication, antiemetics. Provide nutritional support: hyperalimentation as needed.

(Continued on next page)

Table 9-4. Summary of Complications and Management Following Stem Cell Transplantation *(Continued)*		
Complication	**Manifestation**	**Intervention/Management**
Psychological complications	The intense experience of SCT and the associated acute and chronic complications are distressing and traumatic and have the potential to cause prolonged psychosocial distress for both patient and family/caregiver.	Identify vulnerable patients (e.g., patients with existing psychiatric comorbidity, those who lack a strong support system). Administer antidepressants as ordered. Assess patient using the National Comprehensive Cancer Network distress thermometer. Identify support groups and facilitate or coordinate referral. Provide complementary and alternative therapies as available.

Note. Based on information from AABB et al., 2007; Cooke et al., 2009; Cornelissen, 2004; Gorak et al., 2005; Mitchell, 2004; National Comprehensive Cancer Network, 2009a; Saria & Gosselin-Acomb, 2007.

REFERENCES

AABB, America's Blood Centers, American Association of Tissue Banks, American Red Cross, American Society for Apheresis, American Society for Blood and Marrow Transplantation, ... National Marrow Donor Program. (2007). *Circular of information for the use of cellular therapy products.* Retrieved from http://www.aabb.org/Documents/About_Blood/ Circulars_of_Information/coi_ct0607.pdf

Arora, M., Burns, L.J., Barker, J.N., Miller, J.S., Defor, T.E., Olujohungbe, A.B., & Weisdorf, D.J. (2004). Randomized comparison of granulocyte colony-stimulating factor versus granulocyte-macrophage colony-stimulating factor plus intensive chemotherapy for peripheral blood stem cell mobilization and autologous transplantation in multiple myeloma. *Biology of Blood and Marrow Transplantation, 10,* 395–404. doi:10.1016/j. bbmt.2004.02.001

Bakken, A.M. (2006). Cryopreserving human peripheral blood progenitor cells. *Current Stem Cell Research and Therapy, 1,* 47–54. doi:10.2174/157488806775269179

Basquiera, A.L., Abichain, P., Damonte, J.C., Ricchi, B., Sturich, A.G., Palazzo, E.D., & Garcia, J.J. (2006). The number of CD34(+) cells in peripheral blood as a predictor of the CD34(+) yield in patients going to autologous stem cell transplantation. *Journal of Clinical Apheresis, 21,* 92–95. doi:10.1002/jca.20062

Cooke, L., Gemmil, R., Kravits, K., & Grant, M. (2009). Psychological issues of stem cell transplant. *Seminars in Oncology Nursing, 25,* 139–150. doi:10.1016/j.soncn.2009.03.008

Cornelissen, J.J. (2004). Hematopoietic reconstitution after hematopoietic stem cell transplantation. In K. Atkinson, R. Champlin, J. Ritz, W.E. Fibbe, P. Ljungman, & M.K. Brenner (Eds.), *Clinical bone marrow and blood stem cell transplantation* (3rd ed., pp. 160–193). New York, NY: Cambridge University Press.

Corso, A., Arcaini, L., Caberlon, S., Zappasodi, P., Mangiacavalli, S., Lorenzi, A., ... Lazzarino, M. (2002). A combination of dexamethasone, cyclophosphamide, etoposide and etoposide is less toxic and more effective than high dose cyclophosphamide for peripheral stem cell mobilization in multiple myeloma. *Haematologica, 87,* 1041–1045.

DeMeyer, E.S. (2009). Emerging immunology of stem cell transplantation. *Seminars in Oncology Nursing, 25,* 100–104. doi:10.1016/j.soncn.2009.03.001

Flowers, M.E.D., & Sullivan, K.M. (2004). Management of patients undergoing marrow or blood stem cell transplantation. In K. Atkinson, R. Champlin, J. Ritz, W.E. Fibbe, P. Ljungman, & M.K. Brenner (Eds.), *Clinical bone marrow and blood stem cell transplantation* (3rd ed., pp. 313–226). New York, NY: Cambridge University Press.

Goldberg, S.L., Mangan, K.F., Klumpp, T.R., Macdonald, J.S., Thomas, C., Mullaney, M.T., & Au, F.C. (1995). Complications of peripheral blood stem cell harvesting: A review of 554 PBSC leukaphereses. *Journal of Hematotherapy, 4,* 85–90.

Gorak, E., Geller, N., Srinivasan, R., Espinoza-Delgado, I., Donohue, T., Barrett, A.J., ... Childs, R. (2005). Engraftment syndrome after non-myeloablative allogeneic hematopoietic stem cell transplantation: Incidence and effects on survival. *Biology of Blood and Marrow Transplantation, 11,* 542–550. doi:10.1016/j.bbmt.2005.04.009

Korbling, M. (2004). Mobilization regimens for harvesting autologous and allogeneic peripheral blood stem cells. In K. Atkinson, R. Champlin, J. Ritz, W.E. Fibbe, P. Ljungman, & M.K. Brenner (Eds.), *Clinical bone marrow and blood stem cell transplantation* (3rd ed., pp. 383–403). New York, NY: Cambridge University Press.

Lefrere, F., Zohar, S., Ghez, D., Delarue, R., Audat, F., Suarez, F., ... Varet, B. (2006). The VAD chemotherapy regimen plus a G-CSF dose of 10 μg/kg is as effective and less toxic than high-dose cyclophosphamide plus a G-CSF dose of 5 μg/kg for progenitor cell mobilization: Results from a monocentric study of 82 patients. *Bone Marrow Transplantation, 37,* 725–729. doi:10.1038/sj.bmt.1705308

Lerro, K.A., Medoff, E., Wu, Y., Seropian, S.E., Snyder, E., Krause, D., & Cooper, D.L. (2003). A simplified approach to stem cell mobilization in multiple myeloma patients not previously treated with alkylating agents. *Bone Marrow Transplantation, 32,* 1113–1117. doi:10.1038/sj.bmt.1704286

Liseth, K., Ersvaer, E., Abrahamsen, J.F., Nesthus, I., Ryningen, A., & Bruserud, O. (2009). Long-term cryopreservation of autologous stem cell grafts: A clinical and experimental study of hematopoietic and immunocompetent cells. *Transfusion.* Advance online publication. doi:10.1111/j.1537-2995.2009.02180.x

McAdams, F.W., & Burgunder, M.R. (2004) Transplant course. In S. Ezzone (Ed.), *Hematopoietic stem cell transplantation: A manual for nursing practice* (pp. 43–59). Pittsburgh, PA: Oncology Nursing Society.

Mitchell, S.A. (2004). Graft versus host disease. In S. Ezzone (Ed.), *Hematopoietic stem cell transplantation: A manual for nursing practice* (pp. 85–131). Pittsburgh, PA: Oncology Nursing Society.

National Comprehensive Cancer Network. (2009a, October 15). *NCCN Clinical Practice Guidelines in Oncology™: Distress management* [v.1.2010]. Retrieved from http://www.nccn. org/professionals/physician_gls/PDF/distress.pdf

National Comprehensive Cancer Network. (2009b, July 1). *NCCN Clinical Practice Guidelines in Oncology™: Multiple myeloma* [v.2.2010]. Retrieved from http://www.nccn.org/professionals/ physician_gls/PDF/myeloma.pdf

Niess, D., & Duffy, K.M. (2004). Basics concepts of transplantation. In S. Ezzone (Ed.), *Hematopoietic stem cell transplantation: A manual for nursing practice* (pp. 13–21). Pittsburgh, PA: Oncology Nursing Society.

Reddy, R.L. (2005). Mobilization and collection of peripheral blood progenitor cells for transplantation. *Transfusion and Apheresis Science, 32,* 63–72. doi:10.1016/j.transci.2004.10.007

Rodriguez, A.L., Tariman, J.D., Enecio, T., & Estrella, S.M. (2007). The role of high-dose chemotherapy supported by hematopoietic stem cell transplantation in patients with multiple myeloma: Implications for nursing. *Clinical Journal of Oncology Nursing, 11,* 579–589. doi:10.1188/07.CJON.579-589

Saria, M.G., & Gosselin-Acomb, T.K. (2007). Hematopoietic stem cell transplantation: Implications for critical care nurses. *Clinical Journal of Oncology Nursing, 11,* 53–63. doi:10.1188/07.CJON.53-63

Schmit-Pokorny, K. (2004). Stem cell collection. In S. Ezzone (Ed.), *Hematopoietic stem cell transplantation: A manual for nursing practice* (pp. 23–42). Pittsburgh, PA: Oncology Nursing Society.

Socinski, M.A., Cannistra, S.A., Elias, A., Antman, K.H., Schnipper, L., & Griffin, J.D. (1988). Granulocyte-macrophage colony stimulating factor expands the circulating haemopoietic progenitor cell compartment in man. *Lancet, 1,* 1194–1198. doi:10.1016/S0140-6736(88)92012-0

Szer, J. (2004). Cryopreservation and functional assessment of harvested bone marrow and blood stem cells. In K. Atkinson, R. Champlin, J. Ritz, W.E. Fibbe, P. Ljungman, & M.K. Brenner (Eds.), *Clinical bone marrow and blood stem cell transplantation* (3rd ed., pp. 450–456). New York, NY: Cambridge University Press.

To, L.B., Roberts, M.M., Haylock, D.N., Dyson, P.G., Branford, A.L., Thorp, D., ... Juttner, C.A. (1992). Comparison of haematological recovery times and supportive care requirements of autologous recovery phase peripheral blood stem cell transplants, autologous bone marrow transplants and allogeneic bone marrow transplant. *Bone Marrow Transplantation, 9,* 277–284.

Tricot, G., Barlogie, B., Zangari, M., van Rhee, F., Hoering, A., Szymonifka, J., & Cottler-Fox, M. (2008). Mobilization of peripheral blood stem cells in myeloma with either pegfilgrastim or filgrastim following chemotherapy. *Haematologica, 93,* 1739–1742. doi:10.3324/haematol.13204

Vogel, W., Kopp, H.G., Kantz, L., & Einsele, H. (2002). Correlations between hematopoietic progenitor cell counts as measured by Sysmex and CD34+ cell harvest yields following mobilization with different regimens. *Journal of Cancer Research and Clinical Oncology, 128,* 380–384. doi:10.1007/s00432-002-0351-4

Management and Evaluation of Patients Receiving Novel Agents

Kena Miller, RN, MSN, FNP

INTRODUCTION

Multiple myeloma is a malignancy of plasma cell origin and currently is incurable. Increasing knowledge of the underlying biologic pathogenesis of this disease has resulted in the development of new therapies for its treatment. New treatments have demonstrated an increase in overall and complete response rates when compared to standard treatment, but more promising is their combination with existing antimyeloma treatments, which has further improved responses. The combination of novel agents with existing conventional therapies increases the treatment options available for patients with multiple myeloma, thus leading to better clinical outcomes. More than 20,500 individuals were diagnosed with multiple myeloma in the United States in 2009 (Jemal et al., 2009). Nurses will be at the forefront of evaluating and managing the associated side effects of these therapeutic modalities to maintain patient quality of life.

THALIDOMIDE

Thalidomide (Thalomid®, Celgene Corp.) is a derivative of glutamic acid, consisting of a chiral (an atom in a molecule that is bonded to four different chemical species) center and two amide (a group of chemical compounds containing nitrogen) rings. It is pharmacologically classified as an immuno-modulatory agent (IMiD) and possesses anti-inflammatory and antiangiogenic properties. Thalidomide was used initially as a sedative and was found to be effective for treating morning sickness associated with pregnancy. However, it was withdrawn from the market in the early 1960s because of its teratogenic effects as evidenced by phocomelia, a deformity in which babies are born with missing limbs (Lenz, Pfeiffer, Kosenow, & Hayman, 1962).

In 1998, the U.S. Food and Drug Administration (FDA) approved thalidomide for the treatment of erythema nodosum leprosum (Singhal & Mehta, 2003), and in 2006, the FDA approved thalidomide in combination with high-dose dexamethasone for the treatment of newly diagnosed multiple myeloma (Celgene Corp., 2006b). The antitumor activity of thalidomide in patients with multiple myeloma was first reported by Singhal et al. (1999). It has been used in HIV wasting syndrome, graft-versus-host disease, and Behcet disease (a rare disorder that causes chronic inflammation of the blood vessels). Thalidomide has demonstrated some activity in Kaposi sarcoma, renal cell carcinoma, agnogenic myeloid metaplasia (a condition that occurs when the bone marrow is scarred, causing problems in erythropoiesis), Waldenström macroglobulinemia, and myelodysplastic syndrome (Bertolini et al., 2001; Ghobrial & Rajkumar, 2003).

Dosing

Thalidomide is not available as an IV preparation because of its insolubility in water. It is available in capsules of 50 mg, 100 mg, and 200 mg. In 200 mg dosing, maximum serum concentration is reached, on average, in four hours (with a mean half-life of four to nine hours), and the drug undergoes spontaneous, nonenzymatic, hydrolytic cleavage to its metabolites, which are rapidly excreted in the urine, while the unabsorbed drug is excreted in the feces (Chen et al., 1989; Stirling, 2000).

Thalidomide's optimum dose for multiple myeloma has not been formally evaluated in a phase I clinical trial. Generally, starting at a lower dose of 50 mg daily with a slow escalation by 50 mg per week has shown improved tolerability of side effects (Chanan-Khan & Miller, 2006). Barlogie et al. (2001) suggested there is a dose response effect, with higher response rates (54%) observed in patients who receive greater than or equal to 42 g (approximately 400 mg/day) over three months and a higher two-year survival rate (63%) than patients who received less than or equal to 42 g (21% and 45%, respectively). With increased dosing is the potential for intensified side effects. Patients receiving doses of less than or equal to 200 mg seem to tolerate the medication with fewer side effects. A similar correlation exists with duration of therapy (more than six months); peripheral neuropathy (PN) and hypothyroidism increase in frequency, while constipation and sedation actually decrease, likely related to tolerance and dose modification (Ghobrial & Rajkumar, 2003).

Evaluation and Management of Side Effects

Teratogenicity: Thalidomide is contraindicated during pregnancy. Teratogenicity is the most preventable adverse event with thalidomide. Patients treated in the United States are required to be enrolled in the S.T.E.P.S.® (System for Thalidomide Education and Prescribing Safety) program (Zeldis, Williams, Thomas, & Elsayed, 1999). This is a comprehensive program implemented to counsel patients on serious complications of thalidomide therapy, including potentially devastating consequences that occur with pregnancy. Women of childbearing potential, or women who have not been postmenopausal for at least two years, are required to have a negative pregnancy test prior to receiving thalidomide and for each subsequent month while on medication, and they must maintain *two* effective forms of birth control. Men who are on therapy with thalidomide must either abstain from intercourse with women of childbearing potential (as outlined previously) or use a latex condom.

Neurologic manifestations: Multiple studies have shown that neurologic manifestations may account for more than 80% of thalidomide's major toxicities (Ghobrial & Rajkumar, 2003). Although PN is the most common neurologic manifestation, other neurologic side effects may occur, including somnolence, fatigue, dizziness, tremors, confusion, and incoordination (ataxia). Less commonly reported neurologic manifestations include agitation, anxiety, psychosis, amnesia, insomnia, confusion, depression, euphoria, circumoral paresthesia, hyperesthesia, neuralgia, peripheral neuritis, and vasodilation. Seizures also have been reported, and patients with preexisting seizure disorders should be monitored with diligence.

The exact etiology of thalidomide-associated sensory neuropathy remains unknown (Isoardo et al., 2004). PN may present as motor or sensory symptoms often described as numbness, tingling, pain in the feet or hands, or weakness. Symptoms may present after cessation of therapy and may or may not be reversible. Patients with multiple myeloma have up to an estimated 13% underlying presentation of PN prior to any treatment (as reviewed in Kelly, Kyle, Miles, O'Brien, & Dyck, 1981). Therefore, a comprehensive baseline assessment and ongoing evaluation of PN are imperative. Electrophysiologic testing at baseline and every six months may be helpful in patients who are at higher risk for progressive PN, such as patients with diabetes. Control of comorbid disease that may contribute to underlying neuropathy is essential (i.e., diabetes), and concurrent medications known to cause neuropathy should be avoided when possible. Oncology nurses should use the Common Terminology Criteria for Adverse Events developed by the National Cancer Institute Cancer Therapy Evaluation Program (2009) and the thalidomide package insert (Celgene Corp., 2006b) for dose reduction (Tariman, Love, McCullagh, & Sandifer, 2008).

Interventions such as vitamin supplementation (B complex, folic acid, vitamin E), alpha-lipoic acid, L-carnitine, glutamate, and acupuncture have been reported to prevent PN or decrease the severity of PN in some patients. Pharmacologic interventions such as gabapentin, pregabalin, duloxetine, and tricyclic antidepressants such as desipramine and amitriptyline may also have some efficacy (Colson, Doss, Swift, Tariman, & Thomas, 2004).

Autonomic neuropathy may be manifested as dizziness or orthostatic hypotension. Interventions include evaluation and management of concomitant medication (i.e., antihypertensives) and patient teaching for adequate precautions, such as slow movement or rising from a recumbent position to a sitting, and then to a standing position. Adequate fluid intake should be encouraged and diuretics avoided when possible. For severe cases of orthostatic hypotension, clinicians should consider IV fluid supplementation and hold thalidomide until resolution of signs and symptoms.

Fatigue: Somnolence, weakness, and fatigue are debilitating and often underreported side effects. Bedtime dosing of thalidomide is therefore recommended. Nurses should advise patients and their families of the possibility of impairment of mental and physical abilities. Patients should avoid hazardous tasks and operate a motor vehicle with careful consideration until tolerance of the medication is stabilized.

Tremors: Mild tremors may occur in approximately 35% of patients, and ataxia may occur in 15% of patients. Hearing loss has been reported in 3% of patients (Rajkumar, 2001a, 2001b).

Sinus bradycardia: The mechanism of the sinus bradycardia phenomenon is unknown. This side effect may occur in approximately 25% of patients (Ghobrial & Rajkumar, 2003). Concomitant use of medications that may decrease heart rate should be used with caution or discontinued.

Deep vein thrombosis: Patients treated with IMiDs, thalidomide and its analog, lenalidomide, are at a higher risk of developing vascular thrombosis (Chanan-Khan & Miller, 2006). Thrombosis has been reported in arterial and venous circulation (Scarpace et al., 2005). In single-agent thalidomide, the incidence of deep vein thrombosis (DVT) or pulmonary embolism is only about 1%–3% (Buadi & Rajkumar, 2008). However, when thalidomide is combined with dexamethasone, DVT incidence increases to 10%–12% if no prophylaxis is used (Cavenagh & Oakervee, 2003; Rajkumar et al., 2002). There is an increased incidence of DVT of up to 26% when thalidomide is used with other chemotherapy (Barbui & Falanga, 2003; Bennett et al., 2002; Camba et al., 2001; Cavo et al., 2002; Schutt et al., 2005; Zangari et al., 2001).

Consideration of prophylaxis needs to take into account individual patient risk factors, including concomitant medications, procedure-related factors, disease-related factors, genetic factors, demographics, and antimyeloma therapy, which may increase the probability of thrombolytic events (Rome, Doss, Miller, & Westphal, 2008). Although no consensus exists regarding prophylaxis to prevent DVT, many investigators have reported benefits of aspirin (Baz et al., 2004, 2005), low-dose warfarin, low-molecular-weight heparin (Zangari et al., 2004), and weight-based warfarin (Chanan-Khan et al., 2005; Miller et al., 2006). Therapeutic anticoagulation should be strongly considered if multiple risk factors are present. Nurses should evaluate for signs and symptoms of DVT, including calf pain or tenderness, leg pain or cramping, warmth, increased tissue turgor, or swelling in the lower extremities. Increased resistance or pain with dorsiflexion of the foot (Homans sign) is an unreliable diagnostic sign to rule out DVT. Diagnosis is made by D-dimer and Doppler ultrasound. Shortness of breath, tachypnea, abnormal breath sounds, and chest pain may be indicative of pulmonary embolism, which may be life threatening and requires immediate intervention.

Upon diagnosis of DVT or pulmonary embolism, initial therapy should be with unfractionated heparin or low-molecular-weight heparin by subcutaneous (SC) injection (Creager & Dzau, 2001). Depending on the specific preparation, low-molecular-weight heparin is administered SC once or twice daily; for example, the dose of enoxaparin is 1 mg/kg SC twice daily. Warfarin may be initiated as early as the first day of anticoagulant therapy if active partial thromboplastin time is therapeutic, but it is important to overlap heparin treatment with warfarin, as its anticoagulant effect is delayed. The dose of warfarin should be adjusted to maintain the prothrombin time at an international normalized ratio of two to three seconds. Anticoagulant therapy should continue for three to six months. For patients with proximal DVT, incidence of pulmonary embolism may occur in up to 50% if untreated (Mose, Fedullo, LittleJohn, & Crawford, 1994). If treatment with anticoagulants is contraindicated because of bleeding, diathesis, or risk of hemorrhage, protection from pulmonary embolism may be achieved by placement of a percutaneous filter in the inferior vena cava.

Constipation: All patients should be advised of the side effect of constipation and appropriate interventions including high-fiber diet, oral hydration, and an escalating cathartic regimen, and further recommendation and evaluation as necessary. Other gastrointestinal manifestations reported include xerostomia (dry mouth), elevated liver enzymes, increased appetite, weight gain, anorexia, vomiting, dyspepsia, eructation, and flatulence.

Rash: Rashes may occur in more than 46% of patients on thalidomide and may present as a macular or papular eruption, acne, dry skin, or eczematous rash (Hall, El-Azhary, Bouwhuis, & Rajkumar, 2003). Rashes, in most instances, will resolve with symptomatic interventions such as the use of unscented moisturizing lotions, topical corticosteroids, or antihistamines or dose reduction. The presence of pruritic rash, fever, eosinophilia, or reduced blood pressure may indicate a more serious reaction to thalidomide. More severe dermatologic reactions, such as Stevens-Johnson syndrome or toxic epidermal necrolysis syndrome, may occur (Horowitz & Stirling, 1999; Rajkumar, Gertz, & Witzig, 2000). Possible symptoms include sore throat, malaise, fever, and erosions of mucous membranes by small blisters on purpuric lesions, subsequently followed by detachment of the outer epidermal layer of the skin (Stern, Chosidow, & Wintroub, 2001). If rashes are exfoliative, purpuric, or bullous, thalidomide should not be resumed.

Peripheral edema: Mild dependent peripheral edema occurs in approximately 15% of patients (Rajkumar et al., 2000). Patients with previously underlying edema or patients who are at increased risk for edema, such as those with renal impairment, congestive heart failure, and systemic amyloidosis, may manifest the symptom more readily. Cautious use of diuretics, thromboembolic stockings, and elevation of extremities may be appropriate in most patients.

Myelosuppression: Approximately 15%–25% of patients will develop mild neutropenia while on thalidomide therapy. The general recommendation is to not start thalidomide if the absolute neutrophil count is less than 750/mm^3. Nurses should monitor complete blood counts and consider the use of growth factors or reduction of thalidomide dose when the absolute neutrophil count drops below 750/mm^3 (Miceli, Colson, Gavino, & Lilleby, 2008). Anemia and thrombocytopenia should be monitored closely, although these side effects are less common.

Effect on Stem Cell Harvest

In clinical trials, thalidomide induction therapy caused no significant adverse effect on stem cell mobilization, and engraftment was not impaired (Abdelkefi et al., 2005; Cavo et al., 2004; Rajkumar et al., 2002). It is currently recommended that patients be taken off thalidomide two to four weeks prior to stem cell mobilization.

Use in Patients With Renal Insufficiency

Pharmacokinetic studies have demonstrated that dose reduction of thalidomide is not necessary in patients with renal impairment (Eriksson et al., 2003).

LENALIDOMIDE

Lenalidomide (Revlimid®, Celgene Corp.) is a 4-amino substituted second-generation analog of thalidomide. Lenalidomide is approved for the treatment of deletion 5q myelodysplastic syndrome with doses starting at 5–10 mg/day and for patients with multiple myeloma after one line of treatment failure in combination with high-dose dexamethasone (Celgene Corp., 2006a). It has activity against the myeloma cell directly, as well as in the bone marrow microenvironment. It has direct cytotoxic activity against myeloma cells and induces apoptosis and cell cycle growth arrest. As suggested by its classification as an IMiD, its effects on the immune system likely contribute to its antimyeloma activity. Several studies are ongoing to evaluate the utility of lenalidomide in the front-line setting.

Dosing

Lenalidomide is available in 5, 10, 15, and 25 mg capsules. It is rapidly absorbed, with maximum plasma concentrations at a median of 0.6–1.5 hours and no trend in maximum concentration with increased dose or multiple doses (Chen et al., 2007). Pharmacokinetic analysis of lenalidomide shows that following maximum concentration, there is a decline in a monophasic manner, with the elimination phase starting at 1–8 hours after the dose and a mean terminal elimination half-life of 3.1–4.2 hours (Richardson et al., 2002).

Evaluation and Management of Side Effects

Teratogenicity: Lenalidomide is contraindicated during pregnancy, as it is an analog of thalidomide and has the potential for teratogenicity. Teratogenicity is the most preventable adverse event. Patients treated in the United States are required to be enrolled in Celgene Corp.'s RevAssist® program, which is a comprehensive program implemented to counsel patients of the potentially devastating consequences of becoming pregnant while on lenalidomide therapy. Women of childbearing potential or women who have not been postmenopausal for at least two years are required to have a negative pregnancy test prior to lenalidomide being prescribed and for each subsequent month while on medication, and they must maintain *two* effective forms of birth control. Men who are on therapy with lenalidomide must either abstain from intercourse with women of childbearing potential or use a latex condom. The restricted distribution of lenalidomide and pregnancy prevention strategies are similar to those for patients taking thalidomide.

Myelosuppression: Myelosuppression is the most common side effect associated with lenalidomide. In the original phase I trial, 12 of 13 patients developed grade 3 and 4 myelosuppression at 50 mg/day dosing. Therefore, 25 mg/day was determined to be the maximum tolerated dose (Richardson et al., 2002). Introduction of growth factors and dose reduction when appropriate have improved this side effect. Side effects that occur with thalidomide, such as somnolence, constipation, and neuropathy, were not as prevalent.

In phase II studies, nonhematologic toxicities, including DVT, fatigue, muscle weakness, anxiety, pneumonitis, light-headedness, and leg cramps, occurred. From the published data, side effects of treatment with lenalidomide are predictable and manageable (Rajkumar et al., 2007).

In a phase III clinical trial conducted through the Eastern Cooperative Oncology Group in patients with newly diagnosed multiple myeloma, lenalidomide 25 mg given on days 1–21 of a 28-day cycle in combination with high-dose dexamethasone (40 mg on days 1–4, 9–12, and 17–20) for four induction cycles was compared to the same dose of lenalidomide in combination with low-dose dexamethasone 40 mg/day on days 1, 8, 15, and 22 of a 28-day cycle. Planned interim analysis of this trial led to an early closure, as a demonstrated one-year survival benefit from the lower-dose dexamethasone arm was at 96.5% versus 86% with the standard-dose dexamethasone arm. The low-dose treatment appeared to diminish side effects while maintaining response rates. The one-year survival seen with lenalidomide and low-dose dexamethasone was remarkably higher than what had been historically observed with other approaches, including those using stem cell transplant–based therapies (Rajkumar et al., 2007).

Thromboembolic events: Single-agent lenalidomide has not been associated with an increased incidence of thromboembolic events. However, when used in combination with dexamethasone, rates increased significantly over use of either agent alone. Higher rates of thromboembolic complications in phase III trials of relapsed multiple myeloma were noted, especially when lenalidomide was used concurrently with erythropoietic growth factors. The rate of venous thromboembolic events was higher in the high-dose dexamethasone arm than in the low-dose arm (18.2% versus 3.7%) (Rajkumar et al., 2007).

Use in Patients With Renal Insufficiency

As creatinine clearance decreases, causing mild to severe impairment, the half-life of lenalidomide increases and drug clearance decreases linearly. Patients with moderate or severe renal impairment have a threefold increase in drug half-life and a 66%–75% decrease in drug clearance compared to healthy subjects. Patients on hemodialysis (n = 6) who were given a single dose of lenalidomide 25 mg had an approximate 4.5-fold increase in drug half-life and an 80% decrease in drug clearance compared to healthy volunteers. Approximately 40% of the administered dose was removed from the body during a single dialysis session. Therefore, adjustment of the starting dose of lenalidomide is recommended in patients with moderate or severe (creatinine clearance less than 60 ml/min) renal impairment (Celgene Corp., 2006a). Impaired renal function is associated with a higher incidence of grade 3 or 4 thrombocytopenia (creatinine clearance less than 50 ml/min, 13.8%; greater than 50 ml/min, 4.6%).

Effect on Stem Cell Harvest

A trend is seen toward decreased peripheral blood stem cell yield with increasing duration of lenalidomide therapy as well as with increasing patient age. However, there was no demonstrated effect on the quality of peripheral blood stem cells collected across all groups who proceed to stem cell transplantation (Kumar, 2008).

BORTEZOMIB

Bortezomib (Velcade®, Millennium Pharmaceuticals, Inc.) is a selective inhibitor of proteasome, which is responsible for the degradation of cellular products, including short-lived proteins, regulatory cyclins, and cyclin-dependent kinase inhibitors that control cell cycle progression.

Dosing

As a single agent and in variable combinations with other agents such as dexamethasone, bortezomib typically is given as an IV push over three to five seconds at 1.3 mg/m^2 on days 1, 4, 8, and 11 of a 21-day cycle (Jagannath et al., 2004; Richardson et al., 2003). Laboratory studies have shown synergy with bortezomib and a number of conventional cytotoxic agents, showing that even chemoresistant multiple myeloma cell lines were sensitive to combinations of bortezomib with melphalan, doxorubicin, and mitoxantrone (Ma et al., 2003). Bortezomib has also been used in clinical trials with combinations such as 17-N-allylamino-17-demethoxygeldanamcyin and heat shock protein 90 inhibitors. The concept behind the study designs is that these combination regimens involve pairing bortezomib with drug classes that may neutralize molecular pathways, which can confer resistance to proteasome inhibition. The combination of bortezomib with other chemotherapeutic agents enables more potent or more accelerated proapoptotic effects of bortezomib on multiple myeloma cells.

Evaluation and Management of Side Effects

Fatigue: Asthenia, which is described as weakness and profound fatigue, developed in significant numbers of patients treated with bortezomib (Dispenzieri, 2005; Jagannath et al., 2004; Richardson et al., 2003). Patients should be apprised of this side effect and counseled to intersperse activity and exercise with periods of rest. Fatigue is a debilitating and often underreported and underevaluated symptom that directly affects patients' quality of life and their ability to continue therapy. Clinicians should evaluate patients' fatigue level with each cycle of therapy and implement interventions as necessary. These may include an exercise program, physical therapy, and, in some cases, dose reduction of bortezomib.

Hematologic effects: Neutropenia, anemia, and thrombocytopenia are transient and predictably cyclic in nature. Introduction of hematologic growth factors is helpful in count recovery where appropriate. Ongoing monitoring of complete blood count and differential and evaluation for bleeding and bruising are appropriate. Thrombocytopenia typically is lowest at day 11, with rebound usually occurring by the start of the next cycle. It is recommended to hold bortezomib dosing if the patient's platelet count is less than or equal to $30 \times 10^9/L$ or absolute neutrophil count is less than or equal to $0.75 \times 10^9/L$ (other than day 1). If several doses in consecutive cycles are withheld because of toxicity, bortezomib should subsequently be administered at a 25% reduction (Millennium Pharmaceuticals, Inc., 2009). Bortezomib may induce thrombocytopenia via a reversible effect on megakaryocytic platelet production (possibly by inhibiting platelet budding) versus a direct cytotoxic effect (Lonial et al., 2005). Given the reversible nature of thrombocytopenia, platelet transfusion rather than dose reduction would be most prudent.

Peripheral neuropathy: In patients with multiple myeloma, PN is associated not only with anticancer agents but also with the disease itself (Ropper & Gorson, 1998). PN in multiple myeloma is usually axonal, mixed sensorimotor, symmetrical, distal, and possibly progressive (Tariman et al., 2008). The exact mechanism is unknown. Neuropathy resulting from bortezomib therapy is thought to have a mechanism of action that is distinct from the neuropathy seen with thalidomide or platinum drugs. Its pattern of treatment-emergent neuropathy appears to be a small-fiber neuropathy starting in the lower extremities, oftentimes requiring pain medication. Comprehensive baseline evaluation of neuropathy is imperative, including consideration of electrophysiologic testing, and a neurotoxicity tool may be helpful. Ongoing evaluation of neuropathy and dose reduction when appropriate should be performed to ensure success of therapy (Tariman et al., 2008). The evaluation of concomitant drugs (e.g., antihypertensives), patient teaching with change in position, liberal oral fluid intake, and IV fluid hydration and dose reduction of bortezomib when appropriate may improve manifestations of autonomic neuropathy, such as postural hypotension.

Anecdotal interventions for the management of bortezomib-induced PN, such as vitamin B complex, folic acid, vitamin E, alpha-lipoic acid, and L-carnitine have been implemented (Colson et al., 2004). Further study would certainly be warranted to optimize supportive care.

Pharmacologic interventions with medications such as gabapentin, pregabalin, tricyclic antidepressants, and pain medications have been helpful in managing PN. Trials have reported improvement or resolution in PN after cessation of therapy (Richardson et al., 2006).

Gastrointestinal effects: Gastrointestinal toxicity presents as nausea, vomiting, constipation, and diarrhea (more common) and usually is mild and easily treated symptomatically. Clinicians should check for *Clostridium difficile* in this immune-compromised population if diarrhea is persistent. Diet restrictions, nutritional supplementations, electrolyte replacement, and the use of antidiarrheal agents, stool softeners, or laxatives may be necessary depending on side effects with individual patients.

Herpes zoster reactivation: A higher incidence of herpes zoster reactivation has occurred in patients with multiple myeloma while on bortezomib therapy in the front-line and relapsed settings (Manochakian, Miller, & Chanan-Khan, 2007). Although the causal mechanism is not yet known, acyclovir or valacyclovir as prophylaxis can reduce the incidence of bortezomib-associated herpes zoster (Mateos et al., 2006; Vickrey, Allen, Mehta, & Singhal, 2009).

Additional side effects: Other effects of bortezomib include rash, hypotension-induced dizziness, pyrexia, headache, cough, back or bone pain, muscle cramps, and lower extremity edema.

Other notable adverse events, including cardiac toxicity such as cardiac failure (Hacihanefioglu, Tarkun, & Gonullu, 2008; Orciuolo et al., 2007), pulmonary complications such as pulmonary fibrosis (Boyer, Batra, Ascensao, & Schechter, 2006), neurogenic bladder (Shimura et al., 2009), and irreversible hearing loss (Engelhardt, Muller, Maier, & Wasch, 2005), have been reported and should be assessed during follow-up of patients receiving bortezomib. Transient and acute elevations in liver function test parameters have been noted. Nurses should evaluate patients' liver function test on a regular basis and hold or discontinue dosing of the drug as indicated.

Use in Patients With Renal Insufficiency

Bortezomib is an essential option for patients with multiple myeloma who also have renal dysfunction. Clinical experience with bortezomib in patients with renal dysfunction demonstrated the drug is not nephrotoxic and is active in patients with light-chain disease (Chanan-Khan et al., 2005; Jagannath et al., 2005). It demonstrated similar response rates, toxicity profiles, and treatment discontinuation rates in patients with or without renal dysfunction (creatinine clearance less than 30 ml/min). In a retrospective review of 24 individuals with chronic renal failure treated with bortezomib-based regimens, the overall response rate was 75%, and 30% of patients achieved complete response or near complete response (Chanan-Khan et al., 2007). Three patients became independent of dialysis following bortezomib-based therapy, and no increase in treatment-related toxicities was noted. Severe renal failure and significant Bence-Jones proteinuria were associated with a lower probability of reversal of renal function (Ailawadhi & Chanan-Khan, 2008b).

Effect on Stem Cell Harvest

Preclinical studies have shown no toxic effects on stem cells, megakaryocytes, or neutrophil precursors (Fitzgerald et al., 2003; Lonial et al., 2005). After front-line therapy with bortezomib, patients have had adequate numbers of stem cells collected for either single or tandem transplants (Badros et al., 2006). Neutrophil and platelet engraftment is as expected and is successful after high-dose therapy and stem cell transplantation.

PEGYLATED LIPOSOMAL DOXORUBICIN

For many years the anthracycline doxorubicin has been part of the standard multiple myeloma induction regimen of vincristine, doxorubicin (Adriamycin®, Bedford Laboratories), and dexamethasone (known as VAD) (Alexanian, Barlogie, & Tucker, 1990). Anthracyclines are naturally occurring antibiotics derived from Actinobacteria *Streptomyces peucetius* var. *caesius*. Pegylated liposomal doxorubicin (PLD) is a unique doxorubicin formulation in which a polyethylene glycol layer surrounds a doxorubicin-containing liposome. This pegylation process protects the liposome from detection by the immune system, thus increasing the half-life of the doxorubicin, which prolongs drug exposure to tumor cells. PLD overcomes multidrug resistance genes that are overexpressed within plasma cells (Chanan-Khan & Lee, 2007).

Dosing

PLD is used in combination with other antimyeloma agents. PLD is an IV infusion approved for use in combination with bortezomib for patients who have not received prior bortezomib therapy and have received at least one prior therapy. In this regimen, PLD is dosed at 30 mg/m² on day 4 in combination with bortezomib 1.3 mg/m² days 1, 4, 8, and 11 of a 21-day cycle. There is strong preclinical rationale for this combination of agents, as they have different and complementary molecular mechanisms of action and, importantly, nonoverlapping toxicity profiles (Manochakian et al., 2007).

Other combinations studied in the relapsed or refractory setting include PLD at 20 mg/m² on days 1 and 15, with bortezomib 1.3 mg/m² on days 1, 4, 15, and 18, and thalidomide 200 mg daily on a 28-day cycle for four to six cycles (Chanan-Khan et al., 2004, 2009; Chanan-Khan & Lee, 2007; Chanan-Khan & Miller, 2006). This regimen currently is being studied in the front line at Roswell Park Cancer Institute in Buffalo, New York. Additional relapsed studies include PLD 30 mg/m² on day 4 with bortezomib dose ranges of 0.9–1.5 mg/m² (Orlowski et al., 2005, 2006). Additional combinations with PLD both in the front-line and relapsed setting have been undertaken, including PLD in combinations with thalidomide or lenalidomide, cyclophosphamide, and melphalan (Ailawadhi & Chanan-Khan, 2008a; Manochakian et al., 2007).

Evaluation and Management of Side Effects

Infusion reactions: Infusion reactions may occur during administration. Patients should be monitored closely, especially with the first dosing. Possible symptoms include flushing, shortness of breath, facial swelling, headaches, chills, back pain, tightness in the chest or throat, and dizziness or lightheadedness. For some patients, slowing the infusion rate improves symptoms. Typically these reactions resolve within several hours to a day once the infusion is stopped. Serious and sometimes life threatening or fatal allergic/anaphylactoid-like infusion reactions have been reported (Ortho Biotech Products, L.P., 2008).

Cardiac toxicity: PLD has a better cardiac toxicity profile in comparison to the standard formulation of doxorubicin. Cardiac toxicities to anthracyclines manifest in several forms, including acute arrhythmias and nonspecific electrocardiogram changes, decreases in left ventricular ejection fraction, congestive heart failure, and cardiomyopathy. Anthracycline-induced cardiotoxicity has been noted extensively in the past (Pai & Nahata, 2000; Swain, Whaley, & Ewer, 2003). In an effort to reduce cardiac toxicity in PLD, a polyethylene glycol layer surrounds the doxorubicin-containing liposome as a result of a process termed *pegylation*. Pegylation protects the liposomes from detection by mononuclear phagocyte system and increases the plasma half-life compared with conventional doxorubicin. Therefore, PLD is associated with lower concentrations of free doxorubicin and limited distribution to the myocardium, suggesting less cardiac toxicity. Many studies have shown PLD to have a better cardiac safety profile when compared to doxorubicin (Berry et al., 1998; Safra et al., 2000; Wigler et al., 2002).

Predisposing risk factors, including previous exposure to anthracycline-based therapy, age (both older adult and very young patients have greater risks), a history of cardiac disease, and previous cancer therapies such as mediastinal radiation therapy and high-dose anthracycline infusion, should be considered before placing patients on PLD combination regimens. Baseline multigated acquisition (MUGA) scan or echocardiogram should be obtained before initiating PLD therapy in patients. As no specific safety data are available for patients with preexisting heart disease, patients with a left ventricular ejection fraction less than 50% at baseline should not be considered appropriate candidates for PLD. Repeat MUGA scan should be performed after cumulative doses of 400 mg/m^2 and again every 100–200 mg/m^2 thereafter. In patients who have received prior anthracycline treatment, a MUGA scan should be performed after every 200 mg/m^2 interval (Safra, 2003). Nurses should monitor patients with each dose of PLD for associated signs and symptoms of cardiac toxicity and promptly report their findings.

Palmar-plantar erythrodysesthesia: Palmar-plantar erythrodysesthesia (PPE), or hand-foot syndrome, is a skin reaction that may manifest as tingling or burning, redness, flaking or peeling of the skin, swelling, small blisters, or small sores on the palms of the hands or soles of the feet. Symptoms usually appear 2–12 days after administration of PLD and may progress into erythematous plaques with violaceous (violet-colored) and edematous patches on the palms, soles, and other high-pressure areas and can resolve in one to two weeks (Lorusso et al., 2007). Although the physiology of PPE is not fully understood, data support the roles of drug excretion in sweat and local pressure as contributors. Dysesthesias (unpleasant abnormal sensation) and erythema may occur on several other body areas where increased pressure and warmth occur such as the axilla, groin, buttocks, under pendulous breasts, and the scrotal and labial areas. PPE may evolve into blistering desquamation, crusting, ulceration, and epidermal necrosis, requiring delay in treatment, dose reduction, or possible cessation of treatment.

Management of PPE includes patient education for prophylaxis, such as wearing loose-fitting clothes (e.g., boxer shorts versus briefs), avoiding hot showers and sun exposure, keeping shoes and socks off when possible, and avoiding tight-fitting shoes or undue pressure or rubbing of the skin. Regional cooling with ice and consuming iced liquids versus hot fluids or food also are recommended. Cooling is theorized to result in vasoconstriction, leading to reduced circulation of the drug to the distal extremities (Lorusso et al., 2007).

Topical preparations to the skin, such as perfume-free moisturizing creams like cocoa butter, aloe vera lotion, Bag Balm® (Dairy Association Co., Inc.) (Chin et al., 2001), and Biafine® (OrthoNeutrogena) emulsion, have been helpful. Dimethyl sulfoxide, a pharmacologic topical agent, has been investigated, as it is thought to have potential free-radical scavenging properties.

It penetrates tissues rapidly and has successfully treated extravasation with conventional doxorubicin (Bertelli et al., 1995).

In a phase I solid tumor trial using PLD with paclitaxel and cisplatin, pyridoxine 50 mg PO three times daily was used on days 2–21 of a cycle as PPE prophylaxis (Eng et al., 2001). Phase III randomized trials of pyridoxine versus placebo for the prevention of PPE are under way. Other studies have investigated dexamethasone alone (Drake et al., 2004; Titgan, 1997) or in combination with pyridoxine (Kollmannsberger et al., 2000) to reduce the frequency and severity of PPE.

Stomatitis: Stomatitis is a mouth irritation characterized by inflammation or sores. The tongue may be dry or swollen. Patients may feel pain or a burning sensation in the mouth and may have difficulty swallowing. Avoiding hot or spicy foods, using ice chips, drinking cool beverages, chewing gum, or using artificial saliva can be helpful. Nurses should monitor for ulceration and possible viral or fungal infections such as herpes zoster, herpes simplex, or candidiasis and treat appropriately.

Hematologic toxicity: Neutropenia is the most common hematologic toxicity. Nurses should monitor patients' complete blood counts with differential on a regular basis and implement growth factors as appropriate. Patients should be taught to monitor for fever and signs of infection and report these manifestations immediately to their clinician.

Gastrointestinal effects: Nausea and vomiting are possible and usually preventable with antiemetics. Patients also may experience anorexia. Appetite stimulants such as megestrol acetate or dronabinol may be helpful. Diarrhea is possible and may be managed with interventions such as loperamide, attapulgite, or diphenoxylate and atropine. If diarrhea is persistent, intermittent evaluation for *Clostridium difficile* is warranted in this immune-compromised population.

Other side effects: DVT is noted with increased incidence when PLD combinations with IMiDs such as thalidomide or lenalidomide are prescribed; therefore, anticoagulation prophylaxis is recommended (Barlogie et al., 2006; Baz et al., 2005; Offidani et al., 2006). Mild alopecia may be noted, albeit to a lesser degree than that seen with doxorubicin.

Use in Patients With Renal Insufficiency

In a retrospective review of the phase III APEX (Assessment of Proteasome Inhibition for Extending Remission) trial, Blade et al. (2008) noted that renal impairment with creatinine clearance less than 60 ml/min and a small subset of patients with creatinine clearance of 40 ml/min did not compromise the efficacy, time to progression, or overall response rate. In fact, steady improvement in renal function occurred in the PLD plus bortezomib and bortezomib-alone arms. Results suggested that in relapsed or refractory myeloma, the combination of PLD and bortezomib appeared to provide greater efficacy over bortezomib alone. The trade-off, however, is a less favorable toxicity profile.

FUTURE NOVEL AGENTS

Although current studies are considering the sequencing of treatments, cytogenetic risk factor stratification, depth of response, targeted therapy, and stem cell transplantation including single, tandem, and allogeneic transplantation, to date multiple myeloma remains incurable. New agents, including antibody therapies, heat shock protein inhibitors, PI3K/Akt, MAPK, and MEK pathway inhibitors, cyclin-dependent kinase inhibitors, histone deacetylase inhibitors, the next-generation proteasome inhibitor carfilzomib and the new oral IMiD pomalidomide are in active study for the treatment of multiple myeloma (Anderson, 2007). The commitment of all clinicians to innovation and research is instrumental to tackle this disease.

CONCLUSION

This is an exciting time in the treatment of multiple myeloma. In this orphan disease, four new pharmaceutical agents have been approved for medical management since 2003, including bortezomib, thalidomide, lenalidomide, and PLD. Many completed and ongoing clinical trials continue to report on their efficacy and medical management of side effects. Many new agents continue to be investigated in ongoing clinical trials. Although not currently curable, multiple myeloma is very treatable with improved prognosis. Nurses and clinicians will remain instrumental in monitoring and managing side effects in the long term to improve overall survival while maintaining quality of life for patients with this disease.

REFERENCES

Abdelkefi, A., Torjman, L., Ben Romdhane, N., Ladeb, S., El Omri, H., Ben Othman, T., … Ben Abdeladhim, A. (2005). First-line thalidomide-dexamethasone therapy in preparation for autologous stem cell transplantation in young patients (< 61 years) with symptomatic multiple myeloma. *Bone Marrow Transplantation, 36,* 193–198. doi:10.1038/sj.bmt.1705050

Ailawadhi, S., & Chanan-Khan, A. (2008a). Current role of anthracyclines in the treatment of multiple myeloma. In S. Lonial (Ed.), *Myeloma therapy: Pursuing the plasma cell* (pp. 113–121). Totowa, NJ: Humana Press.

Ailawadhi, S., & Chanan-Khan, A. (2008b). Management of multiple myeloma patients with renal dysfunction. In S. Lonial (Ed.), *Myeloma therapy: Pursuing the plasma cell* (pp. 499–516). Totowa, NJ: Humana Press.

Alexanian, R., Barlogie, B., & Tucker, S. (1990). VAD-based regimens as primary treatment for multiple myeloma. *American Journal of Hematology, 33,* 86–89. doi:10.1002/ajh.2830330203

Anderson, K.C. (2007). Targeted therapy of multiple myeloma based upon tumor-microenvironmental interactions. *Experimental Hematology, 35*(4, Suppl. 1), 155–162. doi:10.1016/j.exphem.2007.01.024

Badros, A., Goloubeva, O., Fenton, R., Rapoport, A.P., Akpek, G., Harris, C., … Meisenberg, B. (2006). Phase I trial of first-line bortezomib/thalidomide plus chemotherapy for induction and stem cell mobilization in patients with multiple myeloma. *Clinical Lymphoma, Myeloma and Leukemia, 7,* 210–216. doi:10.3816/CLM.2006.n.061

Barbui, T., & Falanga, A. (2003). Thalidomide and thrombosis in multiple myeloma. *Journal of Thrombosis and Haemostasis, 1,* 421–422. doi:10.1046/j.1538-7836.2003.00084.x

Barlogie, B., Desikan, R., Eddlemon, P., Spencer, T., Zeldis, J., Munshi, N., ... Tricot, G. (2001). Extended survival in advanced and refractory multiple myeloma after single-agent thalidomide: Identification of prognostic factors in a phase 2 study of 169 patients. *Blood, 98,* 492–494. doi:10.1182/blood.V98.2.492

Barlogie, B., Tricot, G., Anaissie, E., Shaughnessy, J., Rasmussen, E., van Rhee, F., ... Crowley, J. (2006). Thalidomide and hematopoietic-cell transplantation for multiple myeloma. *New England Journal of Medicine, 354,* 1021–1030. doi:10.1056/NEJMoa053583

Baz, R., Li, L., Kottke-Marchant, K., Srkalovic, G., McGowan, B., Yiannaki, E., ... Hussein, M.A. (2005). The role of aspirin in the prevention of thrombotic complications of thalidomide and anthracycline-based chemotherapy for multiple myeloma. *Mayo Clinic Proceedings, 80,* 1568–1574. doi:10.4065/80.12.1568

Baz, R., Marchant, K., Yiannaki, E.O., Platt, L., Brand, C., Tso, E., & Hussein, M.A. (2004). Aspirin decreases the thrombotic complications (DVT) of liposomal doxorubicin, vincristine, decreased frequency dexamethasone and thalidomide (DVd-T) treatment of multiple myeloma (MM) [Abstract No. 2397]. *Blood, 104.* Retrieved from http://abstracts.hematologylibrary.org/cgi/content/abstract/104/11/2397

Bennett, C.L., Schumock, G.T., Desai, A.A., Kwaan, H.C., Raisch, D.W., Newlin, R., & Stadler, W. (2002). Thalidomide-associated deep vein thrombosis and pulmonary embolism. *American Journal of Medicine, 113,* 603–606. doi:10.1016/S0002-9343(02)01300-1

Berry, G., Billingham, M., Alderman, E., Richardson, P., Torti, F., Lum, B., ... Martin, F.J. (1998). The use of cardiac biopsy to demonstrate reduced cardiotoxicity in AIDS Kaposi's sarcoma patients treated with pegylated liposomal doxorubicin. *Annals of Oncology, 9,* 711–716. doi:10.1023/A:1008216430806

Bertelli, G., Gozza, A., Forno, G.B., Vidili, M.G., Silvestro, S., Venturini, M., ... Dini, D. (1995). Topical dimethylsulfoxide for the prevention of soft tissue injury after extravasation of vesicant cytotoxic drugs: A prospective clinical study. *Journal of Clinical Oncology, 13,* 2851–2855.

Bertolini, F., Mingrone, W., Alietti, A., Ferrucci, P.F., Cocorocchio, E., Peccatori, F., ... Martinelli, G. (2001). Thalidomide in multiple myeloma, myelodysplastic syndromes and histiocytosis. Analysis of clinical results and of surrogate angiogenesis markers. *Annals of Oncology, 12,* 987–990. doi:10.1023/A:1011141009812

Blade, J., Sonneveld, P., San Miguel, J.F., Sutherland, H.J., Hajek, R., Nagler, A., ... Orlowski, R.Z. (2008). Pegylated liposomal doxorubicin plus bortezomib in relapsed or refractory multiple myeloma: Efficacy and safety in patients with renal function impairment. *Clinical Lymphoma, Myeloma, and Leukemia, 8,* 352–355. doi:10.3816/CLM.2008.n.051

Boyer, J.E., Batra, R.B., Ascensao, J.L., & Schechter, G.P. (2006). Severe pulmonary complication after bortezomib treatment for multiple myeloma. *Blood, 108,* 1113. doi:10.1182/blood-2006-03-011494

Buadi, F.K., & Rajkumar, S.V. (2008). Thalidomide: Induction therapy. In S. Lonial (Ed.), *Myeloma therapy: Pursuing the plasma cell* (pp. 229–237). Totowa, NJ: Humana Press.

Camba, L., Peccatori, J., Pescarollo, A., Tresoldi, M., Corradini, P., & Bregni, M. (2001). Thalidomide and thrombosis in patients with multiple myeloma. *Haematologica, 86,* 1108–1109. PMid:11602422

Cavenagh, J.D., & Oakervee, H. (2003). Thalidomide in multiple myeloma: Current status and future prospects. *British Journal of Haematology, 120,* 18–26. doi:10.1046/j.1365-2141.2003.03902.x

Cavo, M., Zamagni, E., Cellini, C., Tosi, P., Cangini, D., Cini, M., ... Baccarani, M. (2002). Deep-vein thrombosis in patients with multiple myeloma receiving first-line thalidomide-dexamethasone therapy. *Blood, 100,* 2272–2273. doi:10.1182/blood-2002-06-1674

Cavo, M., Zamagni, E., Tosi, P., Cellini, C., Cangini, D., Tacchetti, P., ... Baccarani, M. (2004). First-line therapy with thalidomide and dexamethasone in preparation for autologous stem cell transplantation for multiple myeloma. *Haematologica, 89*, 826–831.

Celgene Corp. (2006a). Revlimid (lenalidomide) [Package insert]. Summit, NJ: Author.

Celgene Corp. (2006b). Thalomid (thalidomide) [Package insert]. Summit, NJ: Author.

Chanan-Khan, A., & Miller, K.C. (2006). Supportive care in multiple myeloma. *Clinical Lymphoma Myeloma, 7*, 42–50. doi:10.3816/CLM.2006.n.038

Chanan-Khan, A., Miller, K.C., Musial, L., Padmanabhan, S., Yu, J., Ailawadhi, S., ... Czuczman, M.S. (2009). Bortezomib in combination with pegylated liposomal doxorubicin and thalidomide is an effective steroid independent salvage regimen for patients with relapsed or refractory multiple myeloma: Results of a phase II clinical trial. *Leukemia and Lymphoma, 50*, 1096–1101. doi:10.1080/10428190902912460

Chanan-Khan, A.A., Kaufman, J.L., Mehta, J., Richardson, P.G., Miller, K.C., Lonial, S., ... Singhal, S. (2007). Activity and safety of bortezomib in multiple myeloma patients with advanced renal failure: A multicenter retrospective study. *Blood, 109*, 2604–2606. doi:10.1182/blood-2006-09-046409

Chanan-Khan, A.A., & Lee, K. (2007). Pegylated liposomal doxorubicin and immunomodulatory drug combinations in multiple myeloma: Rationale and clinical experience. *Clinical Lymphoma, Myeloma and Leukemia, 7*(Suppl. 4), S163–S169. doi:10.3816/CLM.2007.s.018

Chanan-Khan, A.A., Miller, K.C., McCarthy, P., DiMiceli, L.A., Yu, J., Bernstein, Z.P., & Czuczman, M.S. (2004). A phase II study of Velcade (V), Doxil (D) in combination with low-dose thalidomide (T) as salvage therapy for patients (pts) with relapsed (rel) or refractory (ref) multiple myeloma (MM) and Waldenstrom macroglobulinemia (WM): Encouraging preliminary results [Abstract No. 2421]. *Blood, 104.* Retrieved from http://abstracts.hematologylibrary.org/cgi/content/abstract/104/11/2421

Chanan-Khan, A.A., Richardson, P., Lonial, S., Siegel, D., Jagannath, S., Mehta, J., ... Singhal, S. (2005). Safety and efficacy of bortezomib in multiple myeloma patients with renal failure requiring dialysis [Abstract No. 2550]. *Blood, 106.* Retrieved from http://abstracts.hematologylibrary.org/cgi/content/abstract/106/11/2550

Chen, N., Lau, H., Kong, L., Kumar, G., Zeldis, J.B., Knight, R., & Laskin, O.L. (2007). Pharmacokinetics of lenalidomide in subjects with various degrees of renal impairment and in subjects on hemodialysis. *Journal of Clinical Pharmacology, 47*, 1466–1475. doi:10.1177/0091270007309563

Chen, T.L., Vogelsang, G.B., Petty, B.G., Brundrett, R.B., Noe, D.A., Santos, G.W., & Colvin, O.M. (1989). Plasma pharmacokinetics and urinary excretion of thalidomide after oral dosing in healthy male volunteers. *Drug Metabolism and Disposition, 17*, 402–405.

Chin, S.F., Chen, N.T., Oza, A.M., Moore, M.J., Warr, D., & Siu, L.L. (2001). Use of "Bag Balm" as topical treatment of palmar-plantar erythrodysesthesia syndrome (PPES) in patients receiving selected chemotherapeutic agents [Abstract No. 1632]. *Proceedings of the American Society of Clinical Oncology, 20.* Retrieved from http://pda.asco.org/ASCOv2/Meetings/Abstracts?&vmview=abst_detail_view&confID=10&abstractID=1632

Colson, K., Doss, D.S., Swift, R., Tariman, J., & Thomas, T.E. (2004). Bortezomib, a newly approved proteasome inhibitor for the treatment of multiple myeloma: Nursing implications. *Clinical Journal of Oncology Nursing, 8*, 473–480. doi:10.1188/04.CJON.473-480

Creager, M.A., & Dzau, V.J. (2001). Vascular diseases of the extremities. In E. Braunwald, A.S. Fauci, D.I. Kasper, S.L. Hauser, D.L. Longo, & J.L. Jameson (Eds.), *Harrison's principles of internal medicine* (15th ed., pp., 1434–1442). New York, NY: McGraw-Hill.

Dispenzieri, A. (2005). Bortezomib for myeloma-much ado about something. *New England Journal of Medicine, 352*, 2546–2548. doi:10.1056/NEJMe058059

Drake, R.D., Lin, W.M., King, M., Farrar, D., Miller, D.S., & Coleman, R.L. (2004). Oral dexamethasone attenuates Doxil-induced palmar-plantar erythrodysesthesias in patients with recurrent gynecologic malignancies. *Gynecologic Oncology, 94*, 320–324. doi:10.1016/j.ygyno.2004.05.027

Eng, C., Mauer, A.M., Fleming, G.F., Bertucci, D., Rotmensch, J., Jacobs, R.H., & Ratain, M.J. (2001). Phase I study of pegylated liposomal doxorubicin, paclitaxel, and cisplatin in patients with advanced solid tumors. *Annals of Oncology, 12*, 1743–1747. doi:10.1023/A:1013574328938

Engelhardt, M., Muller, A.M., Maier, W., & Wasch, R. (2005). Severe irreversible bilateral hearing loss after bortezomib (VELCADE) therapy in a multiple myeloma (MM) patient. *Leukemia, 19*, 869–870. doi:10.1038/sj.leu.2403723

Eriksson, T., Hoglund, P., Turesson, I., Waage, A., Don, B.R., Vu, J., ... & Kaysen, G.A. (2003). Pharmacokinetics of thalidomide in patients with impaired renal function and while on and off dialysis. *Journal of Pharmacy and Pharmacology, 55*, 1701–1706. doi:10.1211/0022357022241

Fitzgerald, M., Fraser, C., Webb, I., Schenkein, D., Esseltine, D., & Weich, N. (2003). Normal hematopoietic stem cell function in mice following treatment with bortezomib [Poster presentation]. *Biology of Blood and Marrow Transplantation, 9*, 193.

Ghobrial, I.M., & Rajkumar, S.V. (2003). Management of thalidomide toxicity. *Journal of Supportive Oncology, 1*, 194–205.

Hacihanefioglu, A., Tarkun, P., & Gonullu, E. (2008). Acute severe cardiac failure in a myeloma patient due to proteasome inhibitor bortezomib. *International Journal of Hematology, 88*, 219–222. doi:10.1007/s12185-008-0139-7

Hall, V.C., El-Azhary, R.A., Bouwhuis, S., & Rajkumar, S.V. (2003). Dermatologic side effects of thalidomide in patients with multiple myeloma. *Journal of the American Academy of Dermatology, 48*, 548–552. doi:10.1067/mjd.2003.87

Horowitz, S.B., & Stirling, A.L. (1999). Thalidomide-induced toxic epidermal necrolysis. *Pharmacotherapy, 19*, 1177–1180. doi:10.1592/phco.19.15.1177.30571

Isoardo, G., Bergui, M., Durelli, L., Barbero, P., Boccadoro, M., Bertola, A., ... Cocito, D. (2004). Thalidomide neuropathy: Clinical, electrophysiological and neuroradiological features. *Acta Neurologica Scandinavica, 109*, 188–193. doi:10.1034/j.1600-0404.2003.00203.x

Jagannath, S., Barlogie, B., Berenson, J., Siegel, D., Irwin, D., Richardson, P.G., ... Anderson, K.C. (2004). A phase 2 study of two doses of bortezomib in relapsed or refractory myeloma. *British Journal of Haematology, 127*, 165–172. doi:10.1111/j.1365-2141.2004.05188.x

Jagannath, S., Barlogie, B., Berenson, J.R., Singhal, S., Alexanian, R., Srkalovic, G., ... Anderson, K.C. (2005). Bortezomib in recurrent and/or refractory multiple myeloma: Initial clinical experience in patients with impaired renal function. *Cancer, 103*, 1195–1200. doi:10.1002/cncr.20888

Jemal, A., Siegel, R., Ward, E., Hao, Y., Xu, J., & Thun, M.J. (2009). Cancer statistics, 2009. *CA: A Cancer Journal for Clinicians, 59*, 225–249. doi:10.3322/caac.20006

Kelly, J.J., Jr., Kyle, R.A., Miles, J.M., O'Brien, P.C., & Dyck, P.J. (1981). The spectrum of peripheral neuropathy in myeloma. *Neurology, 31*, 24–31.

Kollmannsberger, C., Mayer, F., Harstrick, A., Honecker, F., Vanhofer, U., Oberhoff, C., ... Bokemeyer, C. (2000). Reduction of skin toxicity of pegylated liposomal doxorubicin (PDL) by concomitant administration of dexamethasone and pyridoxine in patient (pts) with anthracycline-sensitive malignancies—A phase I/II trial [Abstract No. 623P]. *Annals of Oncology, 11*(1, Suppl. 4), 136.

Kumar, S. (2008). Lenalidomide for initial therapy of newly diagnosed multiple myeloma. In S. Lonial (Ed.), *Myeloma therapy: Pursuing the plasma cell* (pp. 279–288). Totowa, NJ: Humana Press.

Lenz, W., Pfeiffer, R.A., Kosenow, W., & Hayman, D.J. (1962). Thalidomide and congenital abnormalities. *Lancet, 279*(7219), 45–46. doi:10.1016/S0140-6736(62)92665-X

Lonial, S., Waller, E.K., Richardson, P.G., Jagannath, S., Orlowski, R.Z., Giver, C.R., ... Anderson, K.C. (2005). Risk factors and kinetics of thrombocytopenia associated with bortezomib for relapsed, refractory multiple myeloma. *Blood, 106*, 3777–3784. doi:10.1182/blood-2005-03-1173

Lorusso, D., Di Stefano, A., Carone, V., Fagotti, A., Pisconti, S., & Scambia, G. (2007). Pegylated liposomal doxorubicin-related palmar-plantar erythrodysesthesia ("hand-foot" syndrome). *Annals of Oncology, 18,* 1159–1164. doi:10.1093/annonc/mdl477

Ma, M.H., Yang, H.H., Parker, K., Manyak, S., Friedman, J.M., Altamirano, C., ... Berenson, J.R. (2003). The proteasome inhibitor PS-341 markedly enhances sensitivity of multiple myeloma tumor cells to chemotherapeutic agents. *Clinical Cancer Research, 9,* 1136–1144. PMid:12631619

Manochakian, R., Miller, K.C., & Chanan-Khan, A.A. (2007). Clinical impact of bortezomib in frontline regimens for patients with multiple myeloma. *Oncologist, 12,* 978–990. doi:10.1634/theoncologist.12-8-978

Mateos, M.V., Hernandez, J.M., Hernandez, M.T., Gutierrez, N.C., Palomera, L., Fuertes, M., ... San Miguel, J.F. (2006). Bortezomib plus melphalan and prednisone in elderly untreated patients with multiple myeloma: Results of a multicenter phase 1/2 study. *Blood, 108,* 2165–2172. doi:10.1182/blood-2006-04-019778

Miceli, T., Colson, K., Gavino, M., & Lilleby, K. (2008). Myelosuppression associated with novel therapies in patients with multiple myeloma: Consensus statement of the IMF Nurse Leadership Board. *Clinical Journal of Oncology Nursing, 12*(Suppl. 3), 13–20. doi:10.1188/08.CJON.S1.13-19

Millennium Pharmaceuticals, Inc. (2009). Velcade (bortezomib) [Prescribing information]. Retrieved from http://www.velcade.com/full_prescrib_velcade.pdf

Miller, K.C., Padmanabhan, S., Dimicelli, L., Depaolo, D., Landrigan, B., Yu, J., ... Chanan-Khan, A. (2006). Prospective evaluation of low-dose warfarin for prevention of thalidomide associated venous thromboembolism. *Leukemia Lymphoma, 47,* 2339–2343. doi:10.1080/10428190600799631

Moser, K.M., Fedullo, P.F., LittleJohn, J.K., & Crawford, R. (1994). Frequent asymptomatic pulmonary embolism in patients with deep venous thrombosis. *JAMA, 271,* 223–225. doi:10.1001/jama.271.3.223

National Cancer Institute Cancer Therapy Evaluation Program. (2009). *Common terminology criteria for adverse events (CTCAE) and common toxicity criteria (CTC).* Retrieved August 25, 2009, from http://ctep.cancer.gov/protocolDevelopment/electronic_applications/ctc.htm

Offidani, M., Corvatta, L., Piersantelli, M.-N., Visani, G., Alesiani, F., Brunori, M.,... Leoni, P. (2006). Thalidomide, dexamethasone, and pegylated liposomal doxorubicin (ThaDD) for patients older than 65 years with newly diagnosed multiple myeloma. *Blood, 108,* 2159–2164. doi:10.1182/blood-2006-03-013086

Orciuolo, E., Buda, G., Cecconi, N., Galimberti, S., Versari, D., Cervetti, G., ... Petrini, M. (2007). Unexpected cardiotoxicity in haematological bortezomib treated patients. *British Journal of Haematology, 138,* 396–397. doi:10.1111/j.1365-2141.2007.06659.x

Orlowski, R.Z., Peterson, B.L., Sanford, B., Chanan-Khan, A.A., Zehngebot, L.M., Watson, P.R., ... Larson, R.A. (2006). Bortezomib and pegylated liposomal doxorubicin as induction therapy for adult patients with multiple myeloma: Cancer and Leukemia Group B study 10301 [Abstract No. 797]. *Blood, 108.* Retrieved from http://www.cancereducation.com/CancerSysPagesNB/abstracts/mmrf/72/abbr6.pdf

Orlowski, R.Z., Voorhees, P.M., Garcia, R.A., Hall, M.D., Kudrik, F.J., Allred, T., ... Dees, E.C. (2005). Phase 1 trial of the proteasome inhibitor bortezomib and pegylated liposomal doxorubicin in patients with advanced hematologic malignancies. *Blood, 105,* 3058–3065. doi:10.1182/blood-2004-07-2911

Ortho Biotech Products, L.P. (2008). Doxil (doxorubicin HCl liposome injection) [Prescribing information]. Retrieved from http://www.centocororthobiotech.com/cobi/shared/OBI/PI/DOXIL_PI.pdf

Pai, V.B., & Nahata, M.C. (2000). Cardiotoxicity of chemotherapeutic agents: Incidence, treatment and prevention. *Drug Safety, 22,* 263–302. doi:10.2165/00002018-200022040-00002

Rajkumar, S.V. (2001a). Current status of thalidomide in the treatment of cancer. *Oncology, 15,* 867–874.

Rajkumar, S.V. (2001b). Thalidomide in the treatment of multiple myeloma. *Expert Review in Anticancer Therapy, 1,* 20–28. doi:10.1586/14737140.1.1.20

Rajkumar, S.V., Gertz, M.A., & Witzig, T.E. (2000). Life-threatening toxic epidermal necrolysis with thalidomide therapy for myeloma. *New England Journal of Medicine, 343,* 972–973. doi:10.1056/NEJM200009283431315

Rajkumar, S.V., Hayman, S., Gertz, M.A., Dispenzieri, A., Lacy, M.Q., Greipp, P.R., ... Witzig, T.E. (2002). Combination therapy with thalidomide plus dexamethasone for newly diagnosed myeloma. *Journal of Clinical Oncology, 20,* 4319–4323. doi:10.1200/JCO.2002.02.116

Rajkumar, S.V., Jacobus, S., Callander, N., Fonseca, R., Vesole, D., Williams, M., ... Greipp, P. (2007). A randomized trial of lenalidomide plus high-dose dexamethasone versus lenalidomide plus low-dose dexamethasone in newly diagnosed myeloma (E4A03): A trial coordinated by the Eastern Cooperative Oncology Group [Abstract No. 74]. *Blood, 110.* Retrieved from http://abstracts.hematologylibrary.org/cgi/content/abstract/110/11/74?maxtoshow=&HITS=10&hits=10&RESULTFORMAT=&fulltext=rajkumar+and+lenalidomide&searchid=1&FIRSTINDEX=0&sortspec=relevance&resourcetype=HWCIT

Richardson, P., Barlogie, B., Berenson, J., Singhal, S., Jagannath, S., Irwin, D., ... Anderson, K.C. (2003). A phase 2 study of bortezomib in relapsed, refractory myeloma. *New England Journal of Medicine, 348,* 2609–2617. doi:10.1056/NEJMoa030288

Richardson, P., Schlossman, R.L., Weller, E., Hideshima, T., Mitsiades, C.S., Davies, F.E., ... Anderson, K.C. (2002). Immunomodulatory drug CC5013 overcomes drug resistance and is well tolerated in patients with relapsed multiple myeloma. *Blood, 100,* 3063–3067. doi:10.1182/blood-2002-03-0996

Richardson, P.G., Briemberg, H., Jagannath, S., Wen, P.Y., Barlogie, B., Berenson, J., ... Amato, A.A. (2006). Frequency, characteristics, and reversibility of peripheral neuropathy during treatment of advanced multiple myeloma with bortezomib. *Journal of Clinical Oncology, 24,* 3113–3120. doi:10.1200/JCO.2005.04.7779

Rome, S., Doss, D., Miller, K., & Westphal, J. (2008). Thromboembolic events associated with novel therapies in patients with multiple myeloma: Consensus statement of the IMF Nurse Leadership Board. *Clinical Journal of Oncology Nursing, 12*(Suppl. 3), 21–28. doi:10.1188/08.CJON.S1.21-27

Ropper, A.H., & Gorson, K.C. (1998). Neuropathies associated with paraproteinemia. *New England Journal of Medicine, 338,* 1601–1607. doi:10.1056/NEJM199805283382207

Safra, T. (2003). Cardiac safety of liposomal anthracyclines. *Oncologist, 8*(Suppl. 2), 17–24. doi:10.1634/theoncologist.8-suppl_2-17

Safra, T., Muggia, F., Jeffers, S., Tsao-Wei, D.D., Groshen, S., Lyass, O., ... Gabizon, A. (2000). Pegylated liposomal doxorubicin (Doxil): Reduced clinical cardiotoxicity in patients reaching or exceeding cumulative doses of 500 mg/m^2. *Annals of Oncology, 11,* 1029–1033. doi:10.1023/A:1008365716693

Scarpace, S.L., Hahn, T., Roy, H., Brown, K., Paplham, P., Chanan-Khan, A., ... McCarthy, P., Jr. (2005). Arterial thrombosis in four patients treated with thalidomide. *Leukemia and Lymphoma, 46,* 239–242. doi:10.1080/10428190400015675

Schutt, P., Ebeling, P., Buttkereit, U., Brandhorst, D., Opalka, B., Hoiczyk, M., ... Nowrousian, M.R. (2005). Thalidomide in combination with vincristine, epirubicin and dexamethasone (VED) for previously untreated patients with multiple myeloma. *European Journal of Haematology, 74*(1), 40–46. doi:10.1111/j.1600-0609.2004.00349.x

Shimura, K., Shimazaki, C., Taniguchi, K., Inaba, T., Horiike, S., & Taniwaki, M. (2009). Bortezomib-induced neurogenic bladder in patients with multiple myeloma. *Annals of Hematology, 88,* 383–384. doi:10.1007/s00277-008-0614-5

Singhal, S., & Mehta, J. (2003). Treatment of relapsed and refractory multiple myeloma. *Current Treatment Options in Oncology, 4,* 229–237. doi:10.1007/s11864-003-0024-9

Singhal, S., Mehta, J., Desikan, R., Ayers, D., Roberson, P., Eddlemon, P., ... Crowley, J. (1999). Antitumor activity of thalidomide in refractory multiple myeloma. *New England Journal of Medicine, 341,* 1565–1571. doi:10.1056/NEJM199911183412102

Stirling, D.I. (2000). Pharmacology of thalidomide. *Seminars in Hematology, 37*(Suppl. 3), 5–14. doi:10.1016/S0037-1963(00)90077-5

Stern, R.S., Chosidow, O.M., & Wintroub, B.U. (2001). Cutaneous drug reactions. In E. Braunwald, A.S. Fauci, D.I. Kasper, S.L. Hauser, D.L. Longo, & J.L. Jameson (Eds.), *Harrison's principles of internal medicine* (15th ed., pp. 336–342). New York, NY: McGraw-Hill.

Swain, S.M., Whaley, F.S., & Ewer, M.S. (2003). Congestive heart failure in patients treated with doxorubicin: A retrospective analysis of three trials. *Cancer, 97,* 2869–2879. doi:10.1002/cncr.11407

Tariman, J.D., Love, G., McCullagh, E., & Sandifer, S. (2008). Peripheral neuropathy associated with novel therapies in patients with multiple myeloma: Consensus statement of the IMF Nurse Leadership Board. *Clinical Journal of Oncology Nursing, 12*(Suppl. 3), 29–36. doi:10.1188/08.CJON.S1.29-35

Titgan, M.A. (1997). *Prevention of palmar-plantar erythrodysesthesia associated with liposome-encapsulated doxorubicin (Doxil) by oral dexamethasone* [Abstract No. 288]. Retrieved from http://www.asconews.com/ASCOv2/Meetings/Abstracts?&vmview=abst_detail_view&confID=30&abstractID=11113

Vickrey, E., Allen, S., Mehta, J., & Singhal, S. (2009). Acyclovir to prevent reactivation of varicella zoster virus (herpes zoster) in multiple myeloma patients receiving bortezomib therapy. *Cancer, 115,* 229–232. doi:10.1002/cncr.24006

Wigler, N., Inbar, M., O'Brien, M., Rosso, R., Grischke, E.M., Santoro, A., ... Tendler, C.L. (2002). Reduced cardiac toxicity and comparable efficacy in a phase III trial of pegylated liposomal doxorubicin (Caelyx/Doxil) vs. doxorubicin for first-line treatment of metastatic breast cancer [Abstract No. 177]. *Proceedings of the American Society of Clinical Oncology, 21.* Retrieved from http://asco-news.com/ASCOv2/Meetings/Abstracts?&vmview=abst_detail_view&confID=16&abstractID=177

Zangari, M., Anaissie, E., Barlogie, B., Badros, A., Desikan, R., Gopal, A.V., ... Tricot, G. (2001). Increased risk of deep-vein thrombosis in patients with multiple myeloma receiving thalidomide and chemotherapy. *Blood, 98,* 1614–1615. doi:10.1182/blood.V98.5.1614

Zangari, M., Barlogie, B., Anaissie, E., Saghafifar, F., Eddlemon, P., Jacobson, J., ... Tricot, G. (2004). Deep vein thrombosis in patients with multiple myeloma treated with thalidomide and chemotherapy: Effects of prophylactic and therapeutic anticoagulation. *British Journal of Haematology, 126,* 715–721. doi:10.1111/j.1365-2141.2004.05078.x

Zeldis, J.B., Williams, B.A., Thomas, S.D., & Elsayed, M.E. (1999). S.T.E.P.S.: A comprehensive program for controlling and monitoring access to thalidomide. *Clinical Therapeutics, 21,* 319–330. doi:10.1016/S0149-2918(00)88289-2

CHAPTER **11**

Patient Teaching

Sandra Rome, RN, MN, AOCN®, CNS

"At first, I was so scared I let my partner, Peg, look up everything and feed me information about multiple myeloma. I didn't want to start using the Internet, being afraid that I would get more information than I could handle. Later on, even as a teacher, I preferred getting information verbally in person from the nurse or doctor."
—*Linda Morrow, a 68-year-old multiple myeloma survivor diagnosed in 2005*

INTRODUCTION

Patient education begins at diagnosis and should continue along the cancer trajectory in all aspects of care. Patient education should include information about the disease, treatment, and treatment goals. Oncology nurses should prevent and treat acute care problems when they occur and address the prevention of other cancer and non-cancer-related problems to maximize wellness. Additionally, oncology nurses should optimize patients' quality of life and develop a survivorship-focused plan of care, which includes involvement of patients and significant others through teaching. Thorough patient and family education can influence clinical outcomes.

Multiple myeloma can be considered a chronic disease, and there is hope for cure; unfortunately, patients usually experience negative aspects of the disease at different times, thereby requiring the healthcare team to address and provide the appropriate education at each encounter. Furthermore, current and future novel therapies have their own potential side effects, making oncology nurses' ongoing patient and family education essential. Patient teaching should be a permanent part of each patient's plan of care and should be tailored specifically to the patient's phases of illness and treatment.

HOW TO TEACH

Assessment of Educational Needs

The process of patient education is not separate from the nursing process. Experienced clinicians respect the importance of the assessment phase: the assessment of the need to learn, motivation, and cultural, psychosocial, and other variables. These assessment-related activities must be performed before setting goals, performing interventions, and evaluating outcomes. It is important not to assume the learner's willingness and abilities. Correct assessment includes attentive, active listening with patients and caregivers and sensitivity to their responses. Inattentiveness, poor communication, and lack of empathy impair the nurse's ability to assess and reassess the patient's and family's ability to be attentive and absorb essential information (Coon, McBride-Wilson, & Coleman, 2007).

Some general screening questions should be a part of the initial assessment. For example, what does the patient know about the disease, and how does the individual perceive the current problems? The answers to an open-ended question, such as "Tell me your understanding of your diagnosis and the treatment plan you have discussed with your physician," can be very telling in terms of what the patient actually understands or remembers (Redman, 2001). Although creating an unhurried and quiet patient interview environment can be challenging, Gorman and Sultan (2008) have provided helpful guidelines for oncology nurses (see Figure 11-1). Open-ended questions can be helpful at any time during a patient's disease trajectory because the answers may provide information that helps the clinician to provide additional teaching. For example, the nurse might say, "Review for me specific signs and symptoms for which you should go to the emergency room" and "What are less serious signs and symptoms for which you should call the physician?" To ensure that a stem cell transplant (SCT) recipient knows his or her crucial medications, the nurse could state, "Tell me what these medications are for and why they are important to take after your stem cell transplant." The nurse should ask this question before discharge and then on subsequent clinic visits.

Assessment of motivation and readiness prior to educating patients and families is important in maintaining particular patient behaviors. If a patient is in pain, it is not a good time to conduct an in-depth educational session on the impending chemotherapy treatment. Once the pain is under control, the patient may still not be interested in the information. Although lack of motivation and readiness may delay in-depth teaching, certain safety aspects, such as the importance of the patient returning for laboratory visits and calling the healthcare team if fever or acute back pain develops, cannot be omitted. In this situation, the nurse must make sure to include the caregiver in the teaching session, along with making a follow-up call if warranted.

Sociodemographic factors affect an individual's ability to understand health problems and influence one's health beliefs, and thus affect learning outcomes

---

Figure 11-1. Creating an Appropriate Interview Environment

- Ask the patient's permission to be interviewed.
- Create a quiet, private space that is safe for the patient.
- Minimize interruptions if possible.
- Maintain appropriate eye contact.
- Sit at eye level with the patient.
- Ask open-ended questions to encourage the patient to talk.
- Avoid writing a lot of notes during the interview.
- Demonstrate an interest in the patient's concerns.
- Indicate acceptance of the patient by avoiding criticism, frowning, or demonstrating shock.
- Avoid asking more personal questions than are actually needed.
- Determine whether the family can provide information if the patient is unable to communicate.
- Maintain confidentiality.
- Be aware of your own biases and discomforts that could influence the assessment.
- Keep the focus on the patient.

Note. Based on information from Gorman & Sultan, 2008.

(Redman, 2001). Patient information such as primary caregiver, occupation, age, spirituality, culture, primary and secondary spoken and written languages, and highest education level achieved must be considered and assessed. Major personal and family issues caused by multiple myeloma, such as functional limitations, role changes, etc., should be explored (Gorman & Sultan, 2008). No matter what their background may be, patients with cancer value education. Moadel, Morgan, and Dutcher (2007) surveyed an ethnically diverse population of patients from two outpatient oncology clinics in the Bronx, New York, to assess psychosocial needs. They found that patients of Hispanic and African American background seemed to have the greatest need for information and education. Thus, expression of informational needs among patients with cancer cannot be assumed based on ethnographic background; some patients in the Western world do not express the desire to learn about their disease and treatment (Meredith et al., 1996).

Because learning usually requires a change in beliefs and behavior, it normally produces a mild level of anxiety. Mild anxiety is useful in motivating an individual, but severe anxiety is usually incapacitating (Redman, 2001). Thus, before providing education, nurses should assess and consider preexisting personality and emotional disorders and previous coping skills of patients. Because the potential for cure of patients with multiple myeloma is still considered rare, fear and anxiety are expected. An individual's health beliefs and practices need to be explored; culturally influenced ideas such as fatalism can affect a patient's emotional response and thus impact learning (Pesquera, Yoder, & Lynk, 2008). For example, if a patient's religious beliefs oppose receiving blood transfusions, a bloodless SCT can be performed safely, thereby supporting the patient's beliefs while providing an effective therapy (Sloan & Ballen, 2008).

Generally, the experience of illness requires adaptive skills that may vary throughout the cancer experience. Thus, the patient may have an intense emotional response to illness: personality styles that make care difficult, psychiatric disorders, or stresses and family problems that affect the patient's reactions to illness or hospitalization (Gorman & Sultan, 2008). Insufficient adaptation can hinder a patient's ability to learn and, subsequently, the strategy that the clinician may use effectively to educate at any given time. However, education can aid in modification of a patient's behavior for psychological adjustment to cancer. Thus, assistance with adaptation and education can occur simultaneously. For effective learning to occur, the nurse must identify the patient's psychosocial adjustment stage before choosing a particular method (Fredette, 1990). Fredette (1990) presented a model for improving cancer patient education that may provide guidance to oncology nurses; it suggests nursing approaches, topics, and teaching strategies based on a patient's behavioral responses. Fredette believed that this model can improve teaching effectiveness in clinical practice by ensuring that the patient is ready to learn prior to teaching. It provides suggestions for content and teaching strategies appropriate to the stage the patient is experiencing, even if the stages are not particularly linear. Oncology nurses also should assess the family and significant others separately and tailor the education for each individual.

Legal aspects of patient and family education should not be ignored. Because much of the treatment and follow-up are done in an outpatient setting, more and more responsibility for safety relies on the patient and family adhering to instructions. A team approach to patient teaching not only decreases conflicts but also ensures continuity in teaching (Kothare, 2000). The healthcare team should verify and document reliable measures of the patient's and family's understanding of the information given.

Strategies for Promoting and Effecting Behavior Change

Only a few effective strategies exist for promoting and sustaining behavior change in people who have chronic conditions. These strategies include providing basic education (to address health literacy), helping patients to set goals, engendering a sense of control (self-efficacy), arranging for professional or social support, and providing feedback (Dunbar-Jacob, 2007). Application of these strategies to education for patients with multiple myeloma is critical to maintaining a positive change in behavior.

Basic Education (Choosing the Correct Method at the Correct Time)

The concepts of multiple myeloma may be difficult to understand, even for a well-educated and English-speaking adult. Because it constitutes only 1% of all cancers (Tricot, 2009), most Americans have not heard of the disease.

Thus, providing appropriate written information along with a verbal explanation is essential. Of course, a thorough nursing assessment will determine whether any given patient learns best by visual or auditory methods or by a detailed monograph on a particular subject. Nurses and other members of the healthcare team will serve patients best by having a variety of information sources to choose from in their practice setting and by tailoring the methods accordingly for each patient and family member.

A wide variety of written materials are available to patients with multiple myeloma and their significant others. Of course, today the Internet is widely used by patients and families for health information (Hesse et al., 2005). Studies indicate that up to 64% of patients with cancer use the Internet to obtain health information, and it often is the second source of information, after the information given by the healthcare provider (Huang & Penson, 2008). However, clinicians cannot assume that the patient or family is computer savvy and need to direct them to reputable and up-to-date information. This is particularly important in diseases such as multiple myeloma, in which survival rates have improved. Although the majority of studies show that patients with cancer tend to want as much information as possible about their illness (Chen & Siu, 2001; Meredith et al., 1996), patient preference for learning method and literacy level need to be considered. Older patients need to be screened for memory or cognitive problems (White & Cohen, 2008). Additionally, imprudent, often conflicting information could potentially be overwhelming for patients and add to ambivalence and anxiety toward treatment decisions. The medical and health news reported by the media often is sensationalized to draw attention to the news story (Chen & Sui, 2001). Thus, clinicians should encourage patients to bring the information they have obtained with them to their appointments and ask their healthcare providers to clarify it and confirm how it applies to them. However, when patients and family members get information from the Internet, clinicians need to take the extra time that may be needed to review the materials and to answer patients' and family members' questions.

If patients use the Internet, clinicians can recommend they review the National Cancer Institute fact sheet *Evaluating Health Information on the Internet* (www.cancer.gov/cancertopics/factsheet/information/internet). This document provides 13 questions that can help people decide whether the health information they find on the Internet is likely to be reliable. This handout may be helpful to have readily available to give to patients.

Some cancer Web sites offer accurate, detailed, and up-to-date information on multiple myeloma. For example, the site for Cancer *Care* (www.cancercare. org), a national nonprofit organization, provides general information about cancer and also has current, detailed information on multiple myeloma, its sequelae, and treatments. The American Cancer Society is a nationwide nonprofit health organization and provides cancer resources online as well as services within many communities. Its Web site has information on complementary treatment, radiation, multiple myeloma treatment drug specifics, bisphosphonates, and plasmapheresis. It offers planning and survivorship information. Other Web sites also offer survivorship information, particularly the Lance Armstrong Foundation (www.livestrong.org), the National Coalition for Cancer Survivorship (www.canceradvocacy.org), and OncoLink (www.oncolink.org). These sites address practical aspects of living with cancer, such as finances, legal planning, and employment, so that patients can then navigate through hospital-based and local services. Importantly, the National Coalition for Cancer Survivorship has a free Cancer Survival Toolbox® that contains a set of basic skills to help patients with cancer to navigate a diagnosis and special topics on key issues. It is available in both written and audio versions, either online or on CD. The International Myeloma Foundation (IMF, http://myeloma.org) provides information online and free brochures on all aspects of the disease, diagnostic tests, treatments, and treatment side effects. This organization also offers free patient and family seminars and webcasts, as well as a 24-hour hotline staffed by trained information specialists. IMF publishes a quarterly newsletter, *Myeloma Today*, and two disease- and treatment-related handbooks (one is a more concise review, and the other is a simpler patient handbook). While other organizations provide Web sites and written materials in English and Spanish, the IMF has information in several languages (English, Spanish, French, German, Italian, Chinese, Portuguese, Polish, Hebrew, Russian, and Arabic), which visitors can select from the home page. Nurses should bear in mind that not all people who can speak a particular language can read that language or that they may have a limited reading level. Interestingly, even Wikipedia (http://en.wikipedia.org/wiki/Multiple_myeloma) has multiple myeloma disease and treatment information that is referenced and was current as of June 2009; it also has links to many languages, as well as to other links such as the American Cancer Society. If patients are consulting these medical resources, nurses should ensure that the healthcare team explains the patient's situation in reference to the general treatment guidelines and why decisions in his or her case were recommended.

The Multiple Myeloma Research Foundation (MMRF, www.multiplemyeloma .org) has information on multiple myeloma as well as a particular focus on helping patients and healthcare workers find clinical trials. The Leukemia and Lymphoma Society (LLS, www.leukemia-lymphoma.org) also has information on the disease and its treatments. LLS will ship written materials free; it also has education programs that patients can listen to online and an information resource center. Again, because not all patients have access to the Internet, the nurse can, with institution approval, print out information for patients and caregivers and provide phone numbers or addresses to them.

Fertile Hope (www.fertilehope.org) is a national nonprofit organization dedicated to providing reproductive information, support, and hope to patients with cancer and cancer survivors whose medical treatments present the risk of infertility. The nurse should not assume that fertility is not an issue with patients with multiple myeloma. Because many treatments affect fertility and birth control is essential with some therapies, the nurse can assist patients and significant others in addressing fertility-related issues. Although less than 5% of patients diagnosed with multiple myeloma are younger than 40 years (Tricot, 2009), the needs of young adults may require special support from the nurse, such as a referral to a young adult group. Aside from the aforementioned information and local support resources, the nurse could refer the patient to a resource such as the I'm Too Young For This! Cancer Foundation (http:// i2y.com), a national, survivor-led advocacy, support, and research organization working exclusively on behalf of survivors and care providers younger than the age of 40. It has links for support activities, chat rooms, local events, excursions, and retreats, as well as a local chapter finder.

Although Internet usage among physicians is high, they may or may not refer patients to helpful Web sites. Nurses, as part of the collaborative team, can make sure that Web site information is offered as appropriate. For example, a readily available handout on the reputable Web sites could be displayed in the clinic. In this way, the healthcare team could be assured that information provided is prudent and consistent. Many institutions have systems in place that require approval of materials provided to patients because of the potential legal impact. Several of the nonprofit agencies have the same information from their Web site available in print. Figure 11-2 lists reputable Web sites for multiple myeloma information. Specific brochures could be displayed in the cancer clinic or unit or be in a storage area for clinicians to access; many brochures are free, including shipping.

Figure 11-2. Web Sites With Information on Multiple Myeloma

- American Cancer Society: www.cancer.org
- CancerCare: www.cancercare.org
- Cancer.Net (patient information from the American Society of Clinical Oncology): www.cancer.net
- Coalition of Cancer Cooperative Groups: www.CancerTrialsHelp.org
- Fertile Hope: www.fertilehope.org
- I'm Too Young For This! Cancer Foundation: http://i2y.com
- International Association for Hospice and Palliative Care: www.hospicecare.com
- International Myeloma Foundation: www.myeloma.org
- Lance Armstrong Foundation: www.livestrong.org
- Leukemia and Lymphoma Society: www.leukemia-lymphoma.org
- Multiple Myeloma Research Foundation: www.multiplemyeloma.org
- National Cancer Institute: www.cancer.gov
- National Bone Marrow Transplant Link: www.nbmtlink.org
- National Coalition for Cancer Survivorship: www.canceradvocacy.org
- National Marrow Donor Program: www.marrow.org
- OncoLink LiveStrong Care Plan: www.oncolink.com/oncolife
- The Wellness Community: www.thewellnesscommunity.org
- Wikipedia: http://en.wikipedia.org/wiki/multiple_myeloma

Note. Based on information from American Cancer Society, 2009; Braccia, 2009; Ganz et al., 2008; Nau & Lewis, 2008.

The Internet may be helpful in providing information on complementary and alternative medicine and the importance of exercise and nutrition. Again, patients and their families need to be encouraged to bring questions to their healthcare providers, as some incorrect information from the Internet can be harmful.

The use of the Internet for communication between patients and healthcare providers is relatively uncommon (Beckjord et al., 2007). Benefits to ongoing communication and reinforcement of teaching via e-mail are conceivable. However, even as benefits can be appreciated, particularly in scheduling appointments, healthcare providers have concerns regarding confidentiality, reimbursement, and the workload that it would cause (Beckjord et al., 2007).

As previously stated, it is important that cancer clinicians provide sound information that is in accordance with their institution/place of employment. Commercial materials also may be helpful, such as those produced by pharmaceutical companies, as long as they are not promotional in nature.

When developing written materials for the institution, guidelines exist to assist nurses in writing materials. A nurse who is in a position to develop written materials may want to form a team of healthcare professionals such as a physician, social worker, registered dietitian, and physical therapist and look at what is available through Internet services already mentioned and what needs exist within the population they serve. Two online resources to assist the clinician in developing materials may be helpful: *How to Write Easy-to-Read Health Materials* (www.nlm.nih.gov/medlineplus/etr.html) and *Clear and Simple: Developing Effective Print Materials for Low-Literate Readers* (www.cancer.gov/cancerinformation/clearandsimple).

Karten (2007) offered suggestions for creating easy-to-read materials: have one specific main objective, organize the information like a conversation, step back and think about each page's organization, avoid using words with more than one meaning, educate the organization about the goals of creating easy-to-read information, and listen to patient-reviewer feedback. Karten also provided a handout on myeloma for patients and caregivers from the Leukemia and Lymphoma Society that can be used as a template for creating an institution-specific handout and that can be reproduced and copied without obtaining permission as long as the organization and publication date are cited.

Audio methods for educating patients with multiple myeloma are not as numerous as the written methods. IMF and MMRF provide webcasts and teleconferences, which may be helpful in augmenting and reinforcing verbal and written methods of patient education.

Setting Goals and Engendering a Sense of Control

Clinicians need to clearly define the desired change in behavior (e.g., coming to the clinic three times a week for treatment and/or monitoring laboratory values), establish a baseline, and encourage patients to self-monitor their progress. Thus, general statements for expected behaviors like "Monitor yourself for fever" or "Take your medication" need to be more specific: "Do you have a thermometer at home? Take your temperature once a day or if you feel warm or chilled. Call the clinic right away if your temperature is 100.5°F or higher." Patients can help in self-monitoring by learning to understand their laboratory values and keeping a notebook to help follow their clinical course or by keeping a symptom diary or medication log. Additionally, because patients with multiple myeloma may have a "moving target," the goals may change as the patient's disease or treatment changes. Therefore, keeping abreast of how the disease and ramifications of it are changing and why the treatment may be changing may help the patient to cope by remaining engaged in the plan. Studies show that creating a relationship with the patient and including the patient as an integral team member in assessing and controlling symptoms is an important component in patient management (Jakobsson, Ekman, & Ahlberg, 2008; Wolpin et al., 2008).

It is important to help each learner set goals and to provide informative feedback regarding progress toward these goals. Although the patient and healthcare team, along with the patient's significant others, may make these goals together, clinicians need to ensure that priority is given to safety. Patients with multiple myeloma may be at high risk for sepsis and death from infection, have bleeding or clotting disorders, and have or be at risk for pathologic fractures, including spinal cord compression. Weakness, fatigue, and uncontrolled pain, including neuropathies, can contribute to a patient's fall risk, resulting in patient injury and possibly a delay in treatment. Gorman and Sultan (2008) pointed out that even psychosocial care incorporates patient safety measures as a routine part of practice by maintaining open communication with the patient and healthcare team. Thus, safety should always be at the forefront of the education goals. If the nurse feels that the patient or family has misunderstandings of the treatment plan or is concerned about patient behaviors that may affect safety, the nurse should immediately contact the physician.

Arranging for Professional or Social Support

The Internet provides a gateway to an inexhaustible volume of virtual communities, networks, and support groups. Many of these are available through the organizations listed in Figure 11-2. However, even in the age of readily accessible information, simply referring the patient to one of these sites should not replace talking with the patient and his or her significant others. Some patients are not comfortable in a group setting or may feel overwhelmed by too much information. Some patients express loss of hope when they see others with multiple myeloma succumb to the sequelae of the disease. Busy clinics and inpatient settings do not always establish an environment in which the nurse has time to explore all of the emotional and social support needs of patients and families. The nurse needs to know when work should be shared or delegated through referrals. A social worker may help with psychosocial issues and provide referrals to support groups and resources.

Advanced practice nurses, psychologists, social workers, pharmacists, clergy members, dietitians, physical therapists, and pain management or palliative care specialists can augment the nurse's teaching and enhance patient and family education and support.

Providing Feedback

Although it may be difficult in a busy healthcare environment, it is important that the nurse allows the patient and family to demonstrate their understanding of what was taught, give them feedback, and reeducate as needed. This will allow the clinician to further tailor education that needs to be imparted and concepts that need to be clarified. Feedback may consist of verbal comments, modeling, demonstration, charts, or other graphics, such as a list of medications and the times at which they need to be taken, or a treatment trajectory calendar (Dunbar-Jacob, 2007).

The nurse could demonstrate how to find myeloma-related information on the Internet. For patients who do not have a computer, most libraries can assist with access. After reading the information, patients should bring it to their next appointment so that the healthcare team can validate patients' understanding and clarify any outlying aspects. Methods to evaluate recall of information should be tailored for each patient. Some studies have shown that an audiotape of the physician/patient conversation or a question prompt sheet is most effective, although further studies are needed (van Der Meulen, Jansen, van Dulmen, Bensing, & Van Weert, 2008).

Culturally, respect for authority and expertise may influence how a patient responds to evaluation questions. For example, a Hispanic patient may acknowledge that he has understood the information when, in fact, he has not; oftentimes, individuals say this to show respect to the healthcare provider, believing that misunderstanding the information would be insulting (Pesquera et al., 2008). Again, this is where specific evaluation of understanding needs to take place; asking open-ended questions with an interpreter may be warranted.

WHAT TO TEACH

The Disease

The concepts surrounding the disease of multiple myeloma most likely will be foreign to patients and their family, even if a family member is in the healthcare field. Multiple myeloma accounts for only 1% of all malignancies (Tricot, 2009) with an estimated 20,580 new cases diagnosed in the United States in 2009 (Jemal et al., 2009) and is occurring with increasing frequency in older adults (Nau & Lewis, 2008). Although the rate is nearly twice as high in Black people, with an increased risk in those with rheumatoid arthritis or obesity, no clear risk factor can be identified in most patients with the disease (Nau & Lewis, 2008). An estimated 10,580 deaths (50% of multiple myeloma cases) from myeloma were expected to occur in the United States in 2009 (Jemal et al., 2009). Because these statistics appear grim, the nurse can offer hope for long-term quality of life. Hope can be instilled realistically, especially in the setting of newer, targeted therapies, which have enabled many patients to live more than five years and even some more than 10 years. A phenomenal amount of research is being done in multiple myeloma, in both basic science and applied clinical trials, leading researchers to believe that long-term survival is a possibility (Raab, Podar, Breitkreutz, Richardson, & Anderson, 2009). This may not be sufficient for a younger individual to be hopeful; thus, the nurse always needs to address emotional needs and concerns when educating patients about the disease.

Many patients initially present with unexplained backache or bone pain, although some patients may be asymptomatic. Other typical symptoms on diagnosis are malaise, weakness, anorexia, nausea, weight loss, polydipsia, and neuropathy, often related to anemia, renal insufficiency, paraproteinemia, and hypercalcemia (Nau & Lewis, 2008). As with many serious illnesses, general symptoms may at first mimic a common symptom, such as a backache (e.g., pulled back muscle while gardening) or bone pain, thus delaying diagnosis. However, pathologic fracture is the presenting symptom in up to 34% of patients (Nau & Lewis, 2008). Helping patients sort through the diagnostic process often is helpful in correcting misconceptions regarding "missed" diagnoses. Helping them to then understand the appropriate workup and staging, such as laboratory tests, bone marrow biopsy, skeletal radiographs, and magnetic resonance imaging, can help them understand the extent of their disease, what questions to ask, and why the physician may be prescribing a particular treatment. The primary healthcare provider should explain the new International Staging System for multiple myeloma (Nau & Lewis, 2008) and its significance to the patient's particular case. The nurse can then explore the patient's and family's understanding, clarify misconceptions, and make sure they are readdressed as needed.

Furthermore, the concepts of the immune system, plasma cells, bone marrow function, lytic lesions, and diagnostic laboratory tests may be difficult for patients to understand and should be reviewed both in concept and as they relate to the particular case. A basic handout on multiple myeloma may be helpful (see Figure 11-3 for an example). Again, tailoring the education for each individual learner is helpful. Some patients and family members desire more or less information than others or request to have the information explained in very simple concepts. Visual aids of the bone marrow, immunoglobulins versus light chains, and other concepts may be needed, not just the written word. The Internet resources in Figure 11-2 can help clarify these advanced concepts, as many of them provide varying written levels, from basic to advanced, and often include simple visual diagrams and glossaries.

Figure 11-3. What Is Multiple Myeloma?

Multiple myeloma is a cancer of plasma cells. Multiple myeloma cells are abnormal *plasma cells*. Some normal plasma cells are found in the bone marrow (the middle of the bones), and some are in the blood. Normal plasma cells are part of our *immune system*.

The immune system helps our body prevent and fight infection. The immune system has several types of cells that work together to prevent and fight infection. *Lymphocytes* are one type of immune system cells. Two types of lymphocytes exist: T cells and B cells.

B cells change into plasma cells when they react to an infection in our body. The plasma cells make proteins called *antibodies* that attack and kill the germs causing the infection.

When plasma cells grow out of control, they can form a tumor. If only one tumor is formed, it is called a solitary *plasmacytoma*. In most cases, this single tumor will become many tumors. This is called *multiple myeloma*.

Other cells are made in the bone marrow like the lymphocytes. They then go into the blood to do their job. These include red blood cells, white blood cells, and platelets. Thus, when abnormal plasma cells grow in the bone marrow, the bone marrow is unable to make enough of these normal cells. The following problems can occur from the growth of myeloma cells in the bone marrow:
- Anemia: A shortage of red blood cells, which can cause you to be weak, tired, and pale
- Bleeding: A shortage of platelets, which can lead to a lot of bruising or bleeding
- Neutropenia: A shortage of a specific white blood cell (neutrophil), which can increase your risk for infection.

Myeloma cells do not act like normal plasma cells. They make antibodies, but these antibodies do not work to kill germs and fight infection. These antibodies may hurt your kidneys and thicken your blood.

Myeloma cells also affect the cells that help keep bones strong. Myeloma cells cause the bones to soften. The body is not able to replace the bone that is thinned and softened. This makes the bones weak, and they may break more easily.

Talk with your nurses and doctors regarding your specific case of multiple myeloma. Ask
- How has the myeloma affected my body?
- What is the treatment plan?
- What are the side effects of the treatment?
- How is the healthcare team going to reduce or prevent side effects of the treatment?
- What can I do to help with the treatment plan?

Make sure you share all of your concerns with your healthcare team.

Note. Based on information from American Cancer Society, 2009; Nau & Lewis, 2008.

When providing education about myeloma, nurses should inform patients that each case is slightly different and that the written information may not pertain to their case. Thus, reviewing the written information with the patient is essential. This is particularly true in cases in which the patient presents with a variant of multiple myeloma, such as those with a solitary plasmacytoma, nonsecretory multiple myeloma, or a plasma cell leukemia.

Important concepts related to multiple myeloma include the effect of the disease on the bones, the immune system, and renal function. Failure to monitor and/or treat these organs can result in often preventable patient morbidity. As it is clinically apparent in most cases, it is important to inform the patient that plasma cells proliferate and overproduce an abnormal immunoglobulin or "M" protein (IgG, or IGA, or rarely IgM, IgE, or IgD), as well as abnormal smaller or light-chain proteins (kappa or lambda light chain), cytokines (proteins) that stimulate osteoclasts and suppress osteoblasts, and angiogenesis. Therefore, uncontrolled disease leads to excessive proteins, hyperviscosity, osteoporosis, hypercalcemia, bone pain, and end-organ damage, especially in the kidneys, bones, and peripheral nerves. Bone marrow invasion by monoclonal plasma cells leads to anemia and immunologic alternations and contributes to recurrent infections (Raab et al., 2009). The explanations of these abnormalities, again, have to be tailored for each individual.

Medical advances in the past decade have made myeloma a chronic disease with hope for cure. Because it can be considered a chronic condition, teaching about the disease, the manifestations, and sequelae related to the manifestations needs to be ongoing, with respect given to the patient's and family's ability and willingness to learn. For example, a patient may be initially diagnosed after presenting with malaise and change in urine output, and the typical bone pain may not have been present. However, the risk of future bone manifestations and serious fractures, including cord compression, needs to be discussed in a way that informs the patient and caregivers of the potential but without initiating undue anxiety. Therefore, the patient and family will know the importance of reporting any new pain and changes in physical function. Another example of specific teaching is that fever is an uncommon presenting symptom (Nau & Lewis, 2008); however, because of the impact of the disease and treatments on the bone marrow and immune system, the patient and family need to be informed on what to report, hygiene practices, and the importance of immunizations when appropriate.

Nurses need to be aware of their scope of practice when providing patient and family education. The primary care provider (nurse practitioner or physician) should provide basic information on the disease, laboratory tests, treatment plan, diagnostic tests, and prognosis. A thorough review of this information must be provided to patients. Ideally, the nurse should be with the patient when the primary healthcare provider reviews this information so that he or she can augment and document the additional teaching appropriately.

Renal Problems

Even if the patient does not present with renal problems, patient teaching should include the potential complications of renal dysfunction. Instructing the patient to be observant for any changes in urine output or the characteristics of urine or urination (e.g., decreased amount, decreased frequency, cloudy, bloody) is important as part of the teaching plan. Often, it is appropriate to instruct the patient to drink up to three liters of fluids a day to maintain kidney health; this instruction needs to include showing what a liter is and may be done by using a specific water bottle or canister as a visual example of the volume discussed. However, some patients may already have renal disease or comorbid conditions such as congestive heart failure, warranting education on fluid restrictions and special dietary modifications as specified in the primary care provider's plan. Patients should be instructed not to take any over-the-counter medications without letting the doctor know, as they may contribute to renal problems. They also need to know that other prescription medications can affect the kidneys and need to make sure that the doctor is aware of all medications the patient has taken.

Bone Disease

Bone disease occurs in the majority (up to 80%) of patients with multiple myeloma and is associated with bone pain, fractures, and hypercalcemia (Kyle et al., 2003). In addition to the vertebral column, the long bones, ribs, skull, hip, humerus, and pelvis are commonly involved. Pathologic fracture is the presenting symptom in 26%–34% of patients (Nau & Lewis, 2008). Furthermore, more than half of patients with multiple myeloma will experience at least one new fracture, and bone disease has a major impact on quality of life and potentially on patient outcome (Sezer, 2009). For this reason, it is important to educate patients and families regarding the ongoing risk of bone disease. Patients and caregivers need to be instructed to promptly report any new pain or ache and make sure to obtain diagnostic tests. Computed tomography scans may be used in lieu of conventional x-ray imaging. Magnetic resonance imaging can be helpful in distinguishing between benign and malignant compression fractures and particularly for suspected cord compression (Sezer, 2009). Education regarding these diagnostic tests, as always, should be provided. Bisphosphonates are particularly helpful in reducing the risk of bone disease and will be discussed later in this chapter.

Balloon Kyphoplasty and Vertebroplasty

Information on potentially recommended percutaneous balloon kyphoplasty (Dudeney, Lieberman, Reinhardt, & Hussein, 2002) or vertebroplasty can be provided as needed. The nurse can inform patients that percutaneous vertebroplasty is performed under fluoroscopy or computed tomography with the patient under sedation in either the prone or lateral lying position. The vertebroplasty needle is fluoroscopically guided into the diseased bone, and cement is injected into the malignant bone cavity, leading to strengthening of the vertebra and stabilizing against vertebral collapse (Lee et al., 2009).

The procedure has a low rate of complications, which should be explained by the physician, and 80% of patients will experience significant pain relief (Lee et al., 2009). In contrast to vertebroplasty, during a balloon kyphoplasty, a 1 cm incision is made where a working cannula is placed through the pedicle, and an orthopedic balloon is guided into the fractured vertebral body. The balloon is then inflated, reducing the fracture and elevating the superior end plate. The approach is bilateral, using two balloons, to achieve en masse reduction. After reduction of the fracture has taken place, the balloons are deflated and removed. Inflation and deflation of the balloons creates a void that serves as a repository for the bone cement. The void is filled with KyphX® HV-R™ (High-Viscosity Radiopaque) Bone Cement (Kyphon Inc.) under low manual pressure. The procedure typically takes less than one hour for each fracture treated and may necessitate a short stay in the hospital (Medtronic, Inc., 2009).

Many of the Web sites listed in Figure 11-2 provide written and visual information on this procedure, as well as information on bone health and bone pain. The patient may potentially need education and support regarding surgery to stabilize long bone fractures. The nurse, as part of the interdisciplinary team, can ensure that patients with multiple myeloma receive a comprehensive screening to minimize bone complications and include optimal functioning in the plan of care. Before addressing potential activity or referral to an exercise regimen, the nurse should know if the patient has any activity restrictions associated with lytic lesions, especially potential cord compression. Comorbid conditions that are myeloma related (e.g., amyloid cardiac deposition, severe neuropathies) and those that are not myeloma related (e.g., vitamin D deficiency, age-related osteoporosis, arthritis) need to be considered in the teaching plan for bone health.

Treatments also can affect bone health and functioning. For example, fatigue and weakness, either generalized or caused by treatment such as steroid-induced proximal muscle weakness, can occur (Faiman, Bilotti, Mangan, & Rogers, 2008). Gastrointestinal problems, such as nausea and vomiting, can lead to electrolyte imbalances and anemia, affecting a patient's ability to adhere to recommendations regarding maximizing bone health and functioning.

Because of the risks of deep vein thrombosis, pulmonary embolism, and stroke as a result of specific patient and multiple myeloma treatment factors, providing tailored education regarding these risks and minimizing them through activity and/or medications are important (Rome, Doss, Miller, & Westphal, 2008). Rome et al. presented a one-page handout on deep vein thrombosis that can be copied and provided to patients and family members.

A low percentage of multiple myeloma survivors exercise regularly, but those who exercised more during either active-treatment or off-treatment periods reported a higher quality of life (Jones et al., 2004). Additionally, even patients undergoing aggressive treatment can safely participate in an individualized strengthening and endurance exercise program (Coon & Coleman, 2004).

Exploring the patient's baseline activities and, as appropriate, ensuring that specific teaching about exercise and activity such as walking and light weight lifting (no more than 20 lbs) can potentially improve a patient's quality of life. Once the safety and appropriateness of activities have been explored, the nurse can make sure that the physician has provided appropriate referrals and instructions. For example, a Tai Chi or yoga program may be beneficial to an older adult patient to improve balance, whereas more aggressive resistance training with weights may be appropriate for another (DiStasio, 2008). The American Cancer Society provides guidelines on nutrition and physical activity during and after cancer treatment (American Cancer Society, 2009; Doyle et al., 2008). Clinicians can use these guidelines as handouts for patients. In addition, the materials may be helpful in exploring possible referral-based and education-based interventions that maximize patients' bone health. Ongoing assessment and reeducation as to the importance of bone health and functioning should be conducted.

Bisphosphonates

As part of ongoing care for multiple myeloma, patients generally receive bisphosphonates for a period of two years. At two years, the physician may or may not continue this treatment (Kyle et al., 2007). In general, the treatment is pamidronate 90 mg IV delivered over at least two hours or zoledronic acid 4 mg IV delivered over at least 15 minutes every three to four weeks (Kyle et al., 2007). If the patient has renal problems, the doses will be adjusted.

The nurse should provide to the patient a basic explanation of why this medication is indicated, along with the potential side effects. The nurse can explain that the aim is to reduce bone-related events (fractures, pain) in patients with myeloma-related bone disease. It should be explained to the patient that he or she will receive an IV infusion in the office or clinic once every three to four weeks. Laboratory work will also be performed to monitor side effects, such as calcium levels and potential effects on the kidneys.

In general, these infusions are well tolerated. Although some patients may have flu-like symptoms the day after the infusion, these often subside with subsequent infusions. Osteonecrosis of the jaw, a rare and potentially serious complication of IV bisphosphonates, is characterized by the presence of exposed bone in the mouth. It typically occurs after dental extraction (Woo, Hellstein, & Kalmar, 2006). Although the risk ranges from 1%–11% (Kyle et al., 2007), all patients should be informed of this risk up front. Initially, patients need to receive a comprehensive dental examination and appropriate preventive dental work before starting bisphosphonate therapy. Active oral infections should be treated, and sites that are at high risk for infection should be eliminated (Kyle et al., 2007). The potential for osteonecrosis of the jaw, how to reduce one's risk, and signs and symptoms should be reviewed with the patient. While on therapy, patients should avoid undergoing invasive dental procedures, if possible. If they are necessary, the patient should make sure to inform the oncology physician. Nurses can assist in assessing patients' oral health and oral hygiene regimen. Simply instructing a patient to "maintain excellent oral hygiene" is not specific enough. General excellent and consistent oral hygiene, which includes brushing with a soft toothbrush four times a day after meals, using dental floss once daily, and using a alcohol-free rinse, has been shown to improve oral health outcomes in patients with cancer. Most studies have shown that it is primarily the frequency and consistency of mouth care that maximizes oral health (Bensinger et al., 2008; Harris, Eilers, Harriman, Cashavelly, & Maxwell, 2008; Rubenstein et al., 2004). Patients should be informed of the early signs and symptoms of any oral or tooth pain, any change in the oral mucosa, and any swelling in the jaw or gum lines. Instructing the patient to accurately visualize his or her mouth is particularly important, as one study reported that approximately one-third of lesions were painless (Marx, Sawatari, Fortin, & Broumand, 2005). A useful tool for recording pain scores, changes in mobility, and adverse events might be to encourage the patient to keep a diary. The nurse should fill out the diary for laboratory results and treatments given and then compare it to the baseline information before administering treatment (Maxwell, 2007). Patients should also be counseled on the importance of adequate hydration, the need for calcium and vitamin D supplements, as appropriate, and how to best manage potential side effects (Maxwell, 2007).

If the patient has dentures, the nurse should check that the dentures are well fitting and confirm with the patient that they are cleaned regularly. They should be removed, if possible, when the patient is not eating and certainly for sleep, as some cases of jaw osteonecrosis have involved dentures, which are believed to be a possible source of local trauma (Woo et al., 2006). If osteonecrosis of the jaw appears, the nurse should make certain that the patient understands and adheres to the antibiotic therapy and oral care directed by the physician or dentist.

Radiation

Radiation may be effective in relieving metastatic bone disease and related pain. Spinal cord compression often is treated with external beam radiation therapy, but surgical decompression may also be needed for spinal instability (Nau & Lewis, 2008). By first assessing a patient's understanding of the treatment, the nurse can tailor teaching accordingly. The nurse can ensure that the patient understands the specific treatment plan, goal of therapy, length of treatment, and anticipated side effects. As with education about radiation treatment for other malignancies, it is helpful to explain the treatment room equipment and personnel to relieve patients' concerns (Iwamoto & Maher, 2001). For example, a patient may not understand that external beam radiation does not pose a risk of radiation exposure to loved ones. Additionally, aside from constitutional symptoms, the side effects are related to the area and surrounding areas that were irradiated. Patients should be instructed to call their oncologist or radiation oncologist if they have any problems related to the radiation therapy. The side effects most likely will start a week or two after treatment begins and can include skin reactions, urinary problems, and diarrhea, depending on the area irradiated. The National Cancer Institute has a comprehensive booklet on radiation therapy titled *Radiation Therapy and You: Support for People With Cancer* that can be ordered or printed from the Internet (see https://cissecure.nci.nih.gov/ncipubs/detail.aspx?prodid=P123).

Steroids

Steroids are a cornerstone of multiple myeloma treatment, but they can cause a wide range of mild to life-threatening side effects that can affect almost every body system, including weight gain, edema, flushing, sweating, insomnia, skin rash or thinning, endocrine imbalances, gastrointestinal disturbances, infection, proximal myopathy, osteopenia, muscle cramping, cataracts, and mood alterations (Faiman et al., 2008). Thus, patients and family members need to be informed on how to help prevent and manage them. General information on steroids, such as a patient information sheet from the pharmacy or a general Web page, may not be specific enough in describing the rationale for this treatment. A more specific fact sheet may be helpful (see Figure 11-4), such as information provided from IMF's Web site or a printable handout developed by the IMF Nurse Leadership Board (Faiman et al., 2008).

Thalidomide

Patient teaching regarding thalidomide should focus on safety without imposing unwarranted fear. The patient may or may not be aware of the birth defects that arose from its use in Europe as a sleeping aid for pregnant women (Kyle & Rajkumar, 2008). This drug can only be prescribed and distributed through Celgene Corp.'s S.T.E.P.S.® (System for Thalidomide Education and Prescribing Safety) Program to ensure that proper patient instruction is provided regarding the severe, life-threatening birth defects and contraindication in pregnant women (Celgene Corp., 2007b). Nonetheless, patients should understand that thalidomide is an effective drug for many patients with multiple myeloma. The main points of education should include the importance of birth control as well as the risk and prevention of deep venous thrombosis and the potential for neuropathies and somnolence, increasing the risk of injuries and falls. Additionally, although rare, serious Stevens-Johnson syndrome and toxic epidermal necrolysis have occurred (Celgene Corp., 2007b). The patient needs to be watchful for possible skin reactions and report them immediately. For mild skin reactions that are more common, the prescriber can recommend topical steroids and antipruritics, and the nurse can provide education regarding the application or administration of these, as well as recommend oatmeal baths. General good skin care and hygiene can be reinforced by teaching the patient that the skin is the largest part of the

---

Figure 11-4. Patient and Family Instructions for Steroids

This medication is used to treat multiple myeloma and may be used in combination with other medications. You will need to follow these precautions while you are taking this medication.

- Swallow the capsule whole; do not crush, break, or chew it. Drink a full glass of water (about 8 ounces) when you take this medication. You may take it with or without food. Take it early in the morning, if possible.
- Tell your doctor if you have any flushing, sweating, difficulty sleeping or hyperactivity, personality or mood changes, difficulty concentrating, muscle weakness, joint or bone pain, muscle cramps, blurred vision, heartburn, changes in appetite, hiccoughs that do not go away, or skin rashes.
- This medication may cause temporary diabetes. Signs and symptoms of high and low blood sugar include aggressiveness, confusion, difficulty waking, increased thirst, and frequent urination. Call your doctor right away if you have any of these.
- Keep this medication in a secure location so that other people in your home do not accidentally take it.
- Avoid getting an infection by washing your hands frequently and avoiding people who are ill. Stay away from activities where you could be bruised, cut, or injured. Brush and floss your teeth regularly and gently. Be careful when using sharp objects, such as razors and fingernail clippers.
- Make sure to keep all appointments with your doctor as instructed. This medication may affect your blood glucose level.
- Call your doctor right away if you notice any of the following: fever or signs of infection anywhere on or in the body (redness, swelling, pain); swelling of your hands, feet, or ankles; increased or decreased urination; small blisters anywhere on the body; a white coating on the tongue; or aggressiveness, increased thirst, confusion, or difficulty waking.

Note. Based on information from Faiman et al., 2008; Thomson Reuters, 2009b.

---

immune system and that keeping it healthy and intact is an important aspect of infection prevention. Although less likely, neutropenia can occur; patients should be instructed to keep all blood count appointments and to call the physician if any signs or symptoms of infection develop. A patient handout on thalidomide is provided in Figure 11-5.

Lenalidomide

As with thalidomide, patient teaching regarding lenalidomide should focus on safety, without imposing unwarranted fear. As this mediation is only available under Celgene Corp.'s restricted distribution program called RevAssist®, the prescriber as well as the pharmacist must review with patients the high potential for birth defects. The U.S. Food and Drug Administration black box warning reflects this important information, along with the risk of myelosuppression and thromboembolism (Celgene Corp., 2007a). Instructions on how to take the medication should be reviewed: the patient should be told not to break, chew, or open the capsules, to take them with water, and to make sure that

---

Figure 11-5. Patient and Family Instructions for Thalidomide

This medication is used to treat multiple myeloma and may be used in combination with dexamethasone. You will need to follow these precautions while you are taking this medication:

- Use two forms of birth control to prevent pregnancy in yourself and your partner for four weeks before you start using thalidomide, during treatment, and for at least four weeks after your treatment ends. This medication can harm an unborn child and cause serious birth defects. If you are a woman who is able to get pregnant, your doctor will do tests to make sure you are not pregnant before starting thalidomide therapy.
- Tell your doctor if you have any shortness of breath, chest pain, arm or leg swelling, or any new skin rash. Thalidomide may increase your risk of having blood clotting problems, so he or she may prescribe a blood thinning medication.
- Call your doctor right away if you have numbness, tingling, burning, or pain in your hands or feet. Protect your hands and feet from extreme temperature changes. Create a safe environment at home to prevent falls.
- Avoid driving, using machines, or doing anything that could be dangerous if you are not alert. This medication may make you dizzy, drowsy, or light-headed when standing up, so stand up slowly. It may be helpful to take this medication in the evening. Avoid alcohol and other medications that may cause sedation.
- Keep this medication in a secure location so that other people in your home do not accidentally take it.
- Avoid getting an infection by washing your hands frequently and avoiding people who are ill. Stay away from activities where you could be bruised, cut, or injured. Brush and floss your teeth regularly and gently. Be careful when using sharp objects, such as razors and fingernail clippers.
- Make sure to keep all appointments with your doctor as instructed. This medication may affect your blood counts.
- Call your doctor right away if you notice any of the following: fever, itching, hives, or swelling in your face, hands, feet, or ankles; rash; swelling or tingling in your mouth or throat; chest tightness, trouble breathing, coughing up blood, blistering or peeling skin, or change in how much or how often you urinate; absence of menstruation or late or missed menstrual periods; confusion, seizures, or tremors; constipation or diarrhea; yellowing of skin or eyes; dry mouth or increased thirst or hunger; or sudden or severe stomach pain, muscle cramps, nausea, or vomiting.

Note. Based on information from Faiman, 2007; Thomson Reuters, 2009a.

---

they are stored in a very secure place, away from children. As with all medications, written instructions should outline when side effects warrant going to the emergency room versus simply calling the physician (see Figure 11-6).

Bortezomib

Patient education on treatment-related peripheral neuropathy associated with bortezomib is crucial to optimize clinical outcomes. Patients should be instructed to report signs and symptoms of progressive neuropathy to clinicians in order to initiate bortezomib dose delay or modification. The use of a self-report neuropathy assessment tool developed by Calhoun et al. (2003) is highly recommended (Tariman, Love, McCullagh, & Sandifer, 2008).

Safety information to emphasize during patient and family instruction should include calling the physician or 911 right away if the patient has a seizure, chest pain or discomfort, shortness of breath, or irregular heartbeat. The physician should be called if the patient has swelling of the feet, ankles, or legs or numbness, tingling, burning, or pain in the hands or feet. The nurse should provide the physician's preferred or emergency number in writing to the patient.

Other safety points of teaching include instructing the patient to avoid driving, using machines, or doing anything that could be dangerous if he or she

---

Figure 11-6. Patient and Family Instructions for Lenalidomide

This medication is used to treat multiple myeloma and may be used in combination with dexamethasone. You will need to follow these precautions while you are taking this medication:

- Use two forms of birth control to prevent pregnancy in yourself and your partner for four weeks before you start using lenalidomide, during treatment, and for at least four weeks after your treatment ends. This medication can harm an unborn child and cause serious birth defects. If you are a woman who is able to get pregnant, your doctor will do tests to make sure you are not pregnant before starting lenalidomide therapy.
- Swallow the capsule whole; do not crush, break, or chew it. Drink a full glass of water (about 8 oz) when you take this medication. You may take it with or without food.
- Do not take this medication with green tea. Check with your doctor before taking any over-the-counter medications or herbs while taking lenalidomide.
- Tell your doctor if you have any shortness of breath, chest pain, arm or leg swelling, or any new skin rash. Lenalidomide may increase your risk of blood clotting problems, so your doctor may prescribe a blood thinning medication.
- Call your doctor right away if you have numbness, tingling, burning, or pain in your hands or feet. Protect your hands and feet from extreme temperature changes. Create a safe environment at home to prevent falls.
- Avoid driving, using machines, or doing anything that could be dangerous if you are not alert. This medication may make you dizzy, drowsy, or light-headed when standing up, so stand up slowly. It may be helpful to take this medication in the evening. Avoid alcohol and other medications that may cause sedation.
- Keep this medication in a secure location so that other people in your home do not accidentally take it.
- Avoid getting an infection by washing your hands frequently and avoiding people who are ill. Stay away from activities where you could be bruised, cut, or injured. Brush and floss your teeth regularly and gently. Be careful when using sharp objects, such as razors and fingernail clippers.
- Make sure to keep all appointments with your doctor as instructed. This medication may affect your blood counts.
- Call your doctor right away if you notice any of the following: fever, itching, hives, or swelling in your face, hands, feet, or ankles; rash; swelling or tingling in your mouth or throat; chest tightness, trouble breathing, coughing up blood, blistering or peeling skin, or change in how much or how often you urinate; absence of menstruation or late or missed menstrual periods; confusion, seizures, or tremors; constipation or diarrhea; yellowing of skin or eyes; dry mouth or increased thirst or hunger; or sudden or severe stomach pain, muscle cramps, nausea, or vomiting.

Note. Based on information from Faiman, 2007; Tariman, 2007; Thomson Reuters, 2009a.

is not alert. Although rare, a specific cautionary point is that bortezomib can cause extreme drowsiness, confusion, or problems with vision caused by the start of a serious brain condition called *reversible posterior leukoencephalopathy*. Thus, patients who live on their own should have a family or friend check on them regularly. Because bortezomib may cause myelosuppression, particularly low platelets, the patient should be counseled on the importance of follow-up laboratory visits, infection prevention, neutropenia, and potentially thrombocytopenia and bleeding precautions (Miceli, Colson, Gavino, & Lilleby, 2008). Recent literature indicates that ingestion of green tea may block the anticancer activity of bortezomib (Golden et al., 2009), so the patient should be specifically instructed to avoid this drink or any foods, such as ice cream, containing green tea. Because herpes zoster reactivation can occur, patients may be instructed to take a prophylactic antiviral medication as well (Vickrey, Allen, Mehta, & Singhal, 2009). If not, he or she should be informed of the signs and symptoms of herpes zoster. Figure 11-7 shows an example of a patient education handout specific to bortezomib.

Doxorubicin Hydrochloride Liposome Injection

Although doxorubicin hydrochloride liposome injection, or doxorubicin hydrochloride liposomal (Doxil®, Centocor Ortho Biotech Products L.P.), generally is better tolerated than the non-liposomal form of doxorubicin (Chanan-Khan et al., 2009), the patient should be informed that it can create some specific side effects that need to be reported. Doxorubicin hydrochloride liposome injection may cause nausea and vomiting, and the patient should make sure to have medication to prevent nausea and vomiting available. The patient should be instructed to call the doctor if unable to drink enough fluids (eight 8-oz glasses a day). Although cardiac problems are less likely with doxorubicin hydrochloride liposome injection than doxorubicin, the patient should be instructed on what to do regarding potential cardiac problems. Allergic reactions and fluid retention or swelling also may occur; the patient should be informed on reporting these problems.

Figure 11-8 lists specific instructions related to doxorubicin hydrochloride liposomal. The patient should be told that his or her urine may turn red for one to two days after treatment and that this is normal. The delayed effects, such as hand-foot syndrome and myelosuppression, should be emphasized so that the patient keeps follow-up visits and knows what to report from home. Patient monitoring (e.g., weight) and hygiene should be emphasized (Faiman, 2007).

Stem Cell Transplantation

The role of high-dose chemotherapy supported by SCT is an effective therapy for patients with multiple myeloma (Bruno, Giaccone, Sorasio, & Boccadoro, 2009; Rodriguez, Tariman, Enecio, & Estrella, 2007). Because

---

Figure 11-7. Patient and Family Instructions for Bortezomib

This medication is used to treat multiple myeloma. You will receive this medication as an IV infusion in a cancer clinic or in the hospital. You will need to follow these precautions while you are taking this medication:

- Tell your doctor or nurse right away if you have any nausea or vomiting. You will receive medication to prevent this and should have medications at home in case you have nausea or vomiting. Call your doctor if you are unable to drink enough fluids (eight 8-oz glasses a day or as instructed by your doctor).
- Call 911 right away if you have chest pain or discomfort, shortness of breath, irregular heartbeat, or seizures. Call your doctor if you have swelling of the feet, ankles, or legs while you are taking this medication. It can cause serious heart problems.
- Call your doctor right away if you have numbness, tingling, burning, or pain in your hands or feet. Protect your hands and feet from extreme temperature changes. Create a safe environment at home to prevent falls.
- Avoid driving, using machines, or doing anything that could be dangerous if you are not alert. This medication may make you dizzy, drowsy, or light-headed when standing up, so stand up slowly. It may be helpful to take this medication in the evening. Avoid alcohol and other medications that may cause sedation.
- Dangle your feet before standing, and stand up slowly.
- Call your doctor right away if you start having headaches, extreme drowsiness, confusion, or problems with vision while you are taking this medication. This may be the start of a serious, treatable brain condition called reversible posterior leukoencephalopathy.
- Make sure to report any signs of infection or bleeding to your doctor right away. This medication may affect your blood counts. Because of this, you may get an infection or bleed more easily.
- Avoid getting an infection by washing your hands frequently and avoiding people who are ill. Stay away from activities where you could be bruised, cut, or injured. Brush and floss your teeth regularly and gently. Be careful when using sharp objects, such as razors and fingernail clippers.
- Make sure to tell your doctor about any medications and herbal products you are taking. This medication may interact with some of them.
- This medication should not be taken while you are pregnant. Use an effective form of birth control while using this medicine. Do not breast-feed while you are taking this medication.
- Make sure to keep all appointments with your doctor as instructed. This medication may affect your blood counts.
- Call your doctor right away if you notice any of the following: fever, itching, hives, swelling in your face, hands, feet, or ankles; rash; swelling or tingling in your mouth or throat; chest tightness, trouble breathing, coughing up blood, blistering or peeling skin, or change in how much or how often you urinate; absence of menstruation or late or missed menstrual periods; confusion or tremors; constipation or diarrhea; yellowing of skin or eyes; dry mouth or increased thirst or hunger; or sudden or severe stomach pain, muscle cramps, nausea, or vomiting.

Note. Based on information from Colson et al., 2008; Faiman, 2007; Thomson Reuters, 2009a.

---

several transplantation-related strategies exist (tandem autologous SCT, autologous followed by an allogeneic SCT, nonmyeloablative allogeneic SCT, related versus unrelated, etc.), as well as different types of infusions (peripheral stem cells versus bone marrow, versus cord blood), patients will need to understand that not all transplants are alike (Hari, Pasquini, & Vesole, 2006).

Pretransplant education usually begins when the patient is first considered to be a candidate for transplantation. Nursing research coordinators often perform this function, providing the patient with general information on the expected trajectory of the treatment. Basic concepts of stem cells, bone mar-

---

Figure 11-8. Patient and Family Instructions for Doxorubicin Hydrochloride Liposomal

This medication is used to treat multiple myeloma. You will receive this medication as an IV infusion in a cancer clinic or hospital. You will need to follow these precautions while you are taking this medication:

- Tell your doctor or nurse right away if you have any nausea or vomiting. You will receive medication to prevent this and should have medications at home in case you have nausea or vomiting. Call your doctor if you are unable to drink enough fluids (eight 8-oz glasses a day or as instructed by your doctor).
- Call 911 right away if you have chest pain or discomfort, shortness of breath, irregular heartbeat, or seizures. Call your doctor if you have swelling of the feet, ankles, or legs while you are taking this medication. It can cause serious heart problems.
- Tell your nurse if you have back pain, flushing in your face, shortness of breath, headache, swelling in your face, or a tight feeling in your chest or throat while you are having this treatment.
- This medicine may turn your urine red for one to two days after your treatment. This is normal.
- Call your doctor right away if you have numbness, tingling, burning, or pain in your hands or feet. Protect your hands and feet from extreme temperature changes.
- Make sure to report any signs of infection or bleeding to your doctor right away. This medication may affect your blood counts. Because of this, you may get an infection or bleed more easily.
- Avoid getting an infection by washing your hands frequently and avoiding people who are ill. Stay away from activities where you could be bruised, cut, or injured. Brush your teeth with a soft toothbrush four times a day and floss your teeth daily. Let your doctor know if your mouth becomes sore or irritated. Be careful when using sharp objects, such as razors and fingernail clippers.
- Make sure to tell your doctor about any medications and herbal products you are taking. This medication may interact with some of them.
- Doxorubicin hydrochloride liposomal should not be taken while you are pregnant. Use an effective form of birth control while using this medicine. Do not breast-feed while you are taking this medication.
- Make sure to keep all appointments with your doctor as instructed. This medication may affect your blood counts.
- Call your doctor right away if you notice any of the following: fever, itching, hives, swelling in your face, hands, feet, or ankles; rash; swelling or tingling in your mouth or throat; chest tightness, trouble breathing, coughing up blood, blistering or peeling skin, or change in how much or how often you urinate; absence of menstruation or late or missed menstrual periods; confusion or tremors; constipation or diarrhea; yellowing of skin or eyes; dry mouth or increased thirst or hunger; sudden or severe stomach pain, muscle cramps, nausea, or vomiting; or weight gain.

Note. Based on information from Faiman, 2007; Ortho Biotech, 2006; Thomson Reuters, 2009a.

row, cord blood, autologous transplant, matched related allogeneic transplant, and matched unrelated allogeneic transplant should be reviewed with the patient and caregiver as appropriate to the impending treatment. Once the transplant treatment is confirmed, topics should be individualized according to the specific type of transplant, the conditioning regimen, and the expected side effects. For example, high-dose melphalan 200 mg/m^2 supported by previously collected peripheral stem cells is a well-established conditioning chemotherapy regimen (Harousseau & Moreau, 2009). The nurse should not assume that a patient who is a nurse or physician has an understanding of these concepts. Patients often have many questions even before meeting with the transplant physician or transplant coordinator. Several Web sites, including the American Cancer Society (www.cancer.org) and the National Cancer Institute (www.cancer.gov), provide good general information that patients can be initially referred to. The National Bone Marrow Transplant Link (www.nbmtlink.org/index.htm) has detailed information about SCT and bone marrow transplantation online; printed brochures must be paid for but PDF versions are available for download (see www.nbmtlink.org/resources_support/resources.htm). Although it does not have specific information about indications for transplantation in patients with multiple myeloma, it provides a comprehensive explanation of the variety of SCTs, as well as the role of the caregiver, insurance information, an extensive glossary, and 15 pages of Web site and book resources.

Aside from the clinical process of pretransplant harvesting of stem cells, the patient and family will need education and assistance with the process of the diagnostic tests that are required to ensure patient suitability (Rodriguez et al., 2007). Many institutions may refer patients to a larger transplant center. The nurse can either print information or refer the patient and family to several of the previously mentioned Web sites. Specific information that should be discussed with the patient prior to transplant includes the route of administration, dosage, side effects, and administration of all medications, such as chemotherapeutic agents, anti-infectives, immunosuppressives, antiemetics, immunomodulators, analgesics, and growth factors (Niess & Duffy, 2004). Prior to transplant and as part of the informed consent process, serious side effects such as fever, bleeding, uncontrolled diarrhea, nausea, vomiting, and unusual toxicities of high-dose therapy should be reviewed. Adjunctive teaching by the nurse should include the supportive care measures that will be initiated to prevent or minimize these sequelae. The nurse, along with the rest of the healthcare team, can reassure the patient that care will be taken to prevent and minimize side effects as well as toxicities.

It may be helpful to develop a calendar plan for the patient and go over each piece of the treatment and recovery trajectory in a global nature, and then review each part prior to that particular event within the SCT plan. Providing an overview, and then tailoring education to a small session focused on the upcoming and current events, may be helpful in minimizing the potentially overwhelming amount of information. One simple directive might be to tell the patient to inform the nurse or doctor of anything "different"; this may reassure the patient and foster involvement in the plan of care. Table 11-1 provides a list of potential adverse effects of SCT and a few simple patient education goals related to each. This could provide a framework for helping the clinician focus on important aspects of this overwhelming topic.

During the transplantation, the nurse should inform the patient and caregiver of what to expect and should reinforce the potential side effects of the treatment. Again, it may be helpful to instruct the patient and caregivers to report anything different and to provide guidance in daily activities and the plan of care: activity, hygiene, laboratory results, and action plan for the patient, such as the need for electrolyte replacement and blood products. The nurse should reassure the patient and family as side effects occur by giving supportive and educational statements. The nurse should explain that neutropenic fever, "stat" cultures, and the administration of broad-spectrum antibiotics are common and that the team is qualified and prepared to help the patient through the experience.

At discharge, the patient should be instructed on the importance of taking the prescribed medications, as well as making sure to come to the follow-up appointment at the transplant center. Because patients with multiple myeloma may have cellular and humoral immune deficits for some time, even though they have recovered from their neutropenia, they may need to be on acyclovir and fluconazole. Instructions to call the physician or healthcare provider for any signs or symptoms of infection are very important. Additionally, engraftment of platelets may lag behind. Patients may be discharged before full platelet engraftment is achieved, depending on the preference of the primary care provider, and need to adhere to activity restrictions until platelet counts reach 100,000/microliter.

Infection

Patients may still be at risk for infection after transplant whether or not they are neutropenic. Because of their immune deficit (Ludwig & Zojer, 2007), patients with myeloma are always at risk for infection, even if they have not undergone SCT. Infection is the leading cause of death in patients with multiple myeloma (Ludwig & Zojer, 2007). Patients need to be informed not only of the risk of infection, but also of the importance of specific hygiene practices (e.g., hand washing, oral care, care of central lines) and the signs and symptoms of infection, even subtle ones, such as thrush caused by being on steroids alone. Patients need to know what to do, as well as the importance of taking any prescribed antimicrobial agents.

Pain Management

Pain control should be assessed at every encounter. Initially, as in all aspects of care, the patient and family's understanding of pain and the plan to treat

Table 11-1. Potential Adverse Effects of Autologous and Allogeneic Stem Cell Transplant and Education Goal Considerations for Patients and Families

Concept/Potential Problem	Patient/Family Education Goals
	The patient and family will be able to verbalize understanding that:
Nausea and vomiting	Medication will be given to prevent nausea and vomiting and also as needed. Inform the nurse when even mild nausea occurs. Prevention of nausea and vomiting, particularly when platelets are low, is critical to prevent bleeding.
Mucositis (mouth and throat soreness)	Oral sores may not be 100% preventable. Sucking on ice before, during, and after melphalan administration can minimize them. Inflammation of the entire gastrointestinal tract is common, leading to diarrhea.
Diarrhea	You must tell the nurse as soon as you have a change in bowel pattern. Stool samples must be sent to make sure it is from the chemotherapy, not an infection. Medications can be given to minimize diarrhea. Inform the nurse and doctor if you have abdominal pain or if the perirectal area becomes sore or irritated.
Malnutrition/dehydration	Loss of appetite is common. Few patients need high-calorie IV infusions, but blood tests will be done to monitor your nutrition and fluid balance. You can help the healthcare team by letting them know how much you eat and drink and by saving urine and stool as instructed.
Infection	A fever is common and may be the result of an infection. Blood tests will be done to check for infection. IV antibiotics will be given to you even if an infection is not found. Notify the nurse or doctor if you have any chills, redness, swelling, or pain in or on any part of your body.
Bleeding	Minor bleeding may occur because of low platelet counts. You will be given platelet transfusions as needed to prevent this. Tell your nurse or doctor immediately if you notice any bruising, red spots on your skin, or bleeding.
Anemia and fatigue	A low red cell count can cause anemia and contribute to weakness. You will be given red cell transfusions as needed. Tell your nurse or doctor immediately if you feel short of breath or dizzy, or if your heart is pounding or beating very fast.
Graft-versus-host disease	Immune suppression medications must be taken as directed. You must report any signs or symptoms of skin or gastrointestinal problems, or weight gain.

(Continued on next page)

Table 11-1. Potential Adverse Effects of Autologous and Allogeneic Stem Cell Transplant and Education Goal Considerations for Patients and Families *(Continued)*	
Concept/Potential Problem	**Patient/Family Education Goals**
Liver problems	Some chemotherapy and other medications can affect the liver. You will have blood tests done to monitor this, and the doctors will adjust medications if needed.
Skin problems	The skin is the largest organ of the immune system. You and your family need to inform the healthcare team if you have any skin discomfort or notice any skin changes, lesions, etc., and participate as directed in skin care.

Note. Based on information from Ezzone, 2004; Miceli et al., 2008; Rodriguez et al., 2007.

the pain should be assessed. Patients with advanced cancer can even benefit from education to help modify their potentially negative attitudes or beliefs toward pain. Patients and family members should be involved in appropriate pain monitoring and treatment modification; this will establish better pain control (Aubin et al., 2006; Rustoen, Gaardsrud, Leegaard, & Wahl, 2009).

Patients should understand that they may have different types of pain or may need several different methods to control each pain. Education should include what specific over-the-counter drugs can be taken and how much per day can be taken safely, as some patients should not take them at all because of adverse renal effects (Nau & Lewis, 2008). For example, the patient should be informed when it is acceptable to use nonsteroidal anti-inflammatory drugs (NSAIDs) because these drugs usually are contraindicated in patients with multiple myeloma because of their adverse effects on the kidneys. The nurse should explain that if NSAIDs are recommended, they may augment a reduction in inflammation caused by tumors and aid with other pain relief measures, such as radiation and opiates. Opiates are the preferred therapies for pain control, and thus the nurse should explain the importance of taking opiates preventively, as well as the potential side effects. Other modalities that may be part of the pain management regimen in patients with multiple myeloma include interventional procedures such as nerve blocks and kyphoplasty. Steroids may help with reducing pain caused by inflammation as well as treating the tumor; steroids are lympholytic and thus reduce pain caused by direct tumor pressure on nerve endings. Prevention of bone-related problems by administration of bisphosphonates also helps to reduce pain problems because they decrease vertebral fractures (Djulbegovic et al., 2002). It is important to inform the patient of the high potential for peripheral neuropathic pain, which may occur from myeloma or comorbid conditions such as diabetes. Although most neuropathies are not curable, they can be reduced with treatment. Patients may be hesitant to report treatment-related neuropathic pain for fear that an effective treatment may be stopped or dose-reduced. It is important to explore this possibility, reeducate the patient, and offer plausible and hopeful scenarios so that this does not occur (Tariman et al., 2008). Tariman et al. (2008) provided a one-page patient education sheet on preventing peripheral neuropathy from novel agents for multiple myeloma by the IMF Nurse Leadership Board that can be copied and provided to patients.

Partnering with the patient and family optimizes pain management. The education should include the following information (Reeves, 2008).

- Terminology related to pain management
- Assessment of the patient's pain at home (diary, log by the patient/family)
- Facts about medications and the rarity of addiction when opiates are used to relieve pain
- Adjuvant therapies for pain management
- Alternative and complementary therapies for pain management
- Vital nature of communication with the interdisciplinary team, especially related to the pain experience, effectiveness of interventions and medications, side effects, and other modalities. The team may consist of physicians, nurses (including pain specialists), psychologists, social workers, physical therapists, and others.

General handouts on pain are available through many of the Web sites already mentioned. Examples of two simple patient education materials from the National Cancer Institute (www.cancer.gov) cover the chemotherapy side effects of pain (www.cancer.gov/cancertopics/chemo-side-effects/pain.pdf) and nerve changes (www.cancer.gov/cancertopics/chemo-side-effects/nerve.pdf). The National Cancer Institute has pain information for patients available at www.cancer.gov/cancertopics/pdq/supportivecare/pain/patient. It reviews the important aspects of patient self-reporting, which is helpful during a clinician's assessment of a patient's pain. It delineates the aspects of pain that the patient must describe, including the pain itself (e.g., when it started, how long it lasts, if it is worse at certain times), location, pattern, intensity or severity, aggravating and relieving factors, and personal response. It includes an excellent glossary of terms, including clarification of drug abuse, drug addiction, and drug tolerance.

The American Cancer Society (www.cancer.org) has an online *I Can Cope* educational program on relieving cancer pain (www.cancer.org/onlineclasses), as well as a printable and orderable detailed monograph, *Pain Control: A Guide for People With Cancer and Their Families* (see www.cancer.org/docroot/MBC/MBC_7_Pain.asp). It includes specific medications and their actions and side effects. For example, the monograph specifically informs the patient that NSAIDs can irritate the stomach, cause bleeding, reduce fever, and cause kidney problems. Opiate side effects, such as drowsiness, constipation, and nausea and vomiting, are also discussed. Importantly, it has a printable pain diary for patients. Self-report diaries have been used to not only educate and involve patients in their own pain control, but also to monitor physical and emotional symptoms, as well as to measure adherence (Hoekstra, Bindels, van Duijn, & Schade, 2004; Oldenmenger et al., 2007).

The LiveStrong Guidebook (see http://store.store-laf.org/guidebook. html) has a simple health diary format for recording the date, time, and any changes in physical or emotional health that can be used for patient self-report and recording of health status in any setting.

Clinical Trials

Ongoing education regarding the availability of clinical trials, as appropriate, should be discussed by the patient with the healthcare team. The patient should be directed to appropriate Web sites if needed. Although physicians may have discussed the possibility of enrollment in a clinical trial, the nurse should not assume this was done and should, along with the research nurse, assist interested patients and families in exploring this possibility (Fenton, Rigney, & Herbst, 2009). As a patient advocate, the nurse can help to ensure that education regarding clinical trial participation is unbiased (Eggly et al., 2008). The Internet may be helpful as patients investigate the availability of clinical trials. The National Cancer Institute (www.cancer.gov/clinicaltrials) and the Coalition of Cancer Cooperative Groups (www.cancertrialshelp.org) provide information about ongoing clinical trials.

Long-Term and Late Side Effects and Survivorship

Long-term and late side effects of chemotherapy include fatigue, pain (including neuropathic pain), sexual dysfunction, cardiac problems, psychological distress, and many other conditions. The nurse should utilize appropriate referrals for psychosocial support and other previously described resources. Some patients prefer one-on-one counseling, whereas others prefer a support group.

Survivorship care plans should contain a cancer treatment history, potential long-term and late effects of treatment, recommended surveillance for long-term and late effects, and recommended surveillance for recurrence and new cancers. Links to resources for ongoing psychosocial support and general health and wellness should be included (Ganz, Casillas, & Hahn, 2008). Patients with myeloma should continue with regular checkups for cancer and cardiovascular disease, as well as other screenings. A clear timeline would be helpful to these patients. The Cancer Survival Toolbox from the National Coalition for Cancer Survivorship, as mentioned previously, includes a basic skill set that covers communicating, finding information, making decisions, solving problems, negotiating, and standing up for one's rights. Patients who are not able or are not interested in using the Internet can be encouraged to keep a notebook or organized file folder. Healthcare providers should make sure that patients speak to their oncologist about myeloma follow-up as well as regular health screenings. Long-term issues, such as fatigue, weight gain, neurotoxicity, and sexual dysfunction, should be specifically assessed, as patients may not bring up symptom concerns that affect their quality of life.

Palliative Care and Hospice

The quality of end-of-life care is now a central issue in health care (Redman, 2001). Patient and family education regarding the patient's right to accept or refuse medical treatments and even supportive care should be done by the physician; the role of the nurse and the rest of the healthcare team is to work collaboratively with the physician, patient, and family and to maximize the quality of this understanding. Education interventions can increase the rate of advance directive completion; again, the nurse and the rest of the healthcare team should provide the necessary education so that the patient can make the most-informed decision. The International Association for Hospice and Palliative Care Web site (www.hospicecare.com) provides resources for healthcare providers, patients, and families.

CONCLUSION

Multiple myeloma is a complex disease affecting multiple organs of the body. Thus, patient and family education is an important aspect of care for this disease. Thorough and attentive assessment and subsequent tailored education should be done at every patient and family encounter. Reputable educational tools can be developed but also are readily available through the Internet and are available to healthcare providers to assist with their interactions with patients and family members. Education is part of the nurturing relationship nurses have with their patients and the patients' caregivers. Education, and evaluation of its effectiveness as part of the healthcare teams' ongoing support and encouragement, is essential for helping patients to maximize their quality of life as they live with multiple myeloma.

REFERENCES

American Cancer Society. (2009). *Detailed guide: Multiple myeloma.* Retrieved from http://www.cancer.org/docroot/CRI/content/CRI_2_4_1X_What_is_multiple_myeloma_30.asp

Aubin, M., Vezina, L., Parent, R., Fillion, L., Allard, P., Bergeron, R., ... Giguere, A. (2006). Impact of an educational program on pain management in patients with cancer living at home. *Oncology Nursing Forum, 33,* 1183–1188. doi:10.1188/06.ONF.1183-1188

Beckjord, E.B., Finney Rutten, L.J., Squiers, L., Arora, N.K., Volckmann, L., Moser, R.P., & Hesse, B.W. (2007). Use of the Internet to communicate with health care providers in the United States: Estimates from the 2003 and 2005 Health Information National Trends Surveys (HINTS). *Journal of Medical Internet Research, 9*(3), e20. doi:10.2196/jmir.9.3.e20

Bensinger, W., Schubert, M., Ang, K.K., Brizel, D., Brown, E., Eilers, J.G., ... Trotti, A.M., III. (2008). NCCN task force report: Prevention and management of mucositis in cancer care. *Journal of the National Comprehensive Cancer Network, 6*(Suppl. 1), S1–S21.

Braccia, D. (2009). Go online for cancer survivor resources. Retrieved from http://onsconnect .epubxpress.com/wps/portal/conn/c0/04_SB8K8xLLM9MSSzPy8xBz9CP0os3iLkCAP EzcPIwN3P0NLAyM3Vw9jD29PQwN_E_1I_ShznPImBvohIBMz9SNNTI1NQcxi_UgDEF-2gH2loBhbILy1KTtWPLE5NLErO0C_ITkyqSk2qcnRUVAQA3ECOTQ!!/

Bruno, B., Giaccone, L., Sorasio, R., & Boccadoro, M. (2009). Role of allogeneic stem cell transplantation in multiple myeloma. *Seminars in Hematology, 46,* 158–165. doi:10.1053/j. seminhematol.2009.02.001

Calhoun, E.A., Welshman, E.E., Chang, C.-H., Lurain, J.R., Fishman, D.A., Hunt, T.L., & Cella, D. (2003). Psychometric Evaluation of the Functional Assessment of Cancer Therapy/Gynecologic Oncology Group—Neurotoxicity (FACT/GOG-NTX) questionnaire for patients receiving systemic chemotherapy. *International Journal of Gynecological Cancer, 13,* 741–748. doi:10.1111/j.1525-1438.2003.13603.x

Celgene Corp. (2007a). Revlimid (lenalidomide) [Package insert]. Summit, NJ: Author.

Celgene Corp. (2007b). Thalomid (thalidomide) [Package insert]. Summit, NJ: Author.

Chanan-Khan, A., Miller, K.C., Musial, L., Padmanabhan, S., Yu, J., Ailawadhi, S., ... Czuczman, M.S. (2009). Bortezomib in combination with pegylated liposomal doxorubicin and thalidomide is an effective steroid independent salvage regimen for patients with relapsed or refractory multiple myeloma: Results of a phase II clinical trial. *Leukemia and Lymphoma, 50,* 1096–1101. doi:10.1080/10428190902912460

Chen, X., & Siu, L.L. (2001). Impact of the media and the Internet on oncology: Survey of cancer patients and oncologists in Canada. *Journal of Clinical Oncology, 19,* 4291–4297. PMid:11731511

Colson, K., Doss, D.S., Swift, R., & Tariman, J. (2008). Expanding role of bortezomib in multiple myeloma: Nursing implications. *Cancer Nursing, 31,* 239–249. doi:10.1097/01. NCC.0000305733.80592.8e

Coon, S.K., & Coleman, E.A. (2004). Exercise decisions within the context of multiple myeloma, transplant, and fatigue. *Cancer Nursing, 27,* 108–118. doi:10.1097/00002820-200403000-00003

Coon, S.K., McBride-Wilson, J., & Coleman, E.A. (2007). Back to basics: Assessment, communication, caring, and follow-up: A lesson from a couple's journey with multiple myeloma. *Clinical Journal of Oncology Nursing, 11,* 825–829. doi:10.1188/07.CJON.825-829

DiStasio, S.A. (2008). Integrating yoga into cancer care. *Clinical Journal of Oncology Nursing, 12,* 125–130. doi:10.1188/08.CJON.125-130

Djulbegovic, B., Wheatley, K., Ross, H., Clark, O.A.C., Bos, G., Goldschmidt, H., ... Glasmacher, A. (2002). Bisphosphonates in multiple myeloma. *Cochrane Database of Systematic Reviews* 2002, Issue 4. Art. No.: CD003188. doi:10.1002/14651858 .CD003188

Doyle, C., Kushi, L.H., Byers, T., Courneya, K.S., Demark-Wahnefried, W., Grant, B., ... Andrews, K.S. (2008). Nutrition and physical activity during and after cancer treatment: An American Cancer Society guide for informed choices. *CA: A Cancer Journal for Clinicians, 56,* 323–353. doi:10.3322/canjclin.56.6.323

Dudeney, S., Lieberman, I.H., Reinhardt, M.K., & Hussein, M. (2002). Kyphoplasty in the treatment of osteolytic vertebral compression fractures as a result of multiple myeloma. *Journal of Clinical Oncology, 20,* 2382–2387.

Dunbar-Jacob, J. (2007). Models for changing patient behavior. *American Journal of Nursing, 107*(Suppl. 6), 20–25.

Eggly, S., Albrecht, T.L., Harper, F.W.K., Foster, T., Franks, M.M., & Ruckdeschel, J.C. (2008). Oncologists' recommendations of clinical trial participation to patients. *Patient Education and Counseling, 70,* 143–148. doi:10.1016/j.pec.2007.09.019

Ezzone, S. (Ed.). (2004). *Hematopoietic stem cell transplantation: A manual for nursing practice.* Pittsburgh, PA: Oncology Nursing Society.

Faiman, B. (2007). Clinical updates and nursing considerations for patients with multiple myeloma. *Clinical Journal of Oncology Nursing, 11*, 831–840. doi:10.1188/07.CJON.831-840

Faiman, B., Bilotti, E., Mangan, P.A., & Rogers, K. (2008). Steroid-associated side effects in patients with multiple myeloma: Consensus statement of the IMF Nurse Leadership Board. *Clinical Journal of Oncology Nursing, 12*(Suppl. 3), 53–63. doi:10.1188/08.CJON. S1.53-62

Fenton, L., Rigney, M., & Herbst, R.S. (2009). Clinical trial awareness, attitudes, and participation among patients with cancer and oncologists. *Community Oncology, 6*, 207–213, 228.

Fredette, S.L. (1990). A model for improving cancer patient education. *Cancer Nursing, 13*, 207–215. doi:10.1097/00002820-199008000-00001

Ganz, P.A., Casillas, J., & Hahn, E.E. (2008). Ensuring quality care for cancer survivors: Implementing the survivorship care plan. *Seminars in Oncology Nursing, 24*, 208–217. doi:10.1016/j.soncn.2008.05.009

Golden, E.B., Lam, P.Y., Kardosh, A., Gaffney, K.J., Cadenas, E., Louie, S.G., ... Schonthal, A.H. (2009). Green tea polyphenols block the anticancer effects of bortezomib and other boronic acid–based proteasome inhibitors. *Blood, 113*, 5027–5037. doi:10.1182/ blood-2008-07-171389

Gorman, L.M., & Sultan, D.F. (2008). *Psychosocial nursing for general patient care* (3rd ed.). Philadelphia, PA: F.A. Davis.

Hari, P., Pasquini, M.C., & Vesole, D.H. (2006). New questions about transplantation in multiple myeloma. *Oncology, 20*, 1230–1242.

Harousseau, J.-L., & Moreau, P. (2009). Autologous hematopoietic stem-cell transplantation for multiple myeloma. *New England Journal of Medicine, 360*, 2645–2654. doi:10.1056/ NEJMct0805626

Harris, D.J., Eilers, J., Harriman, A., Cashavelly, B.J., & Maxwell, C. (2008). Putting evidence into practice: Evidence-based interventions for the management of oral mucositis. *Clinical Journal of Oncology Nursing, 12*, 141–152. doi:10.1188/08.CJON.141-152

Hesse, B.W., Nelson, D.E., Kreps, G.L., Croyle, R.T., Arora, N.K., Rimer, B.K., ... Viswanath, K. (2005). Trust and sources of health information: The impact of the Internet and its implications for health care providers: Findings from the first Health Information National Trends Survey. *Archives of Internal Medicine, 165*, 2618–2624. doi:10.1001/ archinte.165.22.2618

Hoekstra, J., Bindels, P.J., van Duijn, N.P., & Schade, E. (2004). The symptom monitor. A diary for monitoring physical symptoms for cancer patients in palliative care: Feasibility, reliability and compliance. *Journal of Pain and Symptom Management, 27*, 24–35. doi:10.1016/j.jpainsymman.2003.06.005

Huang, G.J., & Penson, D.F. (2008). Internet health resources and the cancer patient. *Cancer Investigation, 26*, 202–207. doi:10.1080/07357900701566197

Iwamoto, R.R., & Maher, K.E. (2001). Radiation therapy for prostate cancer. *Seminars in Oncology Nursing, 17*, 90–100. doi:10.1053/sonu.2000.23071

Jakobsson, S., Ekman, T., & Ahlberg, K. (2008). Components that influence assessment and management of cancer-related symptoms: An interdisciplinary perspective. *Oncology Nursing Forum, 35*, 691–698. doi:10.1188/08.ONF.691-698

Jemal, A., Siegel, R., Ward, E., Hao, Y., Xu, J., & Thun, M.J. (2009). Cancer statistics, 2009. *CA: A Cancer Journal for Clinicians, 59*, 225–249. doi:10.3322/caac.20006

Jones, L.W., Courneya, K.S., Vallance, J.K.H., Ladha, A.B., Mant, M.J., Belch, A.R., ... Reiman, T. (2004). Association between exercise and quality of life in multiple myeloma cancer survivors. *Supportive Care in Cancer, 12*, 780–788. doi:10.1007/s00520-004-0668-4

Karten, C. (2007). Easy to write? Creating easy-to-read patient education materials. *Clinical Journal of Oncology Nursing, 11*, 506–510. doi:10.1188/07.CJON.506-510

Kothare, V.S. (2000). *Nurse's legal handbook* (4th ed.). Springhouse, PA: Springhouse.

Kyle, R.A., Gertz, M.A., Witzig, T.E., Lust, J.A., Lacy, M.Q., Dispenzieri, A., ... Greipp, P.R. (2003). Review of 1027 patients with newly diagnosed multiple myeloma. *Mayo Clinic Proceedings, 78*, 21–33. doi:10.4065/78.1.21

Kyle, R.A., & Rajkumar, S.V. (2008). Multiple myeloma. *Blood, 111,* 2962–2972. doi:10.1182/blood-2007-10-078022

Kyle, R.A., Yee, G.C., Somerfield, M.R., Flynn, P.J., Halabi, S., Jagannath, S., … Anderson, K. (2007). American Society of Clinical Oncology 2007 clinical practice guideline update on the role of bisphosphonates in multiple myeloma. *Journal of Clinical Oncology, 25,* 2464–2472. doi:10.1200/JCO.2007.12.1269

Lee, B., Franklin, I., Lewis, J.S., Coombes, R.C., Leonard, R., Gishen, P., & Stebbing, J. (2009). The efficacy of percutaneous vertebroplasty for vertebral metastases associated with solid malignancies. *European Journal of Cancer, 45,* 1597–1602. doi:10.1016/j.ejca.2009.01.021

Ludwig, H., & Zojer, N. (2007). Supportive care in multiple myeloma. *Best Practice and Research Clinical Haematology, 20,* 817–835. doi:10.1016/j.beha.2007.10.001

Marx, R.E., Sawatari, Y., Fortin, M., & Broumand V. (2005). Bisphosphonates-induced exposed bone (osteonecrosis/osteopetrosis) of the jaws: Risk factors, recognition, prevention, and treatment. *Journal of Oral and Maxillofacial Surgery, 63,* 1567–1575. doi:10.1016/j.joms.2005.07.010

Maxwell, C. (2007). Role of the nurse in preserving patients' independence. *European Journal of Oncology Nursing, 11*(Suppl. 2), S38–S41. doi:10.1016/j.ejon.2007.07.004

Medtronic, Inc. (2009). *Balloon kyphoplasty: About the procedure.* Retrieved from http://www.kyphon.com/us/Physician.aspx?contentid=60&siteid=1

Meredith, C., Symonds, P., Webster, L., Lamont, D., Pyper, E., Gillis, C.R., & Fallowfield, L. (1996). Information needs of cancer patients in west Scotland: Cross sectional survey of patients' views. *BMJ, 313,* 724–726.

Miceli, T., Colson, K., Gavino, M., & Lilleby, K., (2008). Myelosuppression associated with novel therapies in patients with multiple myeloma: Consensus statement of the IMF Nurse Leadership Board. *Clinical Journal of Oncology Nursing, 12*(Suppl. 3), 13–20. doi:10.1188/08.CJON.S1.13-19

Moadel, A.B., Morgan, C., & Dutcher, J. (2007). Psychosocial needs assessment among an underserved, ethnically diverse cancer patient population. *Cancer, 109,* 446–454. doi:10.1002/cncr.22357

Nau, K.C., & Lewis W.D. (2008). Multiple myeloma: Diagnosis and treatment. *American Family Physician, 78,* 853–859.

Niess, D., & Duffy, K.M. (2004). Basic concepts of transplantation. In S. Ezzone (Ed.), *Hematopoietic stem cell transplantation: A manual for nursing practice* (pp. 13–21). Pittsburgh, PA: Oncology Nursing Society.

Oldenmenger, W.H., Echteld, M.A., de Wit, R., Sillevis Smitt, P.A.E., Stronks, D.L., Stoter, G., & van der Rijt, C.C.D. (2007). Analgesic adherence measurement in cancer patients: Comparison between electronic monitoring and diary. *Journal of Pain and Symptom Management, 34,* 639–647. doi:10.1016/j.jpainsymman.2007.01.015

Ortho Biotech. (2006). Pegylated liposomal doxorubicin (Doxil) [Package insert]. Horsham, PA: Author.

Pesquera, M., Yoder, L., & Lynk, M. (2008). Improving cross-cultural awareness and skills to reduce health disparities in cancer. *Medsurg Nursing, 17,* 114–120.

Raab, M.S., Podar, K., Breitkreutz, I., Richardson, P.G., & Anderson, K.C. (2009). Multiple myeloma. *Lancet, 374,* 324–339. doi:10.1016/S0140-6736(09)60221-X

Redman, B.K. (2001). *The practice of patient education.* St. Louis, MO: Mosby.

Reeves, K. (2008). A cancer pain primer. *Medsurg Nursing, 17,* 413–419.

Rodriguez, A.L., Tariman, J.D., Enecio, T., & Estrella, S.M. (2007). The role of high dose chemotherapy supported by hematopoietic stem cell transplantation in patients with multiple myeloma: Implications for nursing. *Clinical Journal of Oncology Nursing, 11,* 579–589. doi:10.1188/07.CJON.579-589

Rome, S., Doss, D., Miller, K., & Westphal, J. (2008). Thromboembolic events associated with novel therapies in patients with multiple myeloma: Consensus statement of the IMF Nurse Leadership Board. *Clinical Journal of Oncology Nursing, 12*(Suppl. 3), 21–28. doi:10.1188/08.CJON.S1.21-27

Rubenstein, E.B., Peterson, D.E., Schubert, M., Keefe, D., McGuire, D., Epstein, J., ... Sonis, S.T. (2004). Clinical practice guidelines for the prevention and treatment of cancer therapy-induced oral and gastrointestinal mucositis. *Cancer, 100*(Suppl. 9), 2026–2046. doi:10.1002/cncr.20163

Rustoen, T., Gaardsrud, T., Leegaard, M., & Wahl, A.K. (2009). Nursing pain management— A qualitative interview study of patients with pain, hospitalized for cancer treatment. *Pain Management Nursing, 10,* 48–55. doi:10.1016/j.pmn.2008.09.003

Sezer, O. (2009). Myeloma bone disease: Recent advances in biology, diagnosis, and treatment. *Oncologist, 14,* 276–283. doi:10.1634/theoncologist.2009-0003

Sloan, J.M., & Ballen, K. (2008). SCT in Jehovah's witnesses: The bloodless transplant. *Bone Marrow Transplantation, 41,* 837–844. doi:10.1038/bmt.2008.5

Tariman, J.D. (2007). Lenalidomide: A new agent for patients with relapsed or refractory multiple myeloma. *Clinical Journal of Oncology Nursing, 11,* 569–574. doi:10.1188/07. CJON.569-574

Tariman, J.D., Love, G., McCullagh, E., & Sandifer, S. (2008). Peripheral neuropathy associated with novel therapies in patients with multiple myeloma: Consensus statement of the IMF Nurse Leadership Board. *Clinical Journal of Oncology Nursing, 12*(Suppl. 3), 29–36. doi:10.1188/08.CJON.S1.29-35

Thomson Reuters. (2009a). *CareNotes® system.* Retrieved from http://www.micromedex. com/products/carenotes

Thomson Reuters. (2009b). *PDR® electronic library.* Retrieved from http://www.micromedex. com/products/pdrlibrary

Tricot, G. (2009). Multiple myeloma. In R. Hoffman, E.J. Benz Jr., S.J. Shattil, B. Furie, L.E. Silberstein, P. McGlave, & H. Heslop (Eds.), *Hematology: Basic principles and practice* (5th ed., pp. 1387–1423). Philadelphia, PA: Elsevier/Churchill Livingstone.

van der Meulen, N., Jansen, J., van Dulmen, S., Bensing, J., & Van Weert, J. (2008). Interventions to improve recall of medical information in cancer patients: A systematic review of the literature. *Psycho-Oncology, 17,* 857–868. doi:10.1002/pon.1290

Vickrey, E., Allen, S., Mehta, J., & Singhal, S. (2009). Acyclovir to prevent reactivation of varicella zoster virus (herpes zoster) in multiple myeloma patients receiving bortezomib therapy. *Cancer, 115,* 229–232. doi:10.1002/cncr.24006

White, H.K., & Cohen, H.J. (2008). The older cancer patient. *Nursing Clinics of North America, 43,* 307–322. doi:10.1016/j.cnur.2008.03.003

Wolpin, S., Berry, D., Austin-Seymour, M., Bush, N., Fann, J.R., Halpenny, B., ... Mc-Corkle, R. (2008). Acceptability of an electronic self-report assessment program for patients with cancer. *Computers, Informatics, Nursing, 26,* 332–338. doi:10.1097/01. NCN.0000336464.79692.6a

Woo, S.B., Hellstein, J.W., & Kalmar, J.R. (2006). Systematic review: Bisphosphonates and osteonecrosis of the jaws. *Annals of Internal Medicine, 144,* 753–761.

CHAPTER 12

Survivorship Issues

Elizabeth Bilotti, MSN, RN, ANP-BC

> Many patients are "cured" long before they pass the five-year mark, and others go well beyond the five-year point with overt or covert disease that removes them from the rank of the "cured," no matter how well they feel. Survival is a much more useful concept, because it is a generic idea that applies to everyone diagnosed as having cancer, regardless of the course of that illness. Survival, in fact, begins at the point of diagnosis, because that is the time when patients are forced to confront their own mortality and begin to make adjustments that will be part of their immediate, and to some extent, long term future. (Mullan, 1985, p. 271)

INTRODUCTION

Over the past two decades, the incidence of multiple myeloma has increased steadily while the mortality rate has remained stable. It is estimated that 20,580 people in the United States were diagnosed with multiple myeloma in 2009, with approximately 10,580 deaths attributable to the disease (Jemal et al., 2009). The median age at diagnosis is 70 years, although approximately 32% of patients are diagnosed between the ages of 45 and 64 years. The five-year overall survival rate in 1988–2005 was estimated to be 33.8% (National Cancer Institute [NCI], 2009).

Historically, the term *cancer survivor* was used by the insurance companies to describe the loved ones left behind after patients succumbed to their oncologic diagnosis. As treatment options increased and efficacy improved, the term *cancer survivor* evolved to describe an individual who lived beyond five years with no evidence of the disease as defined by strict parameters (Leigh, 2004). The definition of cancer survivorship evolves as clinicians continue to understand the ramifications of treatments and the improvement in survival that they impart. The NCI Office of Cancer

Survivorship was developed in 1996 and revised the definition of a cancer survivor: "An individual is considered a cancer survivor from the time of diagnosis, through the balance of his or her life. Family members, friends, and caregivers are also impacted by the survivorship experience and are therefore included in this definition" (NCI, 2006). Welch-McCaffrey, Hoffman, Leigh, Loescher, and Meyskens (1989) realized and developed the concept that not all cancer survivors would follow the same path throughout the course of their survival. The potential paths described range anywhere from living many years free of disease, dying of a late recurrence, dying from a secondary cancer, living with periods of relapse and remission, living with persistent disease, to surviving after expecting imminent death (Welch-McCaffrey et al., 1989).

According to Kumar et al. (2008), patients diagnosed with multiple myeloma since the advent of novel therapies are experiencing a significant improvement in overall survival. This improvement was noted in both the newly diagnosed patient population as well as the relapsed setting in recent years, providing hope to those people diagnosed with this disease.

The issues of survivorship in patients living with a diagnosis of multiple myeloma and the therapeutic interventions are important components of nursing care. With improvement in treatment modalities and subsequent response rates, there is an ongoing philosophical debate as to the appropriate treatment approach. Should patients be treated with more intense regimens that are inherently accompanied by increased toxicity and complications with the hope of achieving an extended overall survival? Or should the approach be to minimize toxicity in an effort to improve quality of life at the cost of decreased efficacy (Rajkumar, 2008)? No matter which side of the debate one chooses, the issues associated with improvement in overall survival must still be addressed in order to preserve both quality and quantity of life.

CONTINUUM OF CARE

The needs of individuals living with a diagnosis of multiple myeloma are numerous and complex. Throughout the course of their disease, they will require education, treatment, screening, and support (Grant & Economou, 2008). The diagnosis of multiple myeloma often arises later in life, with the majority of new cases occurring in or following the sixth decade (NCI, 2009). This is a patient population prone to comorbid conditions that require both detection and management. The comorbid conditions can affect not only the patient's survival but also the ability to effectively treat the cancer. For this reason, strategies for long-term care of these patients must include close monitoring and intervention not only for their multiple myeloma and its inherent complications but also for treatment-related side effects, both physical and psychological, and overall wellness.

BONE HEALTH AND MOBILITY

Bone destruction is a feature of multiple myeloma that occurs in nearly 80% of diagnosed patients. It can manifest in the form of diffuse osteopenia/osteoporosis, focal lytic lesions, pathologic fractures, cord compression, hypercalcemia, and pain (Yeh & Berenson, 2006). The most common sites of skeletal involvement are the spine, pelvis, and long bones. Bone destruction in multiple myeloma is caused by an increase in osteoclast activity with an accompanying decrease in osteoblast differentiation and function, leading to an inequality in bone turnover. This process is a result of both cytokine release from the bone marrow microenvironment and direct interaction among myeloma cells (Sezer, 2009). Complications of bone loss are cited as major causes of morbidity, mortality, and impaired quality of life in these patients (Kyle, 1975). Patients with disease that is not resistant to antimyeloma therapy can have ongoing skeletal progression without repair of existing osteolytic lesions (Berenson, 2004).

In the United States each year, more than one-third of adults older than age 65 experience a fall accident. In 2005 alone, more than 1.8 million adults older than age 65 were treated in emergency rooms for injuries related to an unintentional fall, with more than 430,000 requiring hospitalization and 15,800 suffering fatal injuries related to the fall (Centers for Disease Control and Prevention, 2009). The psychological impact on adults who experience a fall, even without related injuries, is that they develop a fear of falling that may limit their activity, thereby leading to an increased risk of fall related to reduced strength and mobility (Vellas, Wayne, Romero, Baumgartner, & Garry, 1997). Patients with multiple myeloma are clearly at risk for falling at home as a result of several factors, including multiple drugs and organ dysfunction.

Patients with cancer have unique risk factors with the potential to increase their risk of falling that are not inherent to the aging process. Patients with multiple myeloma, in particular, are more susceptible to bone injury. Chemotherapy and a diagnosis of cancer contribute to fall risk because of the following identified factors: muscle weakness, fatigue, anemia, bone metastasis, polypharmacy, incontinence, sensory deficits, impaired functional status, impaired cognition, and ambulatory limitations (Overcash & Beckstead, 2008). Overcash and Beckstead (2008) found that the fall rate of patients older than age 70 with a malignant diagnosis who were not undergoing chemotherapy was 25%, and the rate increased to 33% for those who were receiving systemic chemotherapy. Although the fall rate was not higher than the general geriatric community (42.2%), the causative factors may have varied. The median number of comorbid conditions in the general geriatric population was 5.9, and the comorbid conditions in the patients with a malignant process were not obtained; previous studies reported a mean of three comorbid conditions in patients with cancer (Overcash & Beckstead, 2008).

As the patients' disease course progresses, there is a constant need to reevaluate their risk for falling. Shumway-Cook, Brauer, and Woollacott (2000) found that the get-up-and-go test (see Figure 12-1) is a simple yet sensitive and specific tool that can be used in the outpatient setting to identify patients who are at risk for falls. Once a patient has been identified as being at risk for a fall, thorough evaluation of fall risks and education about appropriate interventions are warranted. Some of the risk factors for falls found in patients with multiple myeloma include fractures or cord compression, peripheral neuropathy, proximal myopathy, anemia, fatigue, altered mental status related to narcotic analgesics, depression, malnutrition, nocturia, and sleep disturbances.

Because of the numerous acute and chronic complications associated with falls, along with a multitude of risk factors noted in patients with multiple myeloma, it is important to institute mechanisms to prevent falls before they happen. The first step is to perform a risk assessment to determine an individual's chance of having a fall and then determine what deficits exist in order to create an appropriate plan of intervention. It is critical to determine whether a patient has had a fall within the past year, and if so, how many. Once that has been determined, the outcome will either be no intervention or evaluation of any gait or balance problems for those with a single fall. If no falls are noted, no intervention is required. If a patient presents having had multiple falls in one year, it is important to embark on a more thorough assessment. The in-depth assessment should evaluate the patient's history, current medications, vision, gait and balance, lower limb joints, and neurologic and cardiovascular systems. Based on the findings, numerous interventions may be recommended, depending on whether the potential causative factor is modifiable (American Geriatrics Society, British Geriatrics Society, & American Academy of Orthopaedic Surgeons Panel on Falls Prevention, 2001).

Once a fall risk assessment is complete, including known contributing factors, the American Geriatrics Society Panel on Falls Prevention guidelines must be followed. The recommendations are based on 11 randomized, controlled studies performed in community-dwelling older adults that evaluated the efficacy of education, self-management programs, home environment modification, advice about medication use (with or without modification), exercise, medical assessment, and management of cardiac disorders. Although evidence of success of any one of these areas alone was not demonstrated, it appears that a combination approach to minimize risks may lead to a reduction in falls (American Geriatrics Society et al., 2001). Modification of the patient's home environment (see Figure 12-2), use of proper footwear, the use of assistive devices, exercise for muscle strengthening and balance, use of appropriate visual devices, and careful review and modification of medications are areas for further investigation and assessment.

Long-term sequelae of skeletal-related events include pain and impaired mobility. To maintain an independent level of functioning for patients, it is important to take proactive measures to reduce the number of skeletal-related events. Once they have occurred, clinicians must initiate prompt interventions, such as pain management and rehabilitation. These interventions are critical to improve mobility, prevent further disability, and maintain quality of life.

Figure 12-1. Hendrich II Fall Risk Model™

Confusion Disorientation Impulsivity		4	
Symptomatic Depression		2	
Altered Elimination		1	
Dizziness Vertigo		1	
Male Gender		1	
Any Administered Antiepileptics		2	
Any Administered Benzodiazepines		1	
Get Up & Go Test			
Ability to rise in a single movement—No Loss of Balance with Steps		0	
Pushes up, successful in one attempt		1	
Multiple attempts, but successful		3	
Unable to rise without assistance during test (OR if a medical order states the same and/or complete bed rest is ordered) * If unable to assess, document this on the patient chart with the date and time		4	

A Score of 5 or Greater = High Risk   Total Score

Figure 12-2. Home Fall Prevention Checklist for Older Adults

Floors
Look at the floor in each room.
Q. When you walk through a room, do you have to walk around furniture?
   Ask someone to remove the furniture so your path is clear.
Q. Do you have throw rugs on the floor?
   Remove the rugs or use double-sided tape or a nonslip backing so the rugs do not slip.
Q. Are papers, magazines, books, shoes, boxes, blankets, towels, or other objects on the
   floor?
   Pick up the things that are on the floor. Always keep objects off the floor.
Q. Do you have to walk over or around cords or wires (like cords from lamps, extension
   cords, or telephone cords)?
   Coil or tape cords and wires next to the wall so you cannot trip over them. Have an
   electrician put in another outlet.

Stairs and Steps
Look at the stairs you use both inside and outside your home.
Q. Are papers, shoes, books, or other objects on the stairs?
   Pick up things on the stairs. Always keep objects off the stairs.
Q. Are some steps broken or uneven?
   Fix loose or uneven steps.
Q. Are you missing a light over the stairway?
   Have a repair person or an electrician put in an overhead light at the top and bottom of
   the stairs.
Q. Has the stairway light bulb burned out?
   Have a friend or family member change the light bulb.
Q. Do you have only one light switch for your stairs (only at the top or bottom of the stairs)?
   Have a repair person or an electrician put in a light switch at the top and bottom of the
   stairs. You can get light switches that glow.
Q. Are the handrails loose or broken? Is there a handrail on only one side of the stairs?
   Fix loose handrails or put in new ones. Make sure handrails are on both sides of the
   stairs and are as long as the stairs.
Q. Is the carpet on the steps loose or torn?
   Make sure the carpet is firmly attached to every step or remove the carpet and attach
   nonslip rubber treads on the stairs.

Kitchen
Look at your kitchen and eating area.
Q. Are the things you often use on high shelves?
   Move items in your cabinets. Keep things you often use on the lower shelves (about
   waist high).
Q. Is your step stool unsteady?
   Get a new, steady step stool with a bar to hold on to. Never use a chair as a step stool.

Bedrooms
Look at all your bedrooms.
Q. Is the light near the bed hard to reach?
   Place a lamp close to the bed where it is easy to reach.
Q. Is the path from your bed to the bathroom dark?
   Put in a night-light so you can see where you are walking. Some night-lights go on by
   themselves after dark.

(Continued on next page)

Figure 12-2. Home Fall Prevention Checklist for Older Adults *(Continued)*

Bathrooms
Look at all your bathrooms.
Q. Is the tub or shower floor slippery?
 Put a nonslip rubber mat or self-stick strips on the floor of the tub or shower.
Q. Do you have some support when you get in and out of the tub or up from the toilet?
 Have a repair person or a carpenter install a grab bar inside the tub and next to the toilet.

Other Things You Can Do to Prevent Falls
• Exercise regularly. Exercise makes you stronger and improves your balance and coordination.
• Have your doctor or pharmacist look at all the medicines you take, even over-the-counter products. Some medicines can make you sleepy or dizzy.
• Have your vision checked at least once a year by an eye doctor. Poor vision can increase your risk of falling.
• Get up slowly after you have been sitting or lying down.
• Wear sturdy shoes with thin, nonslip soles. Avoid slippers and running shoes with thick soles.
• Improve the lighting in your home. Use brighter light bulbs (at least 60 watts). Use lamp shades or frosted bulbs to reduce glare.
• Use reflective tape at the top and bottom of the stairs so you can see them better.
• Paint doorsills a different color to prevent tripping.

Other Safety Tips
• Keep emergency numbers in large print near each phone.
• Put a phone near the floor in case you fall and cannot get up.
• Think about wearing an alarm device that will bring help in case you fall and cannot get up.

Note. Based on information from Centers for Disease Control and Prevention, 2005.

RENAL FUNCTION

Variation exists in the reports of patients experiencing renal failure with a diagnosis of multiple myeloma. Approximately 20% of patients will be diagnosed with renal failure at presentation based on a serum creatinine level of 2 mg/dl or greater (Dimopoulos, Kastritis, Rosinol, Blade, & Ludwig, 2008). It is possible to develop renal insufficiency later in the disease course, although outside the setting of light-chain disease or a presentation of renal failure, it often is associated with hypercalcemia (Dimopoulos et al., 2008). Renal insufficiency or renal failure often will result from toxic effects to the renal tubules by monoclonal light chains and often is termed *cast nephropathy*. Other disease entities that may cause renal damage include light-chain deposition disease, amyloidosis, and acquired adult Fanconi syndrome. Nonpathologic conditions such as dehydration, nephrotoxic medications, and contrast dye also can contribute to renal complications in patients with a monoclonal gammopathy (Dimopoulos et al., 2008). When considering the patient population that multiple myeloma often afflicts, it is important to note that comorbid conditions such as hypertension, diabetes, and other chronic medical conditions can either cause or contribute to renal insufficiency or failure. When caring for patients with myeloma who present with renal impairment, clinicians must initiate prompt interventions to prevent end-stage renal disease.

Bisphosphonate support is used routinely in the treatment of patients with multiple myeloma. Nephrotoxicity is one of the potential complications of bisphosphonate support that may occur either acutely or over an extended period of time. In the setting of multiple myeloma, the more potent IV form of bisphosphonate is used, and the most commonly prescribed agents in the United States are pamidronate and zoledronate (also known as zoledronic acid). The nephrotoxicity associated with pamidronate has been described as collapsing focal segmental glomerulosclerosis in addition to other patterns of glomerular damage. The clinical finding is often that of nephrotic proteinuria, which is best evaluated by 24-hour urine collection (Perazella & Markowitz, 2008). Some studies have suggested that discontinuation of the offending agent can at least partially reverse nephrotic syndrome. Upon review of renal biopsies in patients receiving zoledronate, it appears that the damage affects the tubules, leading to a toxic form of acute tubular necrosis. The clinical findings in these patients are often not that of proteinuria but rather an increase in serum creatinine levels (Perazella & Markowitz, 2008).

Nephrotoxicity associated with IV bisphosphonates is both dose dependent and infusion time dependent. Guidelines recommend evaluating serum creatinine levels prior to each bisphosphonate administration, withholding therapy in the setting of renal insufficiency, and following package insert guidelines for dose reduction in the setting of preexisting chronic kidney disease (Perazella & Markowitz, 2008).

In 2007, American Society of Clinical Oncology (ASCO) guidelines for the use of bisphosphonates were updated to include specific recommendations for patients with multiple myeloma (Kyle et al., 2007). The guidelines recommend that all patients with evidence of lytic bone disease on plain radiographs or imaging studies, or compression fracture of the spine, be initiated on monthly bisphosphonates with either pamidronate or zoledronate administered per the package insert. They also recommend renal dosage adjustments for zoledronate per the package insert and consideration of pamidronate dose reduction in patients with a creatinine clearance less than 30 ml/min or a serum creatinine greater than 3 mg/dl. Serum creatinine monitoring should occur prior to each dose with drug being withheld if the creatinine is elevated and with resumption of the original dose once the level returns to within 10% of the baseline. Evaluation for nonspecific albuminuria (greater than 500 mg/24 hours) every three to six months also is recommended. A 24-hour urine collection is the most accurate way to evaluate this. If noted, it is recommended that treatment be stopped until the renal abnormality resolves. The recommendation for duration of therapy is monthly for two years, with reevaluation of disease status at that time. If the patient has responsive or stable disease, discontinuation should be considered, with the ultimate decision being at the discretion of the physician. If it is discontinued and a patient relapses with skeletal-related disease, reinitiation is recommended. The International Myeloma Working Group (IMWG) and the Mayo Clinic published specific recommendations for the multiple myeloma patient population, as well (see Table 12-1).

Table 12-1. Comparison of Mayo Clinic Consensus Statement and International Myeloma Working Group (IMWG) Recommendations

Clinical Scenario	Mayo Clinic Consensus Statement	Response From the IMWG
Indication for initiating BP therapy in patients with myeloma	All myeloma patients with lytic bone disease on plain radiographs; patients with osteopenia or osteoporosis on bone mineral density studies	In addition to radiographs, the IMWG recommends other imaging studies including MRI with gadolinium enhancement, CT, and/or whole-body CT/PET to determine the presence or absence of bone lesions that may benefit from BP prophylaxis.
Smoldering myeloma	BPs are not recommended except in the setting of a clinical trial.	BPs are not recommended.
Duration of BP therapy	Monthly for two years After two years: Discontinue if myeloma is in complete response or stable plateau phase. Decrease to every three months if disease is active.	One year After one year: Discontinue if complete response or VGPR occurs and no active bone disease is evident. Continue BP therapy if less than a VGPR occurs and/or ongoing active bone disease is evident. After two years: Discontinue BPs if no active bone disease is evident. If active bone disease is present, further BP use is recommended at the discretion of the primary physician.
Choice of BP	Pamidronate	Pamidronate or clodronate

BP—bisphosphonate; CT—computed tomography; IMWG—International Myeloma Working Group; MRI—magnetic resonance imaging; PET—positron-emission tomography; VGPR—very good partial response

Note. From "Use of Bisphosphonates in Multiple Myeloma: IMWG Response to Mayo Clinic Consensus Statement [Reply to Letter to the Editor]," by M.Q. Lacy and S.V. Rajkumar, 2007, *Mayo Clinic Proceedings, 82,* p. 517. Copyright 2007 by Mayo Foundation for Medical Education and Research. Reprinted with permission.

Because of the incidence of osteonecrosis of the jaw and the potential for serious complications, all patients are advised to undergo thorough dental evaluation and preventive intervention before starting bisphosphonate therapy. Active oral infections should be treated promptly, and high-risk sites should be eliminated. Continued routine dental evaluation should be ongoing, along with avoidance of invasive dental procedures whenever possible (Kyle et al., 2007).

The third highest cause of hypercalcemia associated with malignancy is multiple myeloma, and approximately one-third of all patients with multiple myeloma will develop hypercalcemia during their disease course (Kaplan, 2006). Prompt management of hypercalcemia is imperative to preventing permanent renal damage. The systems most often affected by elevated levels of serum calcium include the central nervous, cardiovascular, gastrointestinal, musculoskeletal, and renal systems. Common early signs and symptoms of hypercalcemia include dehydration, muscle weakness, anorexia, nausea, vomiting, constipation, lethargy, confusion, irritability, arrhythmias, and electrocardiogram changes (Kaplan, 2006). The most effective intervention for hypercalcemia associated with an underlying malignancy is systemic therapy to treat the underlying disease. Supportive care measures include IV hydration with electrolyte repletion as indicated, bisphosphonate infusion, calcitonin injection, and steroids (Kaplan, 2006). The use of furosemide is discouraged in patients with multiple myeloma because of the risk of cast formation in the renal tubules, increasing the risk for renal complications (Dimopoulos et al., 2008).

Additional educational and screening opportunities exist within the context of renal health in patients living with multiple myeloma. Patients should be advised to maintain adequate oral hydration. It is recommended that patients consume between two and three liters of noncarbonated, caffeine-free fluids each day. Prompt intervention for infections is recommended. When possible, the use of nephrotoxic antibiotics, such as aminoglycosides, should be avoided, and they should be used with caution when necessary. Nonsteroidal anti-inflammatory drugs should be avoided for pain management, as their mechanism of action leads to decreased renal blood flow, making the kidneys vulnerable to damage (Kaplan, 2006). The use of IV contrast agents when performing diagnostic procedures such as computed tomography scans and angiograms should be avoided whenever possible. If its use is necessary for diagnostic purposes, the patient should receive IV hydration both before and after the procedure with evaluation of renal function using serum creatinine levels. Gadolinium-induced renal dysfunction has been reported, and caution is advised with the use of all contrast media (ten Dam & Wetzels, 2008). Many agents have been evaluated to provide renal protection in patients who are at high risk for renal compromise during diagnostic and therapeutic procedures that require the use of contrast dye. A meta-analysis reviewed the literature of randomized, controlled trials that utilized N-acetylcysteine, theophylline, fenoldopam, dopamine, iloprost, statins, furosemide, or mannitol given to a treatment group to determine their effect on contrast-induced nephropathy (Kelly, Dwamena, Cronin, Bernstein, & Carlos, 2008). The analysis concluded that N-acetylcysteine is more renoprotective than hydration alone and that the remaining agents did not have any significant effects.

Poor renal function can hinder the healthcare team's ability to use therapeutic and diagnostic interventions for the management of multiple myeloma. In turn, these interventions, as well as poorly controlled disease, can impair renal function. Proper screening and ample management of comorbid conditions that affect the kidneys are a necessity for patients diagnosed with multiple myeloma. Educating patients about ways to protect their kidneys and the potential impact of renal insufficiency on their disease management helps them to actively participate in their plan of care.

HEALTH MAINTENANCE

Patients with multiple myeloma are living longer since the advent of new therapeutic agents and the improvement in supportive care that has occurred over the past decade. For this reason, it is important for both healthcare providers and patients to understand the need for overall health promotion and disease prevention. Many health problems are a result of uninformed decisions and an unhealthy lifestyle. To continue making strides in overall survival, nurses must help patients maintain appropriate therapy and must have the opportunity to provide an ample number of treatment options based on patients' health status.

Inadequate organ system function may limit access to therapeutic agents and investigational agents. The elimination of systemic agents is often accomplished by the renal and hepatic systems, and inadequate clearance will increase the risk and severity of toxicity. Systemic agents also can cause direct or indirect toxicity to almost every major organ system, compromising a patient's functional status, safety, and overall quality of life. To avoid unnecessary toxicity and to ensure access to effective agents, it is imperative that patients maintain a good state of health beginning at the time of diagnosis.

Often, opportunities for risk assessment or screening evaluation are missed because of the illness-based approach to medicine. Patients present when they have a complaint, and healthcare providers diagnose and manage the present problem. The act of prevention will require a shift in the thinking of both healthcare providers and patients. Being proactive and preventing disease before it happens, or diagnosing and intervening before adverse sequelae occur, are the first steps to improving overall wellness. The U.S. Preventive Services Task Force, the Centers for Disease Control and Prevention, and the American College of Physicians provide updated recommendations from evidence-based practice for screening and preventive services for the general population based on age, sex, and risk factor assessment. These include screening for cardiovascular disease (e.g., hypertension, hyperlipidemia), other malignancies (e.g., prostate, breast, colon), endocrine disorders (e.g., type 2 diabetes, thyroid dysfunction, adrenal insufficiency), bone metabolism disorders (e.g., bone density, vitamin D deficiency), vision and hearing changes, depression, and elder abuse (U.S. Preventive Services Task Force, 2008).

Many barriers to health maintenance exist, and it is the responsibility of both the patient and the healthcare provider to overcome them. Barriers include knowledge deficits, cynicism about treatments' effectiveness, time constraints, and the mindset that the patient already has a terminal illness (Frame, 1996).

As stated earlier, maintenance of overall health and wellness can improve the experience of a patient with cancer during treatment by allowing access to more treatment opportunities with an improved ability to minimize and manage toxicity. An understanding of health maintenance and a collaborative approach to achieving it by both the healthcare team and the patient can lead to improved satisfaction with quality of life.

PSYCHOSOCIAL ISSUES

Concerns About the Future

In 1985, Dr. Fitzhugh Mullan described the three phases of survival based on his experience as a cancer survivor. The phases are termed *acute survival, extended survival,* and *permanent survival.* In viewing the course of a person's life following the diagnosis of myeloma, it is both the acute and extended survival phases that are the focus. Multiple myeloma is an incurable disease; thus, an unending phase of survival with long-term secondary effects without the need for disease management is not anticipated.

The acute survival phase encompasses the time period from diagnosis through the completion of initial therapy. The dominant focus of this phase is therapeutic treatment of the myeloma and management of adverse sequelae. The psychosocial aspects that arise include the confrontation of one's mortality, leading to feelings of fear and anxiety (Mullan, 1985).

After the completion of induction therapy, the patient often will transition into the second phase of survival, known as extended survival. This phase may consist of consolidation or intermittent therapy and a period of "watchful waiting" while the disease is monitored at intervals for recurrence (Mullan, 1985). The stressors associated with this phase are both physical and psychological. The physical stress or disability often is attributable to treatment-related toxicity. It can result in failure to return to baseline functioning or can impair patients' ability to care for themselves, rendering them dependent on others, which can, in turn, be a source of psychological distress. Patients also may experience psychological stress related to the fear of recurrence and problems inherent in trying to return to the lifestyle they had before the diagnosis of cancer.

Patients living with myeloma will spend the majority of their cancer trajectory in the extended survival phase. After the initial induction therapy and subsequent period of remission that often follows, the patient will experience numerous remissions and relapses that require either intermittent or continuous treatment with multiple regimens, which bring associated toxicity. Welch-McCaffrey et al. (1989) described the different trajectories that the life of a patient diagnosed with cancer may follow. Patients diagnosed with multiple myeloma often will live a life made up of intermittent periods of active disease, persistent disease, and life after expected death. With the advent of novel therapies, some patients may actually fall into the trajectory of living cancer free for many years (Welch-McCaffrey et al., 1989).

Fatigue

One of the most common and persistent complaints reported by patients with multiple myeloma is fatigue. It often is multifactorial in etiology and must be evaluated and managed as such. Approximately 32% of patients with newly diagnosed multiple myeloma will report fatigue at the time of diagnosis (Kyle et al., 2003). The National Comprehensive Cancer Network (NCCN) has defined cancer-related fatigue as "a distressing persistent, subjective sense of physical, emotional and/or cognitive tiredness or exhaustion related to cancer or cancer treatment that is not proportional to recent activity and interferes with usual functioning" (NCCN, 2009, p. FT-1). Up to 80% of patients receiving chemotherapy and up to 90% of those receiving radiation will report fatigue, with the symptom persisting in one-third of all patients after the completion of therapy (Hofman, Ryan, Figueroa-Moseley, Jean-Pierre, & Morrow, 2007).

Several consequences result for patients with cancer who are experiencing fatigue. The psychological effects can range from depression and anxiety to decreased participation in daily activities, leading to a significantly impaired quality of life. Physical consequences of fatigue contribute to a decrease in activity level that can result in deconditioning and weakness. Fatigue can contribute to an inability to focus and make decisions, leading to decreased cognition. Fatigue also can negatively affect a patient's socioeconomic status by impairing the person's ability to work and participate in social activities (Given, 2008). For these reasons, it is important to identify and treat the causes of cancer-related fatigue in an effort to minimize its consequences (see Figure 12-3).

Fatigue may be a culmination of many factors, including anemia, nutritional deficiencies, anxiety, depression, sleep disturbance, physical activity, and unmanaged side effects. One of the most common causes of fatigue in patients with multiple myeloma is anemia, which is identified in 70% of patients at the time of diagnosis (Rajkumar & Kyle, 2005). Numerous studies have evaluated the role of inflammatory cytokines and their association with fatigue in patients with myeloma. It is well known that interleukin-6 (IL-6) plays a role in the growth and survival of myeloma cells and that its production is dysregulated

Figure 12-3. Evaluation of Cancer-Related Fatigue

Focused History
- Disease status and treatment
  - Rule out recurrence or progression.
  - Current medications/medication changes
  - Prescription drugs, over-the-counter products, and supplements
- Review of systems
- In-depth fatigue history
  - Onset, pattern, duration
  - Change over time
  - Associated or alleviating factors
  - Interference with function

Assessment of Treatable Contributing Factors
- Pain
- Emotional distress
  - Depression
  - Anxiety
- Anemia
- Sleep disturbance (e.g., obstructive sleep apnea, restless legs syndrome, narcolepsy, insomnia)
- Nutritional assessment
  - Weight/caloric intake changes
  - Fluid and electrolyte imbalance: sodium, potassium, calcium, magnesium
- Activity level
  - Decreased activity
  - Decreased physical fitness
- Medication side effect profile (i.e., sedation)
- Comorbidities
  - Infection
  - Cardiac dysfunction
  - Pulmonary dysfunction
  - Renal dysfunction
  - Hepatic dysfunction
  - Neurologic dysfunction
  - Endocrine dysfunction (hypothyroidism, hypogonadism, adrenal insufficiency)

in patients with multiple myeloma (Booker, Olson, Pilarski, Noon, & Bahlis, 2009). C-reactive protein (CRP) is an inflammatory cytokine that has been associated with cancer-related symptoms such as fatigue and poor performance status. Studies have shown that IL-6 increases the production of CRP and decreases the production of hemoglobin, leading to the hypothesis that IL-6 dysregulation may be part of the reason why patients with multiple myeloma experience cancer-related fatigue (Booker et al., 2009). One notable result in the study performed by Booker et al. was that once the effect of inflammation (i.e., CRP) was removed, the hemoglobin level was not a significant predictor of fatigue or quality of life. Ongoing clinical trials are evaluating an anti-IL-6 monoclonal antibody in patients with multiple myeloma. Earlier studies of this monoclonal antibody showed subjective improvements in pain and fatigue in patients with advanced disease (Bataille et al., 1995), with more recent studies confirming the reduction in cancer-related symptoms with only minimal antimyeloma activity (Rossi et al., 2005).

Although studies are ongoing to find additional factors that contribute to fatigue in patients with multiple myeloma and that may be potential therapeutic targets in the future, current recommendations are available from the Oncology Nursing Society and NCCN for the assessment and management of cancer-related fatigue (Mitchell, Beck, Hood, Moore, & Tanner, 2007; NCCN, 2009).

Pain

Pain experienced by a patient with multiple myeloma is often either somatic or neuropathic in origin. Somatic pain is often attributed to lytic bone lesions or pathologic fractures resulting from the disease itself. Neuropathic pain can be either from direct nerve root compression from a plasmacytoma or compression fracture in the spine, a result of treatment-related toxicity from therapeutic agents such as thalidomide, bortezomib, vincristine, and cisplatin, or from postherpetic neuralgia related to herpes zoster virus reactivation (Wickham, 2007; Yeager, McGuire, & Sheidler, 2000).

The pain can be classified as either acute or chronic. Both somatic and neuropathic pain can be acute in onset, and a thorough assessment to determine the etiology is imperative. It is then important to promptly intervene not only with pain management but also with direct treatment of the underlying cause in an effort to alleviate as much pain as possible. See Table 12-2 for pain management techniques put forth by NCCN.

A thorough pain evaluation requires both a detailed history and a physical. The assessment should include inquires about the location, onset, duration, quality, severity, associated symptoms, and aggravating and alleviating factors of the pain; medication history; and how the pain affects the patient's ability to function. The physical examination should include examination of the site using both inspection and palpation. Neurologic examination of the sensory, motor, and autonomic systems should be performed to differentiate between large neuronal fiber and small neuronal fiber damage. A neurologic examination also will provide valuable information about any safety measures that must be taken to prevent further injury. Diagnostic evaluation with radiographic studies may be helpful in determining the etiology and possible treatment interventions (Paice, 2004).

Table 12-2. Recommended Interventions for Adult Cancer Pain

Type of Pain	Intervention
Pain associated with inflammation	Glucocorticoids Nonsteroidal anti-inflammatory drugs should be avoided in patients with multiple myeloma.
Nerve compression or inflammation	Glucocorticoids
Bone pain	Analgesic—titrate to effect. Local bone pain—consider local radiation or nerve block. Diffuse bone pain—consider bisphosphonates, chemotherapy, and glucocorticoids. Consider physical medicine evaluation. For resistant pain, consider referral to pain management or interventional strategies.[a]
Neuropathic pain	Anticonvulsant (e.g., gabapentin, carbamazepine, pregabalin) and/or antidepressant (e.g., nortriptyline, doxepin, desipramine, venlafaxine, duloxetine) Consider topical agents, such as local anesthetics including lidocaine patch. For resistant pain, consider referral to pain management or interventional strategies.[a]
Painful lesions likely to respond to antineoplastic therapies	Radiation Chemotherapy

[a] Regional infusions (e.g., epidural, intrathecal, regional plexus), percutaneous vertebroplasty/kyphoplasty, neurodestruction procedures (e.g., nerve block, neurolysis, plexus block), neurostimulation, radiofrequency ablation

Note. Adapted with permission from The NCCN 1.2009 Adult Cancer Pain Clinical Practice Guidelines in Oncology. © National Comprehensive Cancer Network, 2010. Available at http://www.nccn.org. To view the most recent and complete version of the guideline, go online to www.nccn.org.

These Guidelines are a work in progress that will be refined as often as new significant data becomes available.

The NCCN Guidelines are a statement of consensus of its authors regarding their views of currently accepted approaches to treatment. Any clinician seeking to apply or consult any NCCN guideline is expected to use independent medical judgment in the context of individual clinical circumstances to determine any patient's care or treatment. The National Comprehensive Cancer Network makes no warranties of any kind whatsoever regarding their content, use or application and disclaims any responsibility for their application or use in any way.

These Guidelines are copyrighted by the National Comprehensive Cancer Network. All rights reserved. These Guidelines and illustrations herein may not be reproduced in any form for any purpose without the express written permission of the NCCN.

Cancer pain is likely to affect multiple aspects of an individual's physical and emotional well-being. Studies have shown that patients with pain often have a higher incidence of depression and mood disturbance, as well as functional deficits related to the pain's effect on mobility and performance of daily activities. In addition, many patients with cancer pain are inadequately treated, leading to unnecessary pain (Wells, Murphy, Wujcik, & Johnson, 2003). In addition to the subjective report of pain, there is a component of distress that is associated with pain that encompasses the discomfort, anguish, suffering, or unpleasantness associated with the physical component of pain (Wells et al., 2003). The findings of Wells et al. suggest that the symptom distress may be more limiting and have a greater impact on quality of life than the actual pain or the inadequacy of its management.

Appropriate management of pain includes not only an understanding of the interventions required to treat the pain but also an ability to manage the side effects. Pharmacologic intervention with opioid analgesics can have many side effects, including constipation, nausea, pruritus, delirium, sedation, motor and/or cognitive impairment, and respiratory depression. Educating both the patient and the patient's caregiver about the concepts of chronic and acute pain control and the need to communicate openly with the healthcare provider about inadequate pain relief and side effects is imperative to effective pain management.

Although healthcare professionals understand the need to provide pain relief, obstacles often can arise from the healthcare professionals, patients, family members, and caregivers. Barriers attributable to healthcare professionals include a lack of understanding of pain pathophysiology, the appropriate use and titration of analgesics, lack of follow-up assessment, knowledge deficit of nonpharmacologic interventions, and fear of legal conflicts. Patients and their caregivers may have fears related to addiction or side effects, leading to underreporting of symptoms (Yeager et al., 2000). Appropriate education for both healthcare professionals and patients and caregivers may be useful in overcoming the deficit in the identification and adequate management of cancer pain, thereby leading to an improvement in quality of life.

Insurance/Financial Health

The financial burden of a cancer diagnosis is wide ranging. Approximately 35% of patients diagnosed with multiple myeloma are younger than the age of 65 (NCI, 2009). The multitude of problems include loss of earnings because of reduced work hours or the need to stop working coupled with an increase in expenses, including out-of-pocket costs, copayments, prescription medications, and transportation. The financial burden may affect loved ones, and issues can arise from their need to fulfill the role of caregiver or to change their employment practices to assume the role of provider.

The advances that have occurred in both the therapeutic interventions and supportive care measures for the management of cancer have made it possible for patients to continue to work throughout their treatment. This is often beneficial to maintaining one's household income and insurance benefits, as well as for self-esteem and social support (Institute of Medicine, 2005). Numerous federal and state laws, such as the Americans With Disabilities Act, the Health Insurance Portability and Accountability Act, and the Consolidated Omnibus Budget Reconciliation Act, which were passed within the past two decades, have helped protect disabled employees from unemployment, discrimination, and loss of insurance when changing jobs. The Family and Medical Leave Act, enacted in 1993, provides specific benefits to both employees and dependents for serious medical illness. This act can provide up to 12 weeks of annual leave for either a patient or a caregiver while protecting the position and benefits of the employee. The Employee Retirement Income Security Act was created to protect people from discrimination that prevented employees from collecting benefits, including medical, dental, surgical, unemployment, disability, and death benefits. Numerous programs, including federal, state, and nonprofit organizations, are available to offer guidance and support for cancer care providers and their patients who are navigating the maze of potential benefits and programs.

Cancer care is one of the top three most expensive conditions in the United States. Studies have shown that underinsured or uninsured patients with a diagnosis of cancer often have poor outcomes in comparison to similar patients who have insurance. This is thought to be directly related to the amount and quality of the care these patients receive, as well as their access to physicians, testing, and medication. The Institute of Medicine Committee on Cancer Survivorship is in support of universal insurance coverage to ensure that all individuals with a cancer diagnosis have access to comprehensive, affordable, and continuous coverage (Institute of Medicine, 2005). This is not to say that those who are insured do not experience financial constraints of their own. Most managed care plans have out-of-pocket expenses in the form of deductibles and copays. This outlay of money can add up, depending on the frequency of office visits and the number of prescriptions required. Coverage limitations exist for services, including physical therapy, nutritional counseling, and psychiatric benefits. Many of these services are useful to help patients deal with the sequelae of the diagnosis and treatment interventions.

The paradigm for cancer therapeutics is constantly changing, and the addition of oral chemotherapy agents to the armamentarium is increasing the cost of treatment. Many of these agents are covered only by prescription drug plans, which are not all created equal. Often these medications are expensive, and the cost is prohibitive for most people, especially patients who are on a fixed income (Institute of Medicine, 2005).

Fortunately, numerous nonprofit organizations and patient assistance programs exist to help defray costs for those in need. Financial assistance is available for reimbursement of copay costs and transportation expenditure. See Table 12-3 for resources that are available for patients with multiple myeloma.

Table 12-3. Resources and Contacts for Multiple Myeloma Survivors

Organization	Contact Information	Description
American Cancer Society	www.cancer.org 800-ACS-2345	Offers and funds research, education, patient service, advocacy, and rehabilitation
CancerCare	www.cancercare.org 800-813-HOPE	Provides support services to anyone affected by cancer through counseling, support groups, education, financial assistance, and practical help
Chronic Disease Fund	www.cdfund.org 877-968-7233	Helps underinsured patients with chronic diseases, life-altering conditions, and cancer obtain the medications they need
International Myeloma Foundation	www.myeloma.org 800-452-CURE	International organization that supports research and provides education, advocacy, and support for patients with myeloma, families, researchers, and physicians
Lance Armstrong Foundation	www.livestrong.org 866-467-7205	Focuses on prevention, access to care, and screening, improvement in quality of life, and funding research
Leukemia and Lymphoma Society	www.leukemia-lymphoma.org 800-955-4572	Supports funding for blood cancer research, education, and patient services to search for a cure and improve quality of life
Multiple Myeloma Research Foundation	www.multiplemyeloma.org 203-229-0464	Educates patients and raises funds to provide support for research
National Cancer Institute	www.cancer.gov 800-4-CANCER	Conducts and supports research, training, and health information dissemination with respect to all aspects of cancer from etiology to treatment and beyond
National Coalition for Cancer Survivorship	www.canceradvocacy.org 877-622-7937	Survivor-led cancer advocacy organization that helps bring about changes at the federal level to ensure the delivery of quality cancer care
National Marrow Donor Program	www.marrow.org 800-627-7692	Dedicated to providing individuals who require a bone marrow or umbilical cord blood transplant a donor when they need it

(Continued on next page)

Table 12-3. Resources and Contacts for Multiple Myeloma Survivors *(Continued)*		
Organization	**Contact Information**	**Description**
Oncology Nursing Society	www.cancersymptoms .org 866-257-4667	A source of information for patients with cancer and their caregivers on ways to manage the most common treatment-related symptoms
Partnership for Prescription As- sistance	www.pparx.com 888-4PPA-NOW	Provides access to numerous pub- lic and private patient assistance pro- grams for qualifying patients without prescription coverage

Overall Quality of Life

Quality of life has been defined in many ways, ranging from broad terms that take into account many aspects of life to those that apply the term to a given clinical diagnosis. The definition that is commonly applied to cancer care outcomes measures patients' state of well-being based upon their ability to execute daily activities and their perception of their functional status (Ferrans, 2000). Patients living with a chronic illness can often overcome physical limitations while preserving an overall level of satisfaction with their functional status, disease control, and the management of treatment-related toxicities.

In the past, patients diagnosed with multiple myeloma did not have the life expectancy of the patients who have been diagnosed in recent years. To that end, with improvement in quantity of life, it is important to maintain quality of life. During the course of their treatment, patients will be required to play an active role in the decision-making process. According to Hoffman and Stovall (2006), patients who were informed of their options and felt that they had control over decision making often perceived a higher quality of life than those who felt uninformed and not in control. For a patient to be able to provide informed consent for treatment, both the potential benefits (improvement in quantity of life) and risks (impairment in quality of life) must be presented for consideration.

Numerous assessment tools that address quality of life have been validated in an effort to effectively evaluate what is thought to be a subjective concept. Domains of quality-of-life assessment found to be relevant to the cancer population include health and functioning, psychological and spiritual, social and economic, and family. The European Organisation for Research and Treatment of Cancer (EORTC) has completed an international field study to determine the validity and reliability of a disease-specific quality-of-life questionnaire for patients with multiple myeloma (Cocks et al., 2007). The domains of assessment included disease symptoms, side effects, body image, social support, and future perspectives (see Figure 12-4). The goal of the disease-specific

Figure 12-4. European Organisation for Research and Treatment of Cancer Supplemental Module for Myeloma-Specific Quality of Life

EORTC Multiple Myeloma Module (QLQ-MY20)

Patients sometimes report that they have the following symptoms or problems. Please indicate the extent to which you have experienced these symptoms or problems <u>during the past week</u>. Please answer by circling the number that best applies to you.

During the past week:	Not at All	A Little	Quite a Bit	Very Much
31. Have you had bone aches or pain?	1	2	3	4
32. Have you had pain in your back?	1	2	3	4
33. Have you had pain in your hip?	1	2	3	4
34. Have you had pain in your arm or shoulder?	1	2	3	4
35. Have you had pain in your chest?	1	2	3	4
36. If you had pain did it increase with activity?	1	2	3	4
37. Did you feel drowsy?	1	2	3	4
38. Did you feel thirsty?	1	2	3	4
39. Have you felt ill?	1	2	3	4
40. Have you had a dry mouth?	1	2	3	4
41. Have you lost any hair?	1	2	3	4
42. Answer this question only if you lost any hair: Were you upset by the loss of your hair?	1	2	3	4
43. Did you have tingling hands or feet?	1	2	3	4
44. Did you feel restless or agitated?	1	2	3	4
45. Have you had acid indigestion or heartburn?	1	2	3	4
46. Have you had burning or sore eyes?	1	2	3	4

Please turn to next page

(Continued on next page)

Figure 12-4. European Organisation for Research and Treatment of Cancer Supplemental Module for Myeloma-Specific Quality of Life *(Continued)*

During the past week:	Not at All	A Little	Quite a Bit	Very Much
47. Have you felt physically less attractive as a result of your disease or treatment?	1	2	3	4
48. Have you been thinking about your illness?	1	2	3	4
49. Have you been worried about dying?	1	2	3	4
50. Have you worried about your health in the future?	1	2	3	4

Please check through the questionnaire and ensure that you have answered all the questions. Remember that the results of the questionnaire will help improve the quality of life for present and future patients. The results will be strictly confidential.

Thank you for completing this questionnaire

module was to address both the disease-related and treatment-related factors that affect patients with multiple myeloma. The disease-specific symptoms focused on pain, while the treatment-related side effects addressed peripheral neuropathy and the constellation of subjective symptoms related to steroid use. The social support addressed the relationship between the patient and the healthcare team in terms of support and education, and the future perspectives domain of the questionnaire tried to ascertain the burden of living with a terminal disease.

According to the Surveillance, Epidemiology, and End Results (SEER) Program data, the relative overall survival for a patient diagnosed with multiple myeloma has increased by more than 10% from 1975 to 2006 (Horner et al., 2009) (see Figure 12-5). The novel therapies utilized for the treatment of multiple myeloma have made this progress possible, but it is important to note that the side effects and the regimens can be unique. For this reason and many others, it is imperative to evaluate the quality of the years gained in a population of patients living with a terminal illness. EORTC is currently

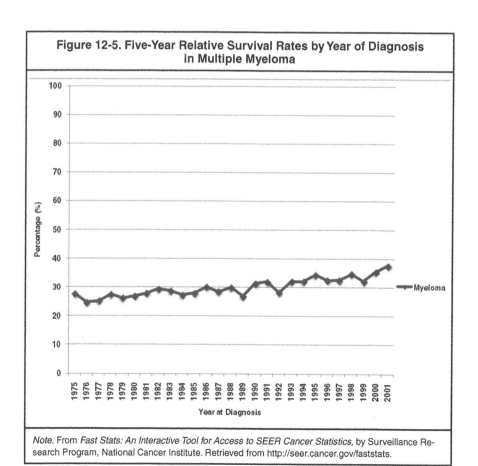

Figure 12-5. Five-Year Relative Survival Rates by Year of Diagnosis in Multiple Myeloma

Note. From *Fast Stats: An Interactive Tool for Access to SEER Cancer Statistics,* by Surveillance Research Program, National Cancer Institute. Retrieved from http://seer.cancer.gov/faststats.

studying additional modules that evaluate adverse events, including peripheral neuropathy, bone metastases, and fatigue, all of which are applicable to patients living with and undergoing therapy for a diagnosis of multiple myeloma.

CONCLUSION

As progress continues in the treatment paradigm of multiple myeloma, nurses will continue to see improvement in overall survival, requiring diligent evaluation and management of not only the disease but also its inherent complications and toxicities from treatment. Providing education and fostering open communication between healthcare professionals and patients will help to ensure that comprehensive quality care is provided. Multiple myeloma is a unique disease with the potential for multisystem organ involvement and significant impairment in functional status. Adequate assessment and prompt intervention by nurses can improve the quality of life experienced by patients living with this disease.

REFERENCES

American Geriatrics Society, British Geriatrics Society, & American Academy of Orthopaedic Surgeons Panel on Falls Prevention. (2001). Guideline for the prevention of falls in older persons. *Journal of the American Geriatrics Society, 49,* 664–672. doi:10.1046/j.1532-5415.2001.49115.x

Bataille, R., Barlogie, B., Lu, Z.Y., Rossi, J.F., Lavabre-Bertrand, T., Beck, T., ... Klein, B. (1995). Biologic effects of anti-interleukin-6 murine monoclonal antibody in advanced multiple myeloma. *Blood, 86,* 685–691.

Berenson, J.R. (2004). Management of skeletal complications. In J.S. Malpas, D.E. Bergsagel, R.A. Kyle, & K.C. Anderson (Eds.), *Myeloma: Biology and management* (3rd ed., pp. 239–249). Philadelphia, PA: Saunders.

Booker, R., Olson, K., Pilarski, L.M., Noon, J.P., & Bahlis, N. (2009). The relationships among physiologic variables, quality of life, and fatigue in patients with multiple myeloma. *Oncology Nursing Forum, 36,* 209–216. doi:10.1188/09.ONF.209-216

Centers for Disease Control and Prevention. (2005). *Check for safety: A home fall prevention checklist for older adults.* Retrieved from http://www.cdc.gov/ncipc/pub-res/toolkit/ Falls_ToolKit/DesktopPDF/English/booklet_Eng_desktop.pdf

Centers for Disease Control and Prevention. (2009). *Falls among older adults: An overview.* Retrieved from http://www.cdc.gov/HomeandRecreationalSafety/Falls/adultfalls .html

Cocks, K., Cohen, D., Wisloff, F., Sezer, O., Lee, S., Hippe, E., ... Brown, J. (2007). An international field study of the reliability and validity of a disease-specific questionnaire module (the QLQ-MY20) in assessing the quality of life of patients with multiple myeloma. *European Journal of Cancer, 43,* 1670–1678. doi:10.1016/j.ejca.2007.04.022

Dimopoulos, M.A., Kastritis, E., Rosinol, L., Blade, J., & Ludwig, H. (2008). Pathogenesis and treatment of renal failure in multiple myeloma. *Leukemia, 22,* 1485–1493. doi:10.1038/ leu.2008.131

Ferrans, E.C. (2000). Quality of life as an outcome of cancer care. In C.H. Yarbro, M.H. Frogge, M. Goodman, & S.L. Groenwald (Eds.), *Cancer nursing: Principles and practice* (5th ed., pp. 243–258). Sudbury, MA: Jones and Bartlett.

Frame, P.S. (1996). Developing a health maintenance schedule. In S.H. Wool, S. Jonas, & R.S. Lawrence (Eds.), *Health promotion and disease prevention in clinical practice* (pp. 467–482). Philadelphia, PA: Lippincott Williams & Wilkins.

Given, B. (2008). Cancer-related fatigue: A brief overview of current nursing perspectives and experiences. *Clinical Journal of Oncology Nursing, 12*(Suppl. 5), 7–9. doi:10.1188/08.CJON.S2.7-9

Grant, M., & Economou, D. (2008). The evolving paradigm of adult cancer survivor care. *Oncology, 22*(4 Suppl., Nurse Ed.), 13–22, 27.

Hoffman, B., & Stovall, E. (2006). Survivorship perspectives and advocacy. *Journal of Clinical Oncology, 24,* 5154–5159. doi:10.1200/JCO.2006.06.5300

Hofman, M., Ryan, J.L., Figueroa-Moseley, C.D., Jean-Pierre, P., & Morrow, G.R. (2007). Cancer-related fatigue: The scale of the problem. *Oncologist, 12*(Suppl. 1), 4–10. doi:10.1634/theoncologist.12-S1-4

Horner, M.J., Ries, L.A.G., Krapcho, M., Neyman, N., Aminou, R., Howlader, N., ... Edwards, B.K. (Eds.). (2009). *SEER cancer statistics review, 1975–2006 (based on November 2008 SEER data submission).* Retrieved from http://seer.cancer.gov/csr/1975_2006

Institute of Medicine. (2005). *From cancer patient to cancer survivor: Lost in transition.* Retrieved from http://www.iom.edu/Reports/2005/From-Cancer-Patient-to-Cancer-Survivor-Lost-in-Transition.aspx

Jemal, A., Siegel, R., Ward, E., Hao, Y., Xu, J., & Thun, M.J. (2009). Cancer statistics, 2009. *CA: A Cancer Journal for Clinicians, 59,* 225–249. doi:10.3322/caac.20006

Kaplan, M. (2006). Hypercalcemia of malignancy. In M. Kaplan (Ed.), *Understanding and managing oncologic emergencies* (pp. 51–97). Pittsburgh, PA: Oncology Nursing Society.

Kelly, A.M., Dwamena, B., Cronin, P., Bernstein, S.J., & Carlos, R.C. (2008). Meta-analysis: Effectiveness of drugs for preventing contrast-induced nephropathy. *Annals of Internal Medicine, 148,* 284–294.

Kumar, S.K., Rajkumar, S.V., Dispenzieri, A., Lacy, M.Q., Hayman, S.R., Buadi, F.K., ... Gertz, M.A. (2008). Improved survival in multiple myeloma and the impact of novel therapies. *Blood, 111,* 2516–2520. doi:10.1182/blood-2007-10-116129

Kyle, R.A. (1975). Multiple myeloma: Review of 869 cases. *Mayo Clinic Proceedings, 50,* 29–40.

Kyle, R.A., Gertz, M.A., Witzig, T.E., Lust, J.A., Lacy, M.Q., Dispenzieri, A., ... Greipp, P.R. (2003). Review of 1027 patients with newly diagnosed multiple myeloma. *Mayo Clinic Proceedings, 78,* 21–33. doi:10.4065/78.1.21

Kyle, R.A., Yee, G.C., Somerfield, M.R., Flynn, P.J., Halabi, S., Jagannath, S., ... Anderson, K. (2007). American Society of Clinical Oncology 2007 clinical practice guideline update on the role of bisphosphonates in multiple myeloma. *Journal of Clinical Oncology, 25,* 2464–2672. doi:10.1200/JCO.2007.12.1269

Leigh, S. (2004). Cancer survivorship: Defining our destiny. In B. Hoffman (Ed.), *A cancer survivor's almanac: Charting your journey* (3rd ed., pp. 8–13). Hoboken, NJ: John Wiley & Sons.

Mitchell, S.A., Beck, S.L., Hood, L.E., Moore, K., & Tanner, E.R. (2007). Putting evidence into practice: Evidence-based interventions for fatigue during and following cancer and its treatment. *Clinical Journal of Oncology Nursing, 11,* 99–113. doi:10.1188/07.CJON.99-113

Mullan, F. (1985). Seasons of survival: Reflections of a physician with cancer. *New England Journal of Medicine, 313,* 270–273.

National Cancer Institute. (2006). About cancer survivorship research: Survivorship definitions. Retrieved from http://dccps.nci.nih.gov/ocs/definitions.html

National Cancer Institute. (2009). SEER stat fact sheets: Myeloma. Retrieved from http://seer.cancer.gov/statfacts/html/mulmy.html

National Comprehensive Cancer Network. (2009). *NCCN Clinical Practice Guidelines in Oncology™: Cancer-related fatigue* [v.1.2009]. Retrieved from https://subscriptions.nccn.org/login.aspx?returnurl=http://www.nccn.org/professionals/physician_gls/PDF/fatigue.pdf

Overcash, J.A., & Beckstead, J. (2008). Predicting falls in older patients using components of a comprehensive geriatric assessment. *Clinical Journal of Oncology Nursing, 12*, 941–949. doi:10.1188/08.CJON.941-949

Paice, J.A. (2004). Pain. In C.H. Yarbro, M.H. Frogge, & M. Goodman (Eds.), *Cancer symptom management* (3rd ed., pp. 77–93). Sudbury, MA: Jones and Bartlett.

Perazella, M.A., & Markowitz, G.S. (2008). Bisphosphonate nephrotoxicity. *Kidney International, 74*, 1385–1393. doi:10.1038/ki.2008.356

Rajkumar, S.V. (2008). Treatment of myeloma: Cure vs. control. *Mayo Clinic Proceedings, 83*, 1142–1145. doi:10.4065/83.10.1142

Rajkumar, S.V., & Kyle, R.A. (2005). Multiple myeloma: Diagnosis and treatment. *Mayo Clinic Proceedings, 80*, 1371–1382. doi:10.4065/80.10.1371

Rossi, J.F., Fegueux, N., Lu, Z.Y., Legouffe, E., Exbrayat, C., Bozonnat, M.C., ... Klein, B. (2005). Optimizing the use of anti-interleukin-6 monoclonal antibody with dexamethasone and 140 mg/m^2 of melphalan in multiple myeloma: Results of a pilot study including biological aspects. *Bone Marrow Transplantation, 36*, 771–779. doi:10.1038/sj.bmt.1705138

Sezer, O. (2009). Myeloma bone disease: Recent advances in biology, diagnosis, and treatment. *Oncologist, 14*, 276–283. doi:10.1634/theoncologist.2009-0003

Shumway-Cook, A., Brauer, S., & Woollacott, M. (2000). Predicting the probability for falls in community-dwelling older adults using the Timed Up & Go Test. *Physical Therapy, 80*, 896–903.

ten Dam, M.A., & Wetzels, J.F. (2008). Toxicity of contrast media: An update. *Netherlands Journal of Medicine, 66*, 416–422.

U.S. Preventive Services Task Force. (2008). *The guide to clinical preventive services* (2nd ed.). Washington, DC: Agency for Healthcare Research and Quality.

Vellas, B.J., Wayne, S.J., Romero, L.J., Baumgartner, R.N., & Garry, P.J. (1997). Fear of falling and restriction of mobility in elderly fallers. *Age and Ageing, 26*, 189–193. doi:10.1093/ageing/26.3.189

Welch-McCaffrey, D., Hoffman, B., Leigh, S.A., Loescher, L.J., & Meyskens, F.L., Jr. (1989). Surviving adult cancers. Part 2: Psychosocial implications. *Annals of Internal Medicine, 111*, 517–524.

Wells, N., Murphy, B., Wujcik, D., & Johnson, R. (2003). Pain-related distress and interference with daily life of ambulatory patients with cancer with pain. *Oncology Nursing Forum, 30*, 977–986. doi:10.1188/03.ONF.977-986

Wickham, R. (2007). Chemotherapy-induced peripheral neuropathy: A review and implications for oncology nursing practice. *Clinical Journal of Oncology Nursing, 11*, 361–376. doi:10.1188/07.CJON.361-376

Yeager, K.A., McGuire, D.B., & Sheidler, V.R. (2000). Assessment of cancer pain. In C.H. Yarbro, M.H. Frogge, M. Goodman, & S.L. Groenwald (Eds.), *Cancer nursing: Principles and practice* (5th ed., pp. 633–656). Sudbury, MA: Jones and Bartlett.

Yeh, H.S., & Berenson, J.R. (2006). Treatment for myeloma bone disease. *Clinical Cancer Research, 12*(20, Pt. 2), 6279s–6284s. doi:10.1158/1078-0432.CCR-06-0681

CHAPTER 13

Nursing Research

Tiffany Richards, MS, ANP-BC, AOCNP®

INTRODUCTION

Multiple myeloma is diagnosed in more than 20,000 patients annually in the United States (Jemal et al., 2009). Most patients will present with disease complications of anemia, lytic bone lesions, renal failure, or hypercalcemia. These symptomatic patients will usually receive treatment with novel agents such as thalidomide, lenalidomide, bortezomib, and liposomal doxorubicin, either as a single agent or in combination with other chemotherapeutic agents. Although these drugs have been successful in prolonging both progression-free and overall survival, they also frequently result in troublesome side effects for the patient (Kumar et al., 2008).

Oncology nurses play an important role in identifying disease- and treatment-related complications and in the management of common side effects from treatment. Because of the paucity of nursing research specifically addressing the management of disease- and treatment-related complications, interventions have predominantly been adapted from research in other malignancies. Although there have been few nurse-led myeloma-related studies in the area of symptom management during and after chemotherapy or in the supportive care arena, a wealth of opportunities exists for well-designed nursing studies to evaluate problems related to complications of myeloma and chemotherapy effects. In the era of novel agents, oncology nurses must be cognizant of the results from current nursing research studies (2000–2009) and continue to explore research areas that need clarification.

A literature review was performed to identify published nursing research related to multiple myeloma. PubMed (1966 to January 2009), CINAHL® (1982 to January 2009), and Google databases were searched to access relevant myeloma-related nursing literature using search terms such as *nursing research, multiple myeloma, nursing, pain, peripheral neuropathy, myelosuppression, autologous stem cell transplantation, diagnosis, fatigue, exercise, supportive care*, and *symptom management*.

NURSING RESEARCH TOPICS IN MULTIPLE MYELOMA

Early Diagnosis

Timely diagnosis is critical to prevent serious complications from myeloma. Nurses have a unique opportunity to contribute to early diagnosis of patients because of differences in interactions between patients and various healthcare professionals. The National Cancer Institute developed the Surveillance, Epidemiology, and End Results (SEER) Program to collect incidence and survival data from regional and state cancer registries, including patient demographics, tumor site, date of treatment initiation, and patient survival (http://seer.cancer.gov). In order to determine the time from initial symptom presentation to diagnosis, a nurse-led study identified 5,483 eligible patients with myeloma diagnosed between 1992 and 2002 from the SEER-Medicare data set (Friese et al., 2009).

Frequent signs and symptoms of multiple myeloma were matched with the ninth edition of the *International Classification of Diseases* (ICD-9) and current procedural terminology codes (Friese et al., 2009). Researchers found that 70% of the patients had a sign or symptom of the disease within six months prior to diagnosis. The median time from onset of symptom to diagnosis was 99 days, and in those patients with a delayed diagnosis, 66% had a delay that exceeded 30 days. Factors that correlated with delayed diagnosis included higher frequency of physician visits, hospital visits, non-Caucasian ethnicity, female sex, increased age, and the presence of one comorbid condition in combination with anemia and back pain. Male patients who were diagnosed during an inpatient stay were less likely to have a delay in their diagnosis compared to female patients. Investigators reported that being diagnosed with myeloma while hospitalized (odds ratio [OR] 2.5, 95% confidence interval [CI] 2.2–2.9) and receiving chemotherapy treatment within six months of diagnosis (OR 1.4, 95% CI 1.2–1.6) were significant predictors of complications; diagnostic delay was not (OR 0.9, 95% CI 0.8–1.1). The researchers concluded that myeloma complications were more strongly associated with health status and disease severity than with diagnostic delays (Friese et al., 2009). These findings may be explained by the need for prompt diagnosis in symptomatic patients and unnecessary early interventions in asymptomatic patients. Furthermore, the findings demonstrate the importance of assessing patients' health status and stage of myeloma during the diagnostic workup to identify patients who are at a higher risk for complications.

Psychosocial Impact of Myeloma Diagnosis

Nurse researchers have investigated the psychosocial impact of receiving a diagnosis of multiple myeloma (Vlossak & Fitch, 2008). The purpose of this qualitative study was to explore the impact that the diagnosis had on patients and their families. Patients were evaluated by telephone interviews lasting 30–90 minutes. Twenty patients were interviewed, and several themes were identified: shock, few treatment options, concern and worry, complex treatment, fatigue, loss of independence, change in self-image, obsession on when life will end, fear of recurrence, and rationalizing their hopes for the future (Vlossak & Fitch, 2008).

All patients expressed the shock of receiving a diagnosis of myeloma. Additionally, many patients expressed disbelief by the negative information on the Internet and the lack of treatment options. Interestingly, many expressed they had entertained the thought of cancer because of frequent physician visits related to chronic pain, infections, and fractures before they received their diagnosis. Although patients expressed surprise as to the lack of treatment options, they felt overwhelmed by the urgency for treatment. In patients older than 65 years of age, health issues of other family members were important when making treatment-related decisions, particularly when it came to autologous stem cell transplantation (ASCT). One thing the authors of the study noted was that once patients had made a treatment decision, they did not deviate from the plan of care (Vlossak & Fitch, 2008).

The concern about family was voiced among both men and women and included a sense of inadequacy, guilt, and uselessness. Patients voiced that the responsibility of appointments and recording of information was typically performed by another family member. In patients with young children, discussing issues surrounding the cancer diagnosis was difficult regardless of the child's age. Patients described the treatment for the disease as long, complex, and requiring frequent office visits. Further complicating the treatment regimens were the multiple modalities used to treat the disease and its complications, including chemotherapy, radiation therapy, and pain medications (Vlossak & Fitch, 2008).

One important aspect that researchers noted was the concept of hope, defined as "living well for as long as possible" (Vlossak & Fitch, 2008). This study demonstrated the importance of not only providing patients with written treatment plans, coordinating physician visits, and patient education but also supporting the goals and hopes of each individual patient. Additionally, nurses should consider complex family dynamics that influence patients when they are making treatment decisions.

Symptom Management and Quality of Life

Patients with multiple myeloma may experience a variety of symptoms either from the disease or from treatment, including pain, neuropathy, bone disease, anemia, fatigue, gastrointestinal symptoms, and myelosuppression. Recommendations for symptom management often come from anecdotal information or single case reports, thus making evidence-based interventions difficult. One study has addressed the potential link between the development of symptoms and subsequent need for hospitalizations.

Most patients, during the course of their disease, will proceed into ASCT either during induction therapy or at first relapse. To determine reasons for unplanned admissions during ASCT, Coleman, Coon, Mattox, and O'Sullivan (2002) conducted a retrospective study of patients who required an unplanned admission and those who completed ASCT without hospitalization. The researchers analyzed symptom development and management in 87 patients with myeloma who were undergoing outpatient ASCT. Of these 87 patients, 16% required hospitalization during their outpatient treatment. The average number of days in the hospital for all 14 patients was 7.3 days with no pattern for admission diagnosis identified (Coleman et al., 2002).

Pain: Lytic bone lesions are present in 67% of patients diagnosed with symptomatic multiple myeloma and may result in somatic or neuropathic pain (Melton, Kyle, Achenbach, Oberg, & Rajkumar, 2005). Stimulation of nociceptive receptors in the musculoskeletal system results in pain, which patients often describe as a dull, achy pain that may be localized but also can radiate to another part of the body (Levy, Chwistek, & Mehta, 2008). Neuropathic pain may result from nerve root compression or as a complication of treatment (Ludwig & Zojer, 2007). Patients with myeloma may develop fractures of vertebral bodies, long bones, and ribs, resulting in decreased mobility and chronic pain (Ludwig & Zojer, 2007). There is a great need to study pain in patients with myeloma, especially in regard to how narcotic and non-narcotic interventions work specifically among the patients who are suffering from treatment-related pain.

Psychological Aspects of Self-Administration of Bisphosphonates: Researchers have evaluated the psychological effects of ambulatory infusion of pamidronate in patients with myeloma. They evaluated the psychological benefits of self-administration of pamidronate in 21 patients who received ambulatory pamidronate via a programmable infusion pump (Johansson, Langius-Eklof, Engervall, & Wredling, 2005). Patients who participated in the study received information related to the drug, step-by-step instruction on disconnection of the pump, removal of the access line, potential complications, staff contact information, and relevant references. After three doses, 12 patients were interviewed about their experiences. While the patients reported a positive experience, they thought that self-administration was not ideal at the time of initial diagnosis but over time would become a consideration. Many of the participants worked either part time or full time, indicating that self-administration is a feasible option for people with limited time schedules. Patients also reported that the program provided not only a greater sense of freedom but also additional time to spend with family (Johansson et al., 2005).

The negatives associated with the self-administration program included lack of written material/group education and patients' concern regarding their venous access device. However, over time, patients felt they had acquired sufficient knowledge to proceed with self-administration (Johansson et al., 2005).

The results of this study indicate that patients may require verbal, or preferably written, educational materials as well as group instruction or return demonstration prior to starting a self-administration program. Additionally, a self-administration program should be avoided in the first few months after diagnosis because of the overwhelming nature of diagnosis and initiation of chemotherapy. Taken further, this study suggests that patient education is most beneficial when repeated and evaluated at each patient encounter.

Peripheral Neuropathy and Neuropathic Pain: Another source of pain in patients with multiple myeloma is chemotherapy-induced neuropathy from bortezomib, thalidomide, vincristine, and, less often, lenalidomide. Approximately 80% of previously treated patients with myeloma report some degree of peripheral neuropathy (Richardson et al., 2009). Unfortunately, no studies have evaluated either pharmacologic or nonpharmacologic agents in relieving or preventing treatment-related neuropathy in this patient population. Although case reports have noted the benefit of supplemental agents such as acetyl L-carnitine, vitamin B complex, or alpha-lipoic acid, no formal studies have been conducted in patients with multiple myeloma (Tariman, Love, McCullagh, & Sandifer, 2008). The role of nurses in recognizing and reporting peripheral neuropathy makes this an ideal topic for nursing research, particularly in evaluating the benefit of nonpharmacologic therapies.

Fatigue: Fatigue in patients with myeloma may be attributed to a variety of factors, including anemia and the secretion of proinflammatory cytokines such as interleukin-6 (IL-6) and nuclear factor-kappa-B. IL-6 is expressed by the bone marrow stromal cells and stimulates myeloma cell growth (Booker, Olson, Pilarski, Noon, & Bahlis, 2009). C-reactive protein (CRP) is synthesized by liver hepatocytes and is reflective of IL-6 concentration (Bataille, Boccadoro, Klein, Durie, & Pileri, 1992; San Miguel, Garcia-Sanz, & Gutierrez, 2008). Studies utilizing an IL-6 monoclonal antibody have found decreased CRP levels and reduction in fever, pain, and cachexia (Booker et al., 2009). Patients with myeloma have described fatigue as a constantly present "inner" tiredness (Vlossak & Fitch, 2008, p. 143).

In a study of 56 patients with multiple myeloma, nurse and physician investigators analyzed the impact of hemoglobin and CRP on fatigue and quality of life (Booker et al., 2009). Patients received a 30-item questionnaire that measured quality of life and a 28-item questionnaire that measured fatigue levels at a single point in time. Additionally, CRP levels were measured at the time of study entry. Although anemia is often thought to be the cause for fatigue in patients with cancer, the median hemoglobin level of patients was 129 g/L, whereas the median fatigue level was 31 (range 7–52) in the Functional Assessment of Cancer Therapy–Fatigue scale and the median quality-of-life score was 4 (range 1–7) in the European Organisation for Research and Treatment of Cancer QLQ-C30 scale. The researchers found that CRP was a predictor of fatigue ($p = 0.003$) and quality of life ($p = 0.020$), but hemoglobin was not predictive of fatigue ($p = 0.237$) or quality of life ($p = 0.412$), as it was codependent with CRP (Booker et al., 2009).

Coleman et al. (2002) measured fatigue in admitted patients compared to outpatients by using the percentage of usual energy. The researchers assessed study participants three days before transplant, on the day of transplant, and on either the day of admission or day 20 for patients not admitted. Both groups of patients exhibited a decline in energy. The average percentage of usual energy for admitted patients before transplant was 84%, compared with 80% for those not admitted. The percentage of usual energy significantly declined the day of transplantation, with both groups reporting a mean of 66%. Following the transplant, the admitted group continued to decline more than the outpatient group: 39% for the admitted group versus 51% for the outpatients. However, in the group of patients admitted to the hospital, energy levels significantly declined when compared with those patients not admitted ($p = 0.017$). Another factor that affected hospital admission was the level of hydration ($p < 0.001$). In those patients who were admitted to the hospital, the level of hydration decreased from 1.2 L/day to 0.73 L/day on the day of transplant to 0.59 L/d on the day of admission. In patients who were not admitted to the hospital, a slight decrease occurred in the amount of oral intake from 1 L/day pretransplant to 0.99 L/day on the day of transplant, but hydration remained fairly consistent at 0.99 L/day for day 20. Interestingly, age was not found to influence whether a person was admitted, which is important given that the median age at diagnosis for patients with myeloma is 70 (Coleman et al., 2002; National Cancer Institute, 2005). Although this study was based on a small number of patients, it raises some interesting points, including the importance of educating patients on oral hydration during treatment and of managing fatigue before, during, and after stem cell transplantation.

A systematic review of research in cancer-related fatigue found that exercise and psychosocial methods (counseling, yoga, massage) were equally effective in reducing fatigue in patients with cancer ($p > 0.05$) (Kangas, Bovbjerg, & Montgomery, 2008). However, fatigue was reduced by 40%–43% in those studies that included a multimodal exercise program. Programs lasting eight weeks or more (effect size = 0.67) had a greater effect in reducing fatigue than those lasting six to eight weeks (effect size = 0.75). Interestingly, exercise demonstrated a greater impact on fatigue during cancer treatment, whereas psychosocial interventions had a greater impact on post-treatment fatigue (Kangas et al., 2008).

Several studies have demonstrated benefit of exercise in improving fatigue levels in patients with myeloma who were undergoing induction therapy. In a study of 24 patients, patients were randomized to an exercise group and a usual care group (Coleman et al., 2003). The exercise program included six months of aerobic activity (walking, cycling, or running) and resistance training (using stretch bands). Prior to the start of the study, patients in the exercise arm met with an exercise physiologist to determine their body mass index and fitness level using the Balke protocol (a method utilized to measure cardiovascular health on a graded treadmill), and they subsequently received a personal exercise program based on their health history. The only statistically significant difference between the two groups was the degree of change in lean body mass (+0.40 kg/month in the exercise group versus –0.44 kg/month in the non-exercise group, $p < 0.01$) (Coleman et al., 2003). Differences between the groups in level of fatigue, daytime sleepiness, and total minutes of sleep were not statistically significant; however, a trend toward improved scores may indicate that aerobic exercise and resistance training may be more significant in a larger patient sample.

In a study of 135 patients with multiple myeloma who were undergoing induction therapy followed by tandem ASCT, patients were randomized to receive epoetin alfa with or without exercise (Coleman et al., 2008). In the exercise group, patients received an individualized exercise plan, exercise stretch bands, and a videotape illustrating the exercises. The usual-care group was advised to follow exercise recommendations provided by their physicians. The exercise group had better exercise performance and less aerobic capacity loss compared to the usual-care group. Interestingly, the exercise group demonstrated a decrease in the number of days required for stem cell collection ($p < 0.025$) and the number of blood or platelet transfusions ($p < 0.025$) compared to the usual-care group (Coleman et al., 2008).

In an attempt to determine patients' feelings, beliefs, and experiences related to exercise, researchers interviewed 21 patients participating in the Coleman et al. (2008) study (Coon & Coleman, 2004). Three themes were identified, including beliefs, social context (culture), and experience. The belief theme included the following ideas: exercise as beneficial; associations between exercise and decreased fatigue; active participants in treatment; and their commitment to keeping their word. The theme of social context included the following: life before cancer; social support (accountability); caregivers' and participants' congruence regarding exercise; and the impact of the social environment on participants' ability to exercise. Regarding experience, many patients reported that they would recommend an exercise program to other patients with multiple myeloma for management of fatigue. Researchers identified factors that created barriers to exercise, including disease and treatment complications, such as fatigue, nausea, vomiting, pain, and chemotherapy administration. However, the investigators found that patients' ability to exercise increased as their disease improved. The weather and schedule demands created barriers to exercise as well (Coon & Coleman, 2004).

Fatigue affects patients' quality of life and interpersonal relationships. These studies provide evidence that an exercise program containing both aerobic and resistance training may counteract the fatigue and muscle loss often experienced by patients receiving treatment for myeloma. Additionally, researchers suggested that when patients begin an exercise program, they are more likely to recommend the program to other patients (Coon & Coleman, 2004). Nurses are in a position to discuss the benefits of exercise with patients, not only at their physician visits but also during treatment time. Providing educational materials on local and home-based exercise programs and other appropriate programs may provide additional incentives for patients to participate.

GAPS IN THE LITERATURE

Overall, myeloma-related nursing studies are few when compared to other cancer specialties. The studies reviewed in this chapter were predominantly in fatigue management, exercise, diagnosis delay, psychological aspects and quality of life, and unexpected admissions during ASCT. Currently, nursing interventions for treatment-related toxicities are based on studies conducted in other malignancies, including pain management and supportive care in patients receiving novel agents, particularly thalidomide and bortezomib. Studies evaluating the efficacy of vitamin supplements in the prevention and treatment of peripheral neuropathy are needed. Research studies in the area of emotional and cognitive dysfunction, end-of-life care, and survivorship issues, as well as interventional studies related to treatment- and disease-related complications, are also direly needed.

As discussed earlier, 80% of previously treated patients with myeloma report some form of neuropathy (Richardson et al., 2009). Studies conducted among patients with neuropathy related to diabetes or other chemotherapy-induced neuropathy indicate that vitamin and mineral supplements may alleviate or prevent neuropathy. Drugs such as bortezomib and thalidomide exert different mechanisms of action than taxanes or platinum-based chemotherapy, and the mechanism by which neuropathy develops may differ between different agents or diabetic neuropathy. Therefore, prospective studies evaluating these regimens among patients with multiple myeloma are needed.

Anecdotal reports on thalidomide's impact on sexual function have been described in the literature (Pouaha, Martin, Reichert-Penetrat, Trechot, & Schmutz, 2002). Additional studies are needed that evaluate sexual function before, during, and after the different treatment regimens, including ASCT. Drugs such as steroids may affect emotional and cognitive function and require further evaluation for appropriate recognition and interventions.

The life expectancy of patients with myeloma has nearly doubled over the past decade (Kumar et al., 2008). This increase in life expectancy has led to consideration of multiple myeloma as a chronic disease. Therefore, survivorship issues associated with disease and long-term treatment-related toxicities such as neuropathy, fatigue, bone health, sexual dysfunction, and renal complications, as well as health maintenance, will need to be addressed in this patient population. Additionally, although patients are living longer with myeloma, they will still require end-of-life care at some point during their care continuum. Studies evaluating the needs of patients at the end of life, as well as symptom management during this period, are needed in order to relieve pain, other symptoms, and caregiver stress that may be experienced by patients and their families.

Culture, religious beliefs, and values influence the way individuals view their lives and the meaning of disease. Therefore, studies should include a broad examination of the cultural influences on diagnosis, treatment, management of side effects, and the end of life in order to provide personalized care.

FUTURE SCENARIO OF NURSING RESEARCH IN MYELOMA

A huge gap exists in the myeloma literature when it comes to nursing care. Additional nursing research is needed to shape the delivery of nursing care of patients with this disease. Oncology nurses can change the current status of nursing research in multiple myeloma and contribute to the currently established evidence-based nursing interventions. The future nursing research scenario in myeloma could be one that is full of research activities or one that remains unstudied or understudied.

CONCLUSION

Although some studies have been conducted in patients with multiple myeloma, more research is needed to better address symptoms both during treatment and at the end of life. Oncology nurses are in an excellent position to design and conduct clinical trials that evaluate the impact of nursing interventions on patient care and clinical outcomes.

REFERENCES

Bataille, R., Boccadoro, M., Klein, B., Durie, B., & Pileri, A. (1992). C-reactive protein and beta-2 microglobulin produce a simple and powerful myeloma staging system. *Blood, 80*, 733–737.

Booker, R., Olson, K., Pilarski, L.M., Noon, J.P., & Bahlis, N.J. (2009). The relationships among physiologic variables, quality of life, and fatigue in patients with multiple myeloma. *Oncology Nursing Forum, 36*, 209–216. doi:10.1188/09.ONF.209-216

Coleman, E.A., Coon, S., Hall-Barrow, J., Richards, K., Gaylor, D., & Stewart, B. (2003). Feasibility of exercise during treatment for multiple myeloma. *Cancer Nursing, 26*, 410–419. doi:10.1097/00002820-200310000-00012

Coleman, E.A., Coon, S.K., Kennedy, R.L., Lockhart, K.D., Stewart, C.B., Anaissie, E.J., & Barlogie, B. (2008). Effects of exercise in combination with epoetin alfa during high-dose chemotherapy and autologous peripheral blood stem cell transplantation for multiple myeloma [Online exclusive]. *Oncology Nursing Forum, 35*, E53–E61. doi:10.1188/08.ONF.E53-E61

Coleman, E.A., Coon, S.K., Mattox, S.G., & O'Sullivan, P. (2002). Symptom management and successful outpatient transplantation for patients with multiple myeloma. *Cancer Nursing, 25*, 452–460. doi:10.1097/00002820-200212000-00009

Coon, S.K., & Coleman, E.A. (2004). Exercise decisions within the context of multiple myeloma, transplant, and fatigue. *Cancer Nursing, 27*, 108–118. doi:10.1097/00002820-200403000-00003

Friese, C.R., Abel, G.A., Magazu, L.S., Neville, B.A., Richardson, L.C., & Earle, C.C. (2009). Diagnostic delay and complications for older adults with multiple myeloma. *Leukemia and Lymphoma, 50*, 392–400. doi:10.1080/10428190902741471

Jemal, A., Siegel, R., Ward, E., Hao, Y., Xu, J., & Thun, M.J. (2009). Cancer statistics, 2009. *CA: A Cancer Journal for Clinicians, 59*, 225–249. doi:10.3322/caac.20006

Johansson, E., Langius-Eklof, A., Engervall, P., & Wredling, R. (2005). Patients' experience of ambulatory self-administration of pamidronate in multiple myeloma. *Cancer Nursing, 28*, 158–165. doi:10.1097/00002820-200503000-00011

Kangas, M., Bovbjerg, D.H., & Montgomery, G.H. (2008). Cancer-related fatigue: A systematic and meta-analytic review of non-pharmacological therapies for cancer patients. *Psychology Bulletin, 134,* 700–741. doi:10.1037/a0012825

Kumar, S.K., Rajkumar, S.V., Dispenzieri, A., Lacy, M.Q., Hayman, S.R., Buadi, F.K., … Gertz, M.A. (2008). Improved survival in multiple myeloma and the impact of novel therapies. *Blood, 111,* 2516–2520. doi:10.1182/blood-2007-10-116129

Levy, M.H., Chwistek, M., & Mehta, R.S. (2008). Management of chronic pain in cancer survivors. *Cancer Journal, 14,* 401–409. doi:10.1097/PPO.0b013e31818f5aa7

Ludwig, H., & Zojer, N. (2007). Supportive care in multiple myeloma. *Best Practice and Research Clinical Haematology, 20,* 817–835. doi:10.1016/j.beha.2007.10.001

Melton, L.J., III, Kyle, R.A., Achenbach, S.J., Oberg, A.L., & Rajkumar, S.V. (2005). Fracture risk with multiple myeloma: A population-based study. *Journal of Bone and Mineral Research, 20,* 487–493. doi:10.1359/JBMR.041131

National Cancer Institute. (2005). Median age of cancer patients at diagnosis, 2000–2003. Retrieved from http://seer.cancer.gov/csr/1975_2003/results_merged/topic_med_age.pdf

Pouaha, J., Martin, S., Reichert-Penetrat, S., Trechot, P., & Schmutz, J.L. (2002). Thalidomide and sexual dysfunction in men. *British Journal of Dermatology, 146,* 1112–1112. doi:10.1046/j.1365-2133.2002.473211.x

Richardson, P.G., Sonneveld, P., Schuster, M., Stadtmauer, E., Facon, T., Harousseau, J.-L., … San Miguel, J. (2009). Reversibility of symptomatic peripheral neuropathy with bortezomib in the phase III APEX trial in relapsed multiple myeloma: Impact of a dose-modification guideline. *British Journal of Haematology, 144,* 895–903. doi:10.1111/j.1365-2141.2008.07573.x

San Miguel, J., Garcia-Sanz, R., & Gutierrez, N. (2008). Prognostic factors and classification in multiple myeloma. In K.C. Anderson & I. Ghobrial (Eds.), *Multiple myeloma: Translational and emerging therapies* (pp. 115–139). New York, NY: Informa Healthcare.

Tariman, J.D., Love, G., McCullagh, E., & Sandifer, S. (2008). Peripheral neuropathy associated with novel therapies in patients with multiple myeloma: Consensus statement of the IMF Nurse Leadership Board. *Clinical Journal of Oncology Nursing, 12*(Suppl. 3), 29–36. doi:10.1188/08.CJON.S1.29-35

Vlossak, D., & Fitch, M.I. (2008). Multiple myeloma: The patient's perspective. *Canadian Oncology Nursing Journal, 18,* 141–151.

CHAPTER 14

On the Horizon: Future Considerations

Joseph D. Tariman, PhC, MN, APRN-BC, OCN®

INTRODUCTION

Novel agents have changed the treatment paradigm for patients with multiple myeloma (Tariman & Estrella, 2005), leading to dramatic improvements in overall response rates and overall survival. In the past decade, therapeutic options have increased, patient outcomes have improved, and further insight has been gained into the biology and genetics of myeloma (Tariman & Faiman, 2010). Since 2003, the U.S. Food and Drug Administration (FDA) has approved thalidomide, bortezomib, lenalidomide, and pegylated liposomal doxorubicin for use in patients with newly diagnosed or relapsed myeloma. Two new drugs, pomalidomide and carfilzomib, have also shown strong clinical activities in patients with relapsed myeloma, leading the way for more potential drugs to be approved by the FDA in the near future. Several advances have also occurred in diagnostics and imaging. The advent of additional novel agents and the optimization of the therapeutic benefits of existing ones can further improve clinical outcomes. Patients' overall survival will continue to improve with new generations of drugs and more breakthroughs in testing and imaging.

ONGOING RESEARCH STUDIES

Biologically based therapeutic agents for multiple myeloma are currently under preclinical and clinical investigation (see Table 14-1). Increased understanding of osteoblast inhibition and improved comprehension of the role of bone marrow microenvironment in the pathophysiology of myeloma have led to the development of several effective therapeutics with promising clinical results (Esteve & Roodman, 2007; Giuliani, Rizzoli, & Roodman, 2006; Mitsiades et al., 2007).

Table 14-1. Novel Agents Currently Under Investigation for Multiple Myeloma	
Drug Classification	**References**
Akt inhibitor	Hideshima et al., 2007; Huston et al., 2008; Podar et al., 2009
Angiogenesis inhibitor	Chauhan et al., 2002; Hou et al., 2005; Mooberry, 2003; Rajkumar et al., 2007; Zhou et al., 2008
Combination of novel agents	Duus et al., 2006; Francis et al., 2006; Huston et al., 2008; Yasui et al., 2007; Zaarur et al., 2006
Farnesyltransferase inhibitor	Alsina et al., 2004; Beaupre et al., 2004; David et al., 2005; Zhu et al., 2005
Heat shock protein inhibitor	Cervantes-Gomez et al., 2009; Davenport et al., 2007; Erlichman, 2009; Huston et al., 2008; Mitsiades et al., 2006; National Institutes of Health, 2009; Patterson et al., 2008; Sydor et al., 2006
Histone deacetylase inhibitor	Catley et al., 2003; Deleu et al., 2009; Galli et al., 2009; Maiso et al., 2006; Siegel et al., 2009
Immunomodulator	Galustian et al., 2009; Lacy et al., 2009; Streetly et al., 2008
Nuclear factor-kappa-B inhibitor	Takatsuna et al., 2005; Tatetsu et al., 2005; Watanabe et al., 2005
Osteoprotegerin	Giuliani et al., 2002; Vanderkerken et al., 2003
Second-generation proteasome inhibitor	Kuhn et al., 2007; Parlati et al., 2009; Zhou et al., 2009
Tyrosine kinase inhibitor	Mitsiades et al., 2004; Sloan & Scheinfeld, 2008; Zangari et al., 2004

PROMISING CLINICAL TRIALS

Carfilzomib

Proteasome inhibition is an attractive anticancer therapy because the ubiquitin-proteasome pathway plays a central role in the targeted destruction of cellular proteins, including cell cycle regulatory proteins (Adams, 2004a). Ubiquitin, a regulatory protein, marks other proteins for proteasomal destruction. Disruption of this pathway alters cell proliferation and survival and, in certain cancer cells, makes the proteasome a suitable antineoplastic target (Adams, 2004b). Carfilzomib is a second-generation proteasome inhibitor that can induce tumor cell death through selective inhibition of the chymotrypsin-like activity (digestion) of the proteasome (Parlati et al., 2009). Specific inhibition of the chymotrypsin-like proteasome and immunoproteasome activities results in the accumulation of ubiquitinated substrates, ultimately leading to apoptosis. Moreover, proteasome inhibition–induced apoptosis is associated with activation of c-Jun-N-terminal kinase, mitochondrial membrane depolarization, release of cytochrome c, and activation of both intrinsic and extrinsic caspase pathways (Kuhn et al., 2007).

Carfilzomib has shown activity in patients with multiple myeloma at first relapse and even in patients who have advanced cancer and have failed bortezomib. It is used in combination with dexamethasone and has an acceptable toxicity profile characterized by a lesser degree of neuropathy than that seen in bortezomib. A phase II trial was conducted with 46 patients, including 78% who had disease progression on or within 60 days of their last therapy and 22% who had no response to their last therapy (Jagannath et al., 2008). Thirty-nine patients initiated treatment, completed at least one cycle of carfilzomib, had measurable monoclonal (M) protein, and were evaluable for response to treatment. The mean number of prior therapies (excluding transplant) was 6.4 (range of 1–18); 100% patients received prior bortezomib, 91% received prior thalidomide, 89% received prior lenalidomide, and 83% had prior stem cell transplantation. Using the Blade criteria (Blade et al., 1998), the overall clinical benefit response was 26% (10 of the 39 evaluable patients), including 5 patients who achieved partial response, 5 patients with minimal response, and 16 additional patients who achieved stable disease (Jagannath et al., 2008).

Pomalidomide

Immunomodulatory drugs (IMiDs) such as pomalidomide and lenalidomide are potent inhibitors of angiogenic response (Anderson, 2007). Pomalidomide's precise mechanism of action is not known; however, preclinical investigations indicate that IMiDs have the following activities in cancer cells:

- Suppression of vascular endothelial growth factor elaboration from myeloma cell lines and cellular response in receptor-competent cells (Crane & List, 2005)
- Inhibition of the proliferation of malignant B cells while expanding CD34+ progenitor cells (Verhelle et al., 2007)
- Downregulation of PU.1 (a transcription factor) causing inhibition of osteoclast formation (Anderson et al., 2006)
- Inhibition of the proliferation and function of T regulatory cells (Galustian et al., 2009).

In a phase I trial, 24 patients with relapsed or refractory myeloma were treated with pomalidomide, resulting in a more than 25% reduction of M spike in 67% of patients, a greater than 50% reduction in M spike in 13 patients (54%), and complete remission (100% reduction of M spike) in 4 (17%) of 24 patients. The maximum tolerated dose (MTD) was determined to be 2 mg/day (Schey et al., 2004). Another phase I study of pomalidomide using an alternate-day dosing schedule showed 10% of patients achieving complete response and 50% of subjects achieving a partial response. In this group of patients, the progression-free survival was 10.5 months and median overall survival was 33 months. The MTD for this group of patients was 5 mg alternate-day dosing (Streetly et al., 2008).

Phase II study results of pomalidomide have recently been reported. Lacy et al. (2009) concluded that the combination of pomalidomide and low-dose dexamethasone is extremely active in the treatment of relapsed disease, with high response rates occurring in patients who were refractory to other novel agents. Overall, 38 patients (63%) achieved confirmed response, including complete response in 3 patients (5%), very good partial response in 17 patients (28%), and partial response in 18 patients (30%) out of 60 patients enrolled in the study. Furthermore, responses were seen in 40% of lenalidomide-refractory patients, 37% of thalidomide-refractory patients, and 60% of bortezomib-refractory patients. Seventy-four percent of patients with high-risk cytogenetic or molecular markers responded to pomalidomide. Side effects were primarily myelosuppression, characterized by grade 3 or 4 anemia (5%), thrombocytopenia (3%), and neutropenia (32%). Only one patient (1.6%) had a thromboembolic event. Lastly, the median progression-free survival time was 11.6 months and was not significantly different in patients with high-risk multiple myeloma compared to those with standard-risk disease (Lacy et al., 2009).

CELLULAR AND MOLECULAR GENETICS

Genetic mutations leading to chromosomal translocations, additions, and deletions play a key role in the development of symptomatic, malignant multiple myeloma. As cellular and molecular tests in myeloma become widely available, clinicians will be able to appropriately diagnose and treat patients specific to their unique presentation of disease (Jagannath, 2008). Molecular diagnostic tools and novel therapeutics now offer the potential for accurate prognostic and individualized treatment pathways. Specifically established negative prognostic factors in patients with myeloma include immunoglobulin heavy-chain (referred to as IgH) translocations such as the t(4;14), t(14;16), chromosome 13 deletion by conventional cytogenetics, and loss of 17p13 by interphase fluorescence in situ hybridization (Stewart & Fonseca, 2005).

Preliminary gene expression profiling studies have demonstrated that individual genes (for example, *CSK1-B*) or groups of genes can define prognosis with greater accuracy than conventional genetic markers (Stewart & Fonseca, 2005). They also can provide pharmacogenomic and biologic insight into the pathophysiology, therapeutics, and future targets of myeloma (Stewart & Fonseca, 2005). Recent clinical trials are now adopting routine genetic testing and risk stratification; however, larger prospective clinical trials are needed to confirm the value of risk stratification based on negative genetic factors (Kapoor et al., 2009).

The systematic application of cytogenetics and molecular genetics, especially gene expression profiling, has led to a molecular classification of multiple myeloma (Zhan, Barlogie, & Shaughnessy, 2003; Zhan et al., 2006). Additionally, molecular-based high-risk stratification is being investigated. Researchers are studying the molecular high-risk signature in order to design clinical trials that can characterize the molecular pathways responsible for the aggressive clinical phenotype of this disease. Once these molecular pathways are identified, determining new therapeutic targets will be critical to improving the outcomes of patients who continue to receive minimal benefit from current therapies (Zhan, Barlogie, Mulligan, Shaughnessy, & Bryant, 2008).

ADVANCES IN IMAGING

Imaging is an important aspect of the general workup of patients with myeloma to determine the effects of myeloma cells on the skeletal system. Traditionally, radiographic skeletal surveys are part of a routine diagnostic workup. Recently, magnetic resonance imaging (MRI) of bone marrow has allowed a direct look at the actual tumor burden within the bone marrow, allowing assessment of the extent of disease in newly diagnosed cases and of the effects of therapy (Angtuaco, Fassas, Walker, Sethi, & Barlogie, 2004). The use of positron-emission tomography (PET) with fluorodeoxyglucose (FDG) aided in detection of unsuspected sites of medullary and extramedullary disease, particularly in patients with recurrent disease not detectable by routine imaging (Schirrmeister et al., 2002).

Recently, PET-FDG with low-dose computed tomography (CT) and whole-body MRI have been investigated as another tool to evaluate response to therapy. A review by Lutje et al. (2009) concluded that both PET-FDG in combination with low-dose CT and whole-body MRI are more sensitive than skeletal survey in screening and diagnosing myeloma. Thus, the combination of PET with low-dose CT can replace the gold-standard conventional skeletal survey. Additionally, whole-body MRI allows assessment of bone marrow involvement but cannot detect bone destruction (affecting myeloma staging at diagnosis) and is less suitable in assessing response to therapy than FDG-PET (Lutje et al., 2009).

Researchers have recently reported that the presence of more than three FDG-avid focal lesions (FLs), related to fundamental features of myeloma biology and genomics, was the leading independent parameter associated with inferior overall and event-free survival in patients with newly diagnosed disease who underwent total therapy 3. Total therapy 3 involves the use of novel agents before, during, and after tandem autologous stem cell transplantation. A complete FDG suppression in FLs before first transplantation conferred significantly better outcomes and was only opposed by gene expression profiling–defined high-risk status, which together accounted for approximately

50% of survival variability. These findings imply that altering treatment can improve survival in patients in whom FDG suppression cannot be achieved after initial induction therapy (Bartel et al., 2009). Future large, prospective, randomized trials are required to test this hypothesis.

The British Committee for Standards in Hematology has issued guidelines for the use of imaging in the management of myeloma: skeletal surveys, MRI, CT, or PET scanning. The committee did not recommend the use of MRI, CT, or PET scans for routine follow-up of treated patients. The committee argued that these imaging techniques are useful only in selected patients who have persistent unexplained symptoms or in whom there is a concern for increased fracture risk or lack of response to therapy. Taken together, the data from imaging studies in patients with multiple myeloma suggest that skeletal surveys are useful in initial diagnostic workup but are not useful for routine follow-up because of their limited reproducibility (Roodman, 2008).

CONCLUSION

Several advances have taken place in the areas of diagnostics and therapeutics for patients with myeloma. In therapeutics, carfilzomib and pomalidomide provide great promise for achieving partial and complete clinical responses. Gene expression profiling and molecular risk stratification could potentially improve the outcome of those patients who do not benefit from current therapies through the identification of new molecular therapeutic targets. The role of MRI and combined PET and CT in the diagnosis and follow-up of patients with multiple myeloma continues to evolve. Large, prospective, randomized trials are needed to establish new standards in diagnostics and therapeutics.

REFERENCES

Adams, J. (2004a). The development of proteasome inhibitors as anticancer drugs. *Cancer Cell, 5,* 417–421. doi:10.1016/S1535-6108(04)00120-5

Adams, J. (2004b). The proteasome: A suitable antineoplastic target. *Nature Reviews Cancer, 4,* 349–360. doi:10.1038/nrc1361

Alsina, M., Fonseca, R., Wilson, E.F., Belle, A.N., Gerbino, E., Price-Troska, T., ... Sebti, S.M. (2004). Farnesyltransferase inhibitor tipifarnib is well tolerated, induces stabilization of disease, and inhibits farnesylation and oncogenic/tumor survival pathways in patients with advanced multiple myeloma. *Blood, 103,* 3271–3277. doi:10.1182/blood-2003-08-2764

Anderson, G., Gries, M., Kurihara, N., Honjo, T., Anderson, J., Donnenberg, V., ... Lentzsch, S. (2006). Thalidomide derivative CC-4047 inhibits osteoclast formation by downregulation of PU.1. *Blood, 107,* 3098–3105. doi:10.1182/blood-2005-08-3450

Anderson, K.C. (2007). Targeted therapy of multiple myeloma based upon tumor-microenvironmental interactions. *Experimental Hematology, 35,* 155–162. doi:10.1016/j.exphem.2007.01.024

Angtuaco, E.J., Fassas, A.B., Walker, R., Sethi, R., & Barlogie, B. (2004). Multiple myeloma: Clinical review and diagnostic imaging. *Radiology*, *231*, 11–23. doi:10.1148/radiol.2311020452

Bartel, T.B., Haessler, J., Brown, T.L.Y., Shaughnessy, J.D., Jr., van Rhee, F., Anaissie, E., ... Barlogie, B. (2009). F18-fluorodeoxyglucose positron emission tomography in the context of other imaging techniques and prognostic factors in multiple myeloma. *Blood*, *114*, 2068–2076. doi:10.1182/blood-2009-03-213280

Beaupre, D.M., Cepero, E., Obeng, E.A., Boise, L.H., & Lichtenheld, M.G. (2004). R115777 induces Ras-independent apoptosis of myeloma cells via multiple intrinsic pathways. *Molecular Cancer Therapeutics*, *3*, 179–186.

Blade, J., Samson, D., Reece, D., Apperley, J., Bjorkstrand, B., Gahrton, G., ... Vesole, D. (1998). Criteria for evaluating disease response and progression in patients with multiple myeloma treated by high-dose therapy and haemopoietic stem cell transplantation. Myeloma Subcommittee of the EBMT. European Group for Blood and Marrow Transplant. *British Journal of Haematology*, *102*, 1115–1123. doi:10.1046/j.1365-2141.1998.00930.x

Catley, L., Weisberg, E., Tai, Y.T., Atadja, P., Remiszewski, S., Hideshima, T., ... Anderson, K.C. (2003). NVP-LAQ824 is a potent novel histone deacetylase inhibitor with significant activity against multiple myeloma. *Blood*, *102*, 2615–2622. doi:10.1182/blood-2003-01-0233

Cervantes-Gomez, F., Nimmanapalli, R., & Gandhi, V. (2009). Transcription inhibition of heat shock proteins: A strategy for combination of 17-allylamino-17-demethoxygeldanamycin and actinomycin d. *Cancer Research*, *69*, 3947–3954. doi:10.1158/0008-5472.CAN-08-4406

Chauhan, D., Catley, L., Hideshima, T., Li, G., Leblanc, R., Gupta, D., ... Anderson, K.C. (2002). 2-Methoxyestradiol overcomes drug resistance in multiple myeloma cells. *Blood*, *100*, 2187–2194. doi:10.1182/blood-2002-02-0376

Crane, E., & List, A. (2005). Immunomodulatory drugs. *Cancer Investigation*, *23*, 625–634. doi:10.1080/07357900500283101

Davenport, E.L., Moore, H.E., Dunlop, A.S., Sharp, S.Y., Workman, P., Morgan, G.J., & Davies, F.E. (2007). Heat shock protein inhibition is associated with activation of the unfolded protein response pathway in myeloma plasma cells. *Blood*, *110*, 2641–2649. doi:10.1182/blood-2006-11-053728

David, E., Sun, S.Y., Waller, E.K., Chen, J., Khuri, F.R., & Lonial, S. (2005). The combination of the farnesyl transferase inhibitor lonafarnib and the proteasome inhibitor bortezomib induces synergistic apoptosis in human myeloma cells that is associated with downregulation of p-AKT. *Blood*, *106*, 4322–4329. doi:10.1182/blood-2005-06-2584

Deleu, S., Lemaire, M., Arts, J., Menu, E., Van Valckenborgh, E., Vande Broek, I., ... Vanderkerken, K. (2009). Bortezomib alone or in combination with the histone deacetylase inhibitor JNJ-26481585: Effect on myeloma bone disease in the 5T2MM murine model of myeloma. *Cancer Research*, *69*, 5307–5311. doi:10.1158/0008-5472.CAN-08-4472

Duus, J., Bahar, H.I., Venkataraman, G., Ozpuyan, F., Izban, K.F., Al-Masri, H., ... Alkan, S. (2006). Analysis of expression of heat shock protein-90 (HSP90) and the effects of HSP90 inhibitor (17-AAG) in multiple myeloma. *Leukemia and Lymphoma*, *47*, 1369–1378. doi:10.1080/10428190500472123

Erlichman, C. (2009). Tanespimycin: The opportunities and challenges of targeting heat shock protein 90. *Expert Opinion in Investigational Drugs*, *18*, 861–868. doi:10.1517/13543780902953699

Esteve, F.R., & Roodman, G.D. (2007). Pathophysiology of myeloma bone disease. *Best Practice in Research and Clinical Haematology*, *20*, 613–624. doi:10.1016/j.beha.2007.08.003

Francis, L.K., Alsayed, Y., Leleu, X., Jia, X., Singha, U.K., Anderson, J., ... Ghobrial, I.M. (2006). Combination mammalian target of rapamycin inhibitor rapamycin and HSP90 inhibitor 17-allylamino-17-demethoxygeldanamycin has synergistic activity in multiple myeloma. *Clinical Cancer Research*, *12*, 6826–6835. doi:10.1158/1078-0432.CCR-06-1331

Galli, M., Salmoiraghi, S., Golay, J., Gozzini, A., Crippa, C., Pescosta, N., & Rambaldi, A. (2009). A phase II multiple dose clinical trial of histone deacetylase inhibitor ITF2357 in patients with relapsed or progressive multiple myeloma. *Annals of Hematology*. Advance online publication. doi:10.1007/s00277-009-0793-8

Galustian, C., Meyer, B., Labarthe, M.C., Dredge, K., Klaschka, D., Henry, J., ... Dalgleish, A.G. (2009). The anti-cancer agents lenalidomide and pomalidomide inhibit the proliferation and function of T regulatory cells. *Cancer Immunology and Immunotherapy, 58*, 1033–1045. doi:10.1007/s00262-008-0620-4

Giuliani, N., Colla, S., Sala, R., Moroni, M., Lazzaretti, M., La Monica, S., ... Rizzoli, V. (2002). Human myeloma cells stimulate the receptor activator of nuclear factor-kappa B ligand (RANKL) in T lymphocytes: A potential role in multiple myeloma bone disease. *Blood, 100*, 4615–4621. doi:10.1182/blood-2002-04-1121

Giuliani, N., Rizzoli, V., & Roodman, G.D. (2006). Multiple myeloma bone disease: Pathophysiology of osteoblast inhibition. *Blood, 108*, 3992–3996. doi:10.1182/blood-2006-05-026112

Hideshima, T., Catley, L., Raje, N., Chauhan, D., Podar, K., Mitsiades, C., ... Anderson, K.C. (2007). Inhibition of akt induces significant downregulation of survivin and cytotoxicity in human multiple myeloma cells. *British Journal of Haematology, 138*, 783–791. doi:10.1111/j.1365-2141.2007.06714.x

Hou, J., Xiong, H., Gao, W., & Jiang, H. (2005). 2-Methoxyestradiol at low dose induces differentiation of myeloma cells. *Leukemia Research, 29*, 1059–1067. doi:10.1016/j.leukres.2005.02.016

Huston, A., Leleu, X., Jia, X., Moreau, A.S., Ngo, H.T., Runnels, J., ... Ghobrial, I.M. (2008). Targeting Akt and heat shock protein 90 produces synergistic multiple myeloma cell cytotoxicity in the bone marrow microenvironment. *Clinical Cancer Research, 14*, 865–874. doi:10.1158/1078-0432.CCR-07-1299

Jagannath, S. (2008). Pathophysiological underpinnings of multiple myeloma progression. *Journal of Managed Care and Pharmacy, 14*(Suppl. 7), 7–11.

Jagannath, S., Vij, R., Stewart, A.K., Somlo, G., Jakubowiak, A., Reiman, T., ... Siegel, D. (2008, December). *Initial results of PX-171-003, an open-label, single-arm, phase II study of carfilzomib (CFZ) in patients with relapsed and refractory multiple myeloma.* Paper presented at the 50th ASH Annual Meeting and Exposition, San Francisco, CA. Abstract retrieved from http://ash.confex.com/ash/2008/webprogram/Paper5718.html

Kapoor, P., Kumar, S., Fonseca, R., Lacy, M.Q., Witzig, T.E., Hayman, S.R., ... Rajkumar, S.V. (2009). Impact of risk stratification on outcome among patients with multiple myeloma receiving initial therapy with lenalidomide and dexamethasone. *Blood*. Advance online publication. doi:10.1182/blood-2009-01-202010

Kuhn, D.J., Chen, Q., Voorhees, P.M., Strader, J.S., Shenk, K.D., Sun, C.M., ... Orlowski, R.Z. (2007). Potent activity of carfilzomib, a novel, irreversible inhibitor of the ubiquitin-proteasome pathway, against preclinical models of multiple myeloma. *Blood, 110*, 3281–3290. doi:10.1182/blood-2007-01-065888

Lacy, M.Q., Hayman, S.R., Gertz, M.A., Dispenzieri, A., Buadi, F., Kumar, S., ... Rajkumar, S.V. (2009). Pomalidomide (CC4047) plus low-dose dexamethasone as therapy for relapsed multiple myeloma. *Journal of Clinical Oncology*. Advance online publication. doi:10.1200/JCO.2009.23.6802

Lutje, S., de Rooy, J.W., Croockewit, S., Koedam, E., Oyen, W.J., & Raymakers, R.A. (2009). Role of radiography, MRI and FDG-PET/CT in diagnosing, staging and therapeutical evaluation of patients with multiple myeloma. *Annals of Hematology*. Advance online publication. doi:10.1007/s00277-009-0829-0

Maiso, P., Carvajal-Vergara, X., Ocio, E.M., Lopez-Perez, R., Mateo, G., Gutierrez, N., ... San Miguel, J.F. (2006). The histone deacetylase inhibitor LBH589 is a potent antimyeloma agent that overcomes drug resistance. *Cancer Research, 66*, 5781–5789. doi:10.1158/0008-5472.CAN-05-4186

Mitsiades, C.S., McMillin, D.W., Klippel, S., Hideshima, T., Chauhan, D., Richardson, P.G., ... Anderson, K. (2007). The role of the bone marrow microenvironment in the pathophysiology of myeloma and its significance in the development of more effective therapies. *Hematology/Oncology Clinics of North America, 21,* 1007–1034. doi:10.1016/j. hoc.2007.08.007

Mitsiades, C.S., Mitsiades, N.S., McMullan, C.J., Poulaki, V., Kung, A.L., Davies, F.E., ... Anderson, K.C. (2006). Antimyeloma activity of heat shock protein-90 inhibition. *Blood, 107,* 1092–1100. doi:10.1182/blood-2005-03-1158

Mitsiades, C.S., Mitsiades, N.S., McMullan, C.J., Poulaki, V., Shringarpure, R., Akiyama, M., ... Libermann, T. (2004). Inhibition of the insulin-like growth factor receptor-1 tyrosine kinase activity as a therapeutic strategy for multiple myeloma, other hematologic malignancies, and solid tumors. *Cancer Cell, 5,* 221–230. doi:10.1016/S1535-6108(04)00050-9

Mooberry, S.L. (2003). New insights into 2-methoxyestradiol, a promising antiangiogenic and antitumor agent. *Current Opinion in Oncology, 15,* 425–430. doi:10.1097/00001622-200311000-00004

National Institutes of Health. (2009). *A study of tanespimycin (KOS-953) in patients with multiple myeloma in first relapse (BMS TIME-1).* Retrieved from http://clinicaltrials.gov/ct2/show/NCT00546780

Parlati, F., Lee, S.J., Aujay, M., Suzuki, E., Levitsky, K., Lorens, J.B., ... Bennett, M.K. (2009). Carfilzomib can induce tumor cell death through selective inhibition of the chymotrypsin-like activity of the proteasome. *Blood, 114,* 3439–3447. doi:10.1182/blood-2009-05-223677

Patterson, J., Palombella, V.J., Fritz, C., & Normant, E. (2008). IPI-504, a novel and soluble HSP-90 inhibitor, blocks the unfolded protein response in multiple myeloma cells. *Cancer Chemotherapy and Pharmacology, 61,* 923–932. doi:10.1007/s00280-007-0546-0

Podar, K., Chauhan, D., & Anderson, K.C. (2009). Bone marrow microenvironment and the identification of new targets for myeloma therapy. *Leukemia, 23,* 10–24. doi:10.1038/leu.2008.259

Rajkumar, S.V., Richardson, P.G., Lacy, M.Q., Dispenzieri, A., Greipp, P.R., Witzig, T.E., ... Gertz, M.A. (2007). Novel therapy with 2-methoxyestradiol for the treatment of relapsed and plateau phase multiple myeloma. *Clinical Cancer Research, 13,* 6162–6167. doi:10.1158/1078-0432.CCR-07-0807

Roodman, G.D. (2008). Skeletal imaging and management of bone disease. *Hematology: American Society of Hematology Education Program, 2008,* 313–319. doi:10.1182/asheducation-2008.1.313

Schey, S.A., Fields, P., Bartlett, J.B., Clarke, I.A., Ashan, G., Knight, R.D., ... Dalgleish, A.G. (2004). Phase I study of an immunomodulatory thalidomide analog, CC-4047, in relapsed or refractory multiple myeloma. *Journal of Clinical Oncology, 22,* 3269–3276. doi:10.1200/JCO.2004.10.052

Schirrmeister, H., Bommer, M., Buck, A.K., Muller, S., Messer, P., Bunjes, D., ... Reske, S.N. (2002). Initial results in the assessment of multiple myeloma using 18F-FDG PET. *European Journal of Nuclear Medicine and Molecular Imaging, 29,* 361–366. doi:10.1007/s00259-001-0711-3

Siegel, D., Hussein, M., Belani, C., Robert, F., Galanis, E., Richon, V.M., ... Rizvi, S. (2009). Vorinostat in solid and hematologic malignancies. *Journal of Hematology and Oncology, 2,* 31. doi:10.1186/1756-8722-2-31

Sloan, B., & Scheinfeld, N.S. (2008). Pazopanib, a VEGF receptor tyrosine kinase inhibitor for cancer therapy. *Current Opinion in Investigational Drugs, 9,* 1324–1335.

Stewart, A.K., & Fonseca, R. (2005). Prognostic and therapeutic significance of myeloma genetics and gene expression profiling. *Journal of Clinical Oncology, 23,* 6339–6344. doi:10.1200/JCO.2005.05.023

Streetly, M.J., Gyertson, K., Daniel, Y., Zeldis, J.B., Kazmi, M., & Schey, S.A. (2008). Alternate day pomalidomide retains anti-myeloma effect with reduced adverse events and evidence of in vivo immunomodulation. *British Journal of Haematology, 141,* 41–51. doi:10.1111/j.1365-2141.2008.07013.x

Sydor, J.R., Normant, E., Pien, C.S., Porter, J.R., Ge, J., Grenier, L., ... Tong, J.K. (2006). Development of 17-allylamino-17-demethoxygeldanamycin hydroquinone hydrochloride (IPI-504), an anti-cancer agent directed against Hsp90. *Proceedings of the National Academy of Sciences of the United States of America, 103,* 17408–17413. doi:10.1073/pnas .0608372103

Takatsuna, H., Asagiri, M., Kubota, T., Oka, K., Osada, T., Sugiyama, C., … Umezawa, K. (2005). Inhibition of RANKL-induced osteoclastogenesis by (–)-DHMEQ, a novel NF-κB inhibitor, through downregulation of NFATc1. *Journal of Bone and Mineral Research, 20,* 653–662. doi:10.1359/JBMR.041213

Tariman, J.D., & Estrella, S.M. (2005). The changing treatment paradigm in patients with newly diagnosed multiple myeloma: Implications for nursing [Online exclusive]. *Oncology Nursing Forum, 32,* E127–E138. doi:10.1188/05.ONF.E127-E138

Tariman, J.D., & Faiman, B. (2010). Multiple myeloma. In C.H. Yarbro, D. Wujcik, & B.H. Gobel (Eds.), *Cancer nursing: Principles and practice* (7th ed., pp. 1513–1545). Sudbury, MA: Jones and Bartlett.

Tatetsu, H., Okuno, Y., Nakamura, M., Matsuno, F., Sonoki, T., Taniguchi, I., … Hata, H. (2005). Dehydroxymethylepoxyquinomicin, a novel nuclear factor-κB inhibitor, induces apoptosis in multiple myeloma cells in an IκBα-independent manner. *Molecular Cancer Therapeutics, 4,* 1114–1120. doi:10.1158/1535-7163.MCT-04-0198

Vanderkerken, K., De Leenheer, E., Shipman, C., Asosingh, K., Willems, A., Van Camp, B., & Croucher, P. (2003). Recombinant osteoprotegerin decreases tumor burden and increases survival in murine model of multiple myeloma. *Cancer Research, 63,* 287–289.

Verhelle, D., Corral, L.G., Wong, K., Mueller, J.H., Moutouh-de Parseval, L., Jensen-Pergakes, K., … Chan, K.W.H. (2007). Lenalidomide and CC-4047 inhibit the proliferation of malignant B cells while expanding normal CD34+ progenitor cells. *Cancer Research, 67,* 746–755. doi:10.1158/0008-5472.CAN-06-2317

Watanabe, M., Dewan, M.Z., Okamura, T., Sasaki, M., Itoh, K., Higashihara, M., … Horie, R. (2005). A novel NF-κB inhibitor DHMEQ selectively targets constitutive NF-κB activity and induces apoptosis of multiple myeloma cells in vitro and in vivo. *International Journal of Cancer, 114,* 32–38. doi:10.1002/ijc.20688

Yasui, H., Hideshima, T., Ikeda, H., Jin, J., Ocio, E.M., Kiziltepe, T., … Anderson, K.C. (2007). BIRB 796 enhances cytotoxicity triggered by bortezomib, heat shock protein (Hsp) 90 inhibitor, and dexamethasone via inhibition of p38 mitogen-activated protein kinase/ Hsp27 pathway in multiple myeloma cell lines and inhibits paracrine tumour growth. *British Journal of Haematology, 136,* 414–423. doi:10.1111/j.1365-2141.2006.06443.x

Zaarur, N., Gabai, V.L., Porco, J.A., Jr., Calderwood, S., & Sherman, M.Y. (2006). Targeting heat shock response to sensitize cancer cells to proteasome and Hsp90 inhibitors. *Cancer Research, 66,* 1783–1791. doi:10.1158/0008-5472.CAN-05-3692

Zangari, M., Anaissie, E., Stopeck, A., Morimoto, A., Tan, N., Lancet, J., … Giles, F.J. (2004). Phase II study of SU5416, a small molecule vascular endothelial growth factor tyrosine kinase receptor inhibitor, in patients with refractory multiple myeloma. *Clinical Cancer Research, 10*(1, Pt. 1), 88–95. doi:10.1158/1078-0432.CCR-0221-3

Zhan, F., Barlogie, B., Mulligan, G., Shaughnessy, J.D., Jr., & Bryant, B. (2008). High-risk myeloma: A gene expression based risk-stratification model for newly diagnosed multiple myeloma treated with high-dose therapy is predictive of outcome in relapsed disease treated with single-agent bortezomib or high-dose dexamethasone. *Blood, 111,* 968–969. doi:10.1182/blood-2007-10-119321

Zhan, F., Barlogie, B., & Shaughnessy, J., Jr. (2003). Toward the identification of distinct molecular and clinical entities of multiple myeloma using global gene expression profiling. *Seminars in Hematology, 40,* 308–320. doi:10.1016/S0037-1963(03)00197-5

Zhan, F., Huang, Y., Colla, S., Stewart, J.P., Hanamura, I., Gupta, S., … Shaughnessy, J.D., Jr. (2006). The molecular classification of multiple myeloma. *Blood, 108,* 2020–2028. doi:10.1182/blood-2005-11-013458

Zhou, H.J., Aujay, M.A., Bennett, M.K., Dajee, M., Demo, S.D., Fang, Y., … Yang, J. (2009). Design and synthesis of an orally bioavailable and selective peptide epoxyketone proteasome inhibitor (PR-047). *Journal of Medicinal Chemistry, 52*, 3028–3038. doi:10.1021/jm801329v

Zhou, L., Hou, J., Fu, W., Wang, D., Yuan, Z., & Jiang, H. (2008). Arsenic trioxide and 2-methoxyestradiol reduce beta-catenin accumulation after proteasome inhibition and enhance the sensitivity of myeloma cells to bortezomib. *Leukemia Research, 32*, 1674–1683. doi:10.1016/j.leukres.2008.03.039

Zhu, K., Gerbino, E., Beaupre, D.M., Mackley, P.A., Muro-Cacho, C., Beam, C., … Sebti, S.M. (2005). Farnesyltransferase inhibitor R115777 (Zarnestra, Tipifarnib) synergizes with paclitaxel to induce apoptosis and mitotic arrest and to inhibit tumor growth of multiple myeloma cells. *Blood, 105*, 4759–4766. doi:10.1182/blood-2004-11-4307

Index

The letter f after a page number indicates that relevant content appears in a figure; the letter t, in a table.

A